Essential Oils & Aromatherapy

2nd Edition

by Kathi Keville
American Herb Association

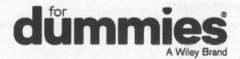

for **dummies**

A Wiley Brand

Essential Oils & Aromatherapy For Dummies® 2nd Edition

Published by: **John Wiley & Sons, Inc.**, 111 River Street, Hoboken, NJ 07030-5774, www.wiley.com

Copyright © 2023 by John Wiley & Sons, Inc., Hoboken, New Jersey

Media and software compilation copyright © 2023 by John Wiley & Sons, Inc. All rights reserved.

Published simultaneously in Canada

For general information on our other products and services, please contact our Customer Care Department within the U.S. at 877-762-2974, outside the U.S. at 317-572-3993, or fax 317-572-4002. For technical support, please visit https://hub.wiley.com/community/support/dummies.

Wiley publishes in a variety of print and electronic formats and by print-on-demand. Some material included with standard print versions of this book may not be included in e-books or in print-on-demand. If this book refers to media such as a CD or DVD that is not included in the version you purchased, you may download this material at http://booksupport.wiley.com. For more information about Wiley products, visit www.wiley.com.

Library of Congress Control Number: 2023937323

ISBN 978-1-119-90451-9 (pbk); ISBN 978-1-119-90453-3 (ebk); ISBN 978-1-119-90452-6 (ebk)

SKY10047428_050923

Contents at a Glance

Table of Contents

Introduction

I f you're like most people, you take the smell of a flower or the scent of freshly baked bread for granted. That's because fragrance is all around — every day and everywhere. Scent may be commonplace, but you'll have to agree that it greatly enhances life. And it does more than provide enjoyment. As its name implies, aromatherapy is indeed a *therapy* that uses *essential oils* for healing. Essential oils offer a way for you to literally smell your way to good health. You can't beat a prescription that reads, "Bathe with scented oils twice a week." *Essential Oils & Aromatherapy For Dummies* is your guide to a new way to stay healthy and fit and to take care of yourself when you do get sick. Aromatherapy works on many levels. It can treat emotional as well as physical problems and even help you think better or improve your athletic performance. "Scentsual" essential oils can improve your love — and your sex — life.

No wonder such a large selection of scented products is now available — everything from candles to facial cream to room freshener is promising to bring essential oils into your life.

About This Book

Essential oils and aromatherapy cover a lot of territory, so I've written this book to guide you through the clouds of wafting aromas. I'll show you how to make real "scents" out of this topic. I've been enjoying the benefits of essential oils for decades — and sharing them with others almost that long. Simply put, I'm impressed. I think you will be, too.

In this book, you discover the world of fragrance along with dozens of ways that aromatherapy can enhance your health and general well-being. *Essential Oils & Aromatherapy For Dummies* helps you understand essential oils so that you can savor and enjoy the pleasures and benefits. It's also a guide to using essential oils effectively and safely.

I show you how to bring essential oils into your home, your work, and wherever you go. One of the best things about aromatherapy is the ease and enjoyment that comes with it. Using essential oils is so simple, I include more than a hundred recipes that I developed so that you can whip up a scent for everything from oily skin to indigestion. Most of these recipes take less than five minutes to make — really!

This book contains so many features you won't find covered in other books on the subject. For starters, you are given an amazing selection of essential oil formulas to treat dozens of physical and emotional conditions in the Symptom Guide. Not only does the Guide describe how you can use them, but it gives you tips on additional treatments to enhance your healing. The detailed descriptions of essential oils in the Essential Oil Guide explain how to use each one. What really makes this book stand out are the guidelines that you'll need for using essential oils effectively and safely. You learn not only about which essential oils you need to use extra carefully or avoid, but also help in making good choices. And, while you're making those choices, here's a book that guides you through the confusion of the botanical names and the many variations and types of each oil. It takes the surprise out of essential oils by explaining how oils can change — for good and bad — with age and different storage conditions.

All of this knowledge is available to you through the easy-access organization of this book, which includes bulleted lists to help you spot exactly what you need to know. Everything you need to know is right there at first glance. Additional information is just a second glance away in sidebars that add a little noteworthy color to what you're reading.

Foolish Assumptions

Probably I do know you at least a little. You're already intrigued by aroma, so you can't help wondering what all the fuss is about essential oils. Maybe you're missing out on something that could really be a plus in your life and help a few physical, and maybe even some emotional, issues that you're working on.

>> You want to spice up your life with fragrance.

>> You want to know if aroma is really a therapy, and if so, how it works.

>> You're interested in the feel-good results provided by using essential oils.

Icons Used in This Book

The Tip icon marks tips and shortcuts that you can use to make using essential oils and aromatherapy even easier. A lot of these are the tips that I've discovered by trial and error, so I save you the expense of learning the hard way.

REMEMBER

It just pays to remember some things. When you spot this icon, I'm telling you something that you'll probably want to know about essential oils in the future. This way, you can pay special attention when you read this information and, just in case you do forget, you're able to quickly locate it again.

TECHNICAL STUFF

The Technical Stuff icon marks information of a highly technical nature that you can normally skip over. (It might be intriguing information to have, but it's not essential.)

WARNING

Essential oils are very concentrated and need to be used with respect. Throughout this book, you find an occasional warning to make sure you play it safe.

Beyond the Book

In addition to the abundance of information and guidance related to essential oils and aromatherapy that I provide in this book, you get access to even more help and information online at Dummies.com. Check out this book's online Cheat Sheet. Just go to www.dummies.com and search for "Essential Oils & Aromatherapy For Dummies Cheat Sheet."

Where to Go from Here

Chances are that you've already experienced aromatherapy even if you haven't used essential oils. If you've ever sipped a cup of chamomile tea, rubbed on rose- or lavender-scented hand lotion, or sniffed a cinnamon roll, you've already enjoyed aromatherapy. Where you go from here is into an adventure that combines enticing fragrances with good health. You hold in your hands a guide that can gently lead you to explore the many facets of this therapy.

Is some ailment bugging you? Then head straight to Chapter 2 to understand how essential oils work and then look up your specific problem in the Symptom Guide. Maybe you're feeling great physically, but you're too tired or need to have a little more focus? Then turn to Chapter 9 to help you stay alert. Want some hints on how to use essential oils? Then browse through Chapter 6. Wherever you turn in this book, you'll find plenty of information that will hopefully spark ideas that will further your involvement with essential oils.

1

Getting Started with Essential Oils

Chapter **1**

Making Sense Out of Scents

How many times have you leaned into a bouquet of flowers to inhale their fragrance? Perhaps you've taken a deep breath of pine or fir while walking in a park or forest or brought a fresh Christmas tree into your home. Stroll through a flower or herb garden, and the scents that waft around you with each step engage your imagination. Maybe you've sat down to a cup of peppermint tea and enjoyed the aroma as much as drinking the tea. With so many different smells surrounding you, you probably don't give them a second thought. Or at least you may not yet.

In this chapter, I begin to explain how all this scent-sation (from a bouquet of flowers, a pine forest, or your cup of tea) is due to essential oils. This chapter gives you just a sniff of essential oil basics and the study and practice of aromatherapy. The rest of the book digs deeper into various subtopics.

Defining Essential Oils

Essential oils are derived from medicinal plants that are commonly referred to as herbs. You may have gone in search of some herbal remedies to take care of a headache or reached for cough syrup or throat lozenges that contains medicinal herbs. Herbs that are aromatic contain essential oils that produce a plant's scent. Not all plants contain essential oils, but the ones that do hold them in special glands. It's easy for you to identify the plants with these oils: Simply smell the plant. If there's a scent, it contains essential oils. Roses, violets, rosemary bushes, and even Christmas trees all owe their distinctive aromas to essential oils.

TECHNICAL STUFF

Essential oils can be extracted from a plant using several methods. Once extracted, a pure essential oil is slightly oily to the touch. Although technically an oil, it is much thinner than vegetable oils used in cooking, such as canola or olive. Essential oils are composed of such tiny compounds that the oils feel thin and seem to disappear when you rub them between your fingers. They also don't leave an oily stain on cloth and evaporate easily into the air. Because they dissipate so quickly, another name for essential oils is *volatile oils*. That's a good description of them because volatile means "vaporous" or to be "like gas." (See Chapter 15 for more on the science behind the oils.)

The scent glands in a plant that produce essential oils can occur anywhere, but they are most likely found in the flowers and leaves. Not all plants need essential oils to survive, yet those that do have them, put them to good use. For a long time, botanists couldn't figure out why plants went to the trouble of producing these oils. Now they know that essential oils play important roles for plants.

>> They attract bees and other pollinators.

>> They repel harmful insects.

FOLLOWING YOUR NOSE

Nowadays, they're sold everywhere, but it's relatively new that you can purchase essential oils. Although they have been distilled for hundreds of years, and quite possibly long before that, they were obtained from aromatic plants only by early chemists — the alchemists. These rare essential oils found their way into a few exclusive cosmetics but were not generally available. Even a few decades ago when I started working as an aromatherapist almost no essential oils were available. I could only find peppermint and birch (sold as wintergreen) essential oils, and that was only in drugstores. I had to search out large essential oil companies distributing to the food and perfume industries for my first set of essential oils. Times have certainly changed.

>> Some repel other plants so that they don't crowd the space.

>> They kill bacterial, viral, and fungal infections.

>> They seal and heal the plant's wounds.

>> They help make the plant waterproof.

>> They increase the plant's immunity to disease.

>> Acting like plant hormones, some influence plant reproduction.

Defining Aromatherapy

Aromatherapy is the technique of using essential oils, which are always aromatic, for healing therapy. The beauty of essential oils is that they are an aroma-based therapy. All those good scents make working with essential oils and using them a wonderful experience. After all, if essential oils have an emphasis, it's that they make you feel great just sniffing them.

What I love about aromatherapy is how it is truly *holistic* (aims to treat the whole person). It embraces the body-mind-spirit concept by working on all these levels. That means the essential oils used in an aromatherapy practice address healing on several levels as they have done in traditional medicine around the world. No matter where your ancestry lies, your people certainly used aromatic plants for healing. In fact, the use of aromatic plants is thought to be one of the oldest forms of healing. A tradition-based practice, it works in our modern world as well as it did ages ago.

TECHNICAL STUFF

As an herbalist and aromatherapist, I always view aromatherapy as a part of herbalism. If you look at the most important types of healing compounds in herbs, essential oils are right at the top because essential oils are responsible for many herbs' healing attributes.

Although most of Western medicine typically relies on medical procedures and pharmaceuticals, modern science has also turned its attention to the healing capabilities of essential oils. When researchers looked for possible candidates to study, they first investigated the uses of aromatic plants that have been recorded in herbal manuscripts and embedded into worldwide folklore. What they discovered is that the old manuscripts were right. Yes, chamomile really does reduce pain. Lavender can help you sleep. Rosemary helps you think better. Some essential oils reduce bruising and inflammation. From these first aromatic findings, research moved on to explore a potpourri of aromatic experiences and provided a scientific foundation for essential oil use.

Aromatherapy is often used in conjunction with other forms of therapies to heal various ailments. This is because it's a perfect, non-intrusive way to balance emotions. For example, incense can be burned during a yoga class. Someone experiencing an anxiety attack can simply spray an essential oil into the air, and a beneficial effect wafts through the room. As an adjunct therapy, aromatherapy can promote relaxation or focus and relieve anxiety and nervousness. I often refer to it as a feel-good therapy to improve almost any situation. (Check out Chapter 6 for many ways to create a mood room with scent.)

In addition to affecting mood, aromatherapy can help to heal a long list of physical problems. Aromatherapy is especially useful when you're dealing with conditions that you normally treat yourself anyway, such as a headache, muscle spasm, or insomnia. Instead of heading to the drugstore, you'll be reaching for rose geranium or peppermint essential oil. To use aromatherapy wisely, read Chapter 4.

There's no denying that certain fragrances from essential oils put your mind into a relaxed focus that promotes prayer and meditation. How aromatherapy addresses the soul is fascinating and a little mysterious. Science hasn't backed this use . . . yet. I like how the essential oils that traditionally have been used in religious settings to inspire devotion are now non-denominational. The scent of essential oils like frankincense, myrrh, sandalwood, and juniper work for everyone. While you may be using frankincense to relax a muscle, its scent floating in the air touches a spiritual aspect, which can help you create or tap into a core of strength to deal with whatever physical and emotional conditions come your way.

Aromatherapy is becoming a household word, and you'll find a large assortment of essential oils readily available online and in brick-and-mortar stores. See chapters in this book that cover more information on individual topics. Refer to Chapter 8 for tips on using aromatherapy to create romance. Chapter 6 explains how to scent your living and workspace. The guides at the end of this book help you find the right oils and scents for your needs.

Using Oils for Healing

Essential oils have a lot in common when it comes to medicine. Due to their general makeup, most essential oils are highly antiseptic and able to kill an assortment of harmful bacterial and viral infections. Many also reduce inflammation to help eliminate pain, which can result when an inflamed or infected area presses on your nerves. Quite a few of these oils also encourage wounds to heal more quickly because they stimulate the repair of cells. All these actions combine into an excellent treatment for your minor injuries, such as cuts, tight or cramped muscles, arthritis, headaches, and inflammation. Over and over, I've seen essential oils quickly knock out an infection, relieve a bruise, or ease a cramping muscle.

Here's a list of essential oils' most important medicinal properties.

>> Kill bacterial, viral, and fungal infections

>> Heal wounds

>> Reduce inflammation

>> Regulate hormones

>> Tone skin

>> Stimulate the immune system

>> Influence reproductive hormones

>> Improve blood circulation and warm the skin

>> Improve digestion

>> Decrease sinus and lung congestion

REMEMBER

Not all essential oils are pros at everything on this list. Some perform better than others doing one thing or another. This book will show you which essential oils do what. Refer to the Essential Oil Guide and the Symptom Guide for help.

Getting Aromas into the Body

There are two main ways to use essential oils. One is by inhaling their aroma through your nose. The other is to dilute them so you can rub them on your skin. Of course, when you rub them on your skin, you also get the benefit of being able to inhale the scent at the same time.

Under your skin

Essential oil molecules are amazingly small. Their tiny size gives them some of their superpowers. An example is their ability to get under your skin when you rub them on. Your skin in very protective about what it lets through. You don't want just anything entering your body and your skin knows that. So, it has a tight structure and protective coating to keep out harmful things like dirt and grime and whatever you touch. After all, anything that's able to penetrate skin reaches blood vessels, moves into the bloodstream, and is then circulated throughout the body to reach all of your cells. It's because they are so small that almost all essential oils are absorbed quickly when applied to the skin and are able to pass through your skin. Some of the oil is absorbed into skin layers; some reach even farther, into underlying tissue. A small amount moves into the bloodstream. On the other hand, some remains on the surface of your skin and evaporates into the air as fragrance.

This absorption doesn't happen all at once. Essential oils are made up of many different compounds, and some pass more quickly through your skin than others. The tiniest, most absorbable components in lavender and clove oils appear in the blood only 20 minutes after being rubbed on the skin. You can detect bergamot, anise, and lemon on the breath 40 to 60 minutes after rubbing them on the skin. Even larger compounds take just a little longer.

Chemists say three things determine how quickly a compound goes through skin: its size, shape, and function. Because some essential oil compounds are tinier than others, it's the small ones with simple shapes that move through the quickest. Function refers to conditions, such as water-solubility. Heat also speeds things up. Warm skin, warm body oil, massage techniques like using hot rocks or compresses, and even a hot day all increase this essential oil migration. Absorption rates are also influenced by your skin type — for example, essential oils penetrate dry, flakey, broken, or freshly washed skin more easily.

Any aromatherapy product that contains vegetable oil — and that includes skin lotion, facial cream, salve, and massage oil — slows the absorption of essential oils into your skin. What's happening is that large molecules in vegetable oils such as almond and olive oil are simply too big to go into your skin, so they slide over the top of your skin. While they're doing all that sliding around, they hold onto some of the essential oil. Eventually most of these suspended essential oil compounds find their way into the skin. This spreads out the essential oil's good effects over time, much like a time-release factor.

TIP

Test this one out at home. Cut a clove of garlic in half and rub the cut side liberally on the bottom of your foot. Put socks on and wait for the results of the experiment. It takes your blood system about 20 minutes to carry the essential oil of garlic throughout your blood system. You'll know because you'll be able to taste it! Not only can you taste garlic, but its powerful antiseptic action is going to work throughout your body! (You may not want to do this experiment before attending a social event.)

TECHNICAL STUFF

Essential oils are derived from aromatic plants, many of which are medicinal herbs that are used for healing. That means the essential oil carries at least some healing properties of the herb from which it was derived. Sometimes, clinical herbalists and aromatherapists turn to the herb and sometimes the oil for a remedy. The decision of which one to use depends on the condition that's being treated and what medicinal properties are needed.

Because aromatic herbs contain the essential oil, there are times when either the herb or oil will do the trick. Take the herb rosemary, for example. If you're want something to relieve sore muscles, you can use a concoction that has the herb rosemary extracted into a base like olive oil or one that has rosemary essential oils added to it.

Essential oils have some advantages over non-aromatic herbs. They're fast to reach their destination. Say that you have a sore muscle. Rub on a massage or body oil that contains the anti-inflammatory essential oil of lavender or chamomile over a sore area, and you'll send the medicine quickly into the underlying area — your tight muscle.

Compare that to using non-aromatic herbs. Drinking an herb tea or downing a pill or extract are all good medicine. However, while herbs do a great job of treating skin disorders and complexion problems on the skin's surface, they rarely go more than skin deep. When applied topically, most herbal compounds lay on the skin's surface. The medicine doesn't reach deep into tissue under the skin to help heal it. This limits herbs to topical use. Our skin is a great protective barrier; otherwise, everything we touch could enter our bodies.

The advantages of having those tiny essential oils pass through your skin via topical application include the following:

>> **Right on target.** Essential oils can be applied right on or over the specific area that needs treatment.

>> **Go deep.** Essential oils penetrate deep into underlying tissue to work their healing magic.

>> **Have a happy liver.** Not only does the problem area get most of the medicinal dose, but less essential oil ends up circulating in your bloodstream. The result is less essential oil has to be processed by your liver. That translates into less work for your liver and a lower chance of too much essential oil producing a toxic reaction in your body.

USING THE "LIZARD BRAIN"

After the nose gathers information about aroma, it sends a report to your brain. That information bypasses the central nervous system and the areas of the brain that control reasoning. Instead, the nose sends its fragrance facts to a very old part of your brain called the limbic system for processing.

The primitive limbic system is sometimes called the "lizard brain" because it works in a similar fashion to the simple brain of a reptile to plug into your basic survival instincts. If you want to understand the limbic system better, think about what a lizard needs: to find food and a mate, be alerted to danger, remember a few survival skills, recognize its territory, and maintain its body's healthy equilibrium. All these requirements are associated with the sense of smell.

Because it is the limbic system's job is to alert your body's warning system of potential danger, it signals the "fight or flight" response. This causes your adrenals to provide a rush of adrenaline with its resulting burst of energy during an emergency. The higher parts of your brain that control long-term memory also receive information about fragrances. The limbic system — and thus our sense of smell — directly communicates with the brain's hypothalamus and pituitary. Both are considered "master glands" because they regulate so many body functions. Through these glands, your sense of smell helps direct various hormone and immune system activity and what regulates appetite, digestion, sexual arousal, memory, body temperature, and heartbeat.

Anthropologists and psychologists are exploring why your sense of smell is closely linked to these areas. They assume that at one time smell played an important role in survival. Perhaps five times more powerful in your ancestors than it is today, this super sense enabled them to smell spoiled food, the potency of their plant medicines, their kin, recognize friend or foe, and to be attracted to a mate. This keen sense of smell also helped treat illnesses. It is likely that the use of aroma as therapy goes back to the earliest uses of plants as medicine. The first recorded uses of aromatherapy are from Egypt, Mesopotamia, and China just after 3000 B.C.

From rose to nose

Certain scents make you think better and faster, while others work on your emotions. Some mood-lifting aromas are antidepressants; some are relaxants; and still others act as stimulants. To learn which oil does what to improve your moods, refer to Chapter 9 and the Essential Oil Guide.

The molecules that produce aromas are too small to see with your eye, yet the air is filled with these microscopic particles of scent. Simply brushing against a fragrant plant or opening a vial of essential oil releases thousands of aromatic molecules into the air where they freely float to your nose (which is happening in Figure 1-1).

Every time you sniff something aromatic — say your favorite fragrant flower or perfume — thousands of tiny scent molecules tumble into your nose. High up in your nose, smell receptors await these compounds. They send information about what you smell to your *olfactory bulb*. (Olfactory is scientific lingo for smell.) These receptors are able to tell the difference between all of the many odor molecules because, much like your fingerprints, each aromatic molecule is unique. One way they differentiate the compounds is according to their shape.

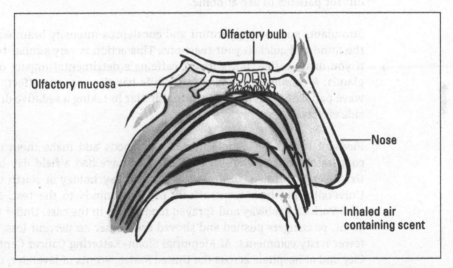

FIGURE 1-1:
Scent captured in the nose and sent to the olfactory bulb in the brain.

Think of essential oil compounds like a child's building blocks that come in all sorts of shapes and sizes. Your brain recognizes the difference. It collects the information and sends it a charge or code to your sense of smell. The higher brain collects the information to relay it to wherever it is needed and alter your body physically or emotionally. All of this happens very rapidly and is why you can smell the difference between a lemon and a lime. It's also why the scent of chamomile makes you dreamy while eucalyptus is a wake-up call.

Capturing the Benefits of Essential Oils

Essential oils can really work some magic on the mind and body. I know this from my clinical and personal experiences, but it's also been proven by various studies.

The Fragrance Research Fund has collaborated with the Psychophysiology Department at Yale University to discover how the aromas of essential oils affect behavior. In one of their programs, they followed more than two thousand people for twenty years. They've found that simply inhaling fragrance helps with a long list of complaints including fatigue, pain, insomnia, depression, nervousness, migraines, and memory loss. Research even points to aromatherapy treating schizophrenia and sexual dysfunction.

Many health providers are turning to aromatherapy to supplement treatment plans. They like its quick action and how it so easily helps with emotions. The Mayo Clinic has trained more than two thousand physicians and nurses so far in using essential oils. They're putting the aroma from essential oils in the air before dispensing medication to patients. For example, Fairview Clinics in Minnesota use ginger and spearmint to alleviate nausea and lemon and Mandarin to ease anxiety and insomnia. The Mayo Clinic also sells inhalation sticks containing essential oils for patients to use at home.

Stimulants such as peppermint and eucalyptus intensify brain waves to sharpen the mind and quicken your reactions. This action is very similar to what happens if you drink coffee, but without caffeine's detrimental impact on your adrenal glands. A calming scent like chamomile has the opposite effect. It slows brain-wave patterns to produce relaxation similar to taking a sedative drug, but without side effects.

Pleasant smells put people into better moods and make them more willing to cooperate and compromise. Psychologists have had a field day testing this out! Dr. Susan Schiffman, professor of Medical Psychology at North Carolina's Duke University, put how scent affects people's minds to the test. She got on the New York City subway and sprayed food scents in the cars. Under the influence of scent, passengers pushed and shoved each other 40 percent less, and they made fewer nasty comments. At Memorial Sloan-Kettering Cancer Center in New York City and at hospitals across the United States, scents of lavender, chamomile, and vanilla have relaxed patients undergoing invasive procedures or MRI (magnetic resonance imaging) scanning.

Other successful treatments are just a sniff away. Researchers are hoping to uncover all the ways in which essential oils heal. They at least want aromatherapy to improve the quality of life for people who suffer from several disorders. Essential oils may offer the ability to take fewer pharmaceutical drugs when the two are used together.

WARNING

REMEMBER

Don't try to reduce your prescription drugs without your doctor's approval. You could end up harming your health more than improving it.

The effect of fragrances on your mind and emotions may be subtle, but the smell alone makes you feel better about yourself. It can improve your mood, reduce stress, cause you to become more energetic, or help you relax or fall asleep more easily. The bottom line is that you are happier. In this way, it achieves the goals set by self-help books and seminars. After all, feeling good about yourself makes you less combative, jealous, and angry. You also feel more in control of your life, and that makes you less frustrated and more satisfied with life. Not bad results for a little sniff of a pleasant fragrance!

A Rose by Any Other Name . . .

The essential oils that are used therapeutically have the same names as the plants from which they're derived. These are called common names and what I use throughout this book. These are the names you already know, such as rose, lavender, and lemon. This keeps it simple and makes easy reading for you. However, plants and their essential oils also have scientific names that are in Latin or Greek. Botanists group plants according to how they look. The more similar the physical characteristics, the closer the relationship.

REMEMBER

Whether you're new to essential oils or already a pro, understanding scientific plant names is very important to you. You won't be able to negotiate through the maze of essential oils for sale without a basic understanding of botany. These names are the only way you can make sure that you're buying the correct essential oils, because some plants and the essential oils derived from them share the same common name.

Why all this fuss about Latin words and classifications? For one thing, go with common names alone, and you will be in for a surprise. Quite a few plants share the same common names. But they don't necessarily share the same medicinal properties or scent. A few examples of common names you may encounter that describe more than one oil are basil, cedarwood, chamomile, fir, and jasmine. There's tee tree from Australia, but there's also a New Zealand tea tree or manuka. While both trees are in the same botanical family — the Myrtle family — they are distinctly different. The same thing occurs with chamomile. The essential oil could be German chamomile or perhaps Roman chamomile. or maybe its gold or Cape chamomile. German chamomile is far more anti-inflammatory than the less popular Roman chamomile so more valuable to use on a condition like inflamed skin. I sniff either one for a relaxing effect.

To toss in even more confusion, if you buy bergamot or spikenard essential oils, it won't be the common garden bergamot, or the herb called spikenard. There are also many variations of lavender and rosemary. To help you sort all of this out, these differences are further explained in the Essential Oil Guide.

Breaking down the system

The organizational system that essential oils fall into is officially called *plant taxonomy*. The full scientific names of plants come from a combination of different information. Some are named after the botanist who identified them, in honor of a person or place, or according to what a plant looks like.

When you go to purchase an essential oil, you'll first see the plant's common name. It is followed by the scientific botanical name, which is written in italics to distinguish it as a non-English name. Some aromatherapy products pass on giving you the common name and only list the botanical names of the essential oils on their ingredient list.

Each botanical name has two parts. The first part of the name is called the *genus*. A lot of related plants are included in this. The genus is followed by the *species*, which designates a specific plant. Together, these are called the *binomials* or "two names." Here's another way to look at botanical names. Say your name is Anne Smith. In botany that would be written *Smith anne*. This designates the Smiths as being related and thus, having similarities. It also shows that there's just one of you.

You can see how this essential oil naming works if you look at two aromatic plants in the same genus. Let's take *Citrus*. Among the members of this genus are lemon (*Citrus limonum*) and bergamot (*Citrus bergamia*). They are in the same *Citrus* genus. You can tell just by their botanical names that they're related. The fact that they have different species names shows they aren't the same plant. Because they're in the same genus, it is likely that they share some medicinal properties and may have a similar scent . . . and they do!

TECHNICAL STUFF

When chemists get involved in this naming game, they sometimes add yet another category that's called a chemotype. You'll also encounter them when purchasing essential oils. *Chemotypes* are subspecies of plants. They look alike but have different chemical components in their essential oils. This usually occurs when the same plant grows in different locations. This means its aroma and use are also slightly different. See Chapter 15 for more on chemotypes and their differences and uses.

Specifying species

Most essential oils that you'll see for sale come from the most common species of herb used medicinally. These aromatic herbs are the ones that are grown for production or, in some cases, harvested from the wild. There's often more species in the genus that aren't being distilled commercially to be turned into essential oils, because there's not enough demand for them.

Species that are in the same genus have similar botanical characteristics and usually have related DNA. The closer species are related, the better the chance that they have a similar chemistry and use, as well as aroma. Even so, they are rarely exactly alike. Even slight chemical alterations can make a difference in how you use the essential oils. The downside is it can be confusing to sort out which oil you need. The upside is that this offers an opportunity to explore new essential oils and fine-tune the aromatherapy formulas you create.

Following are the essential oils that are available in several different species or varieties. Sometimes their effects on the brain and mind are similar, sometimes not.

>> **Chamomile** essential oil is produced from several different plants that are not even in the same genus. Some uses are similar yet not necessarily interchangeable. The most popular oil is German chamomile, which reduces inflammation and muscle pain better than Roman chamomile. Other oils include Cape chamomile, which is another good anti-inflammatory and muscle relaxant somewhat similar to German chamomile. There is also a "gold" chamomile that is more akin to Roman chamomile.

>> **Cinnamon** essential oil can be from the less expensive species cassia or true, but much hotter cinnamon.

>> **Eucalyptus** essential oil has so many species that are distilled. Lemon eucalyptus contains so much of the compound called citronellal that it is a great bug repellent with a delightful lemony scent. *Radiata* is specific to treat sinus and herpes infections, while *australiana* takes care of lung congestion and sore throat. *Smithii* is a gentle version so it's used for children and sensitive individuals. These are the most common species of eucalyptus that are sold today.

>> **Fir** essential oil comes as Balsam fir, Canadian fir, and Siberian fir, which tend to be used interchangeably, although a good nose can detect their slightly different scent.

>> **Lavender** essential oil is most often the standard English lavender or one of its many "Lavandin" hybrids, such as those named Provence and Grosso. There's also Spike, French, Spanish, and various specialty lavenders from different regions. Spike lavender is especially good for treating sinus and lung congestion and acne. The camphorus-smelling Spanish lavender *(Lavendula stoechas)* is a strong wound-healer that helps to ease sore muscles.

>> **Sage** essential oil is the common cooking sage. Spanish sage and a few other sages are also produced, which have a distinctive lavender fragrance and are less irritating to skin. Both are strong antiseptics. Clary sage is a species that is designated as "clary," which is less antiseptic, but its scent produces more of a heavy, relaxing effect than common sage.

>> **Tea tree** essential oil is derived from a few similar species, such as MQV *(Melaleuca quinquenervia)*. MQV is considered the most antiviral species. It has sweeter, more pleasant scent, so it is easier to mix with other essential oils into a nice-smelling blend. The harsher cajeput is another species, but one that is rarely used.

Dealing with name changes

The classifications of plants in modern botany are being influenced and changed according to DNA reports on the plants themselves. This is changing the world of botany from being solely based on physical appearances to paying attention to genetics. Some plants are being moved from one category to another based solely on their DNA. As a result, numerous botanical names have changed because a plant is no longer in the same genus. These changes are creating a more accurate system of plant relatives, but also causing some confusion.

WARNING

When you read older aromatherapy references, you're bound to encounter some outdated names. Make sure you double-check the names you find in older books with updated information you can find online.

One well-known herb that has had a name change in recent years is rosemary. It has now joined the Salvia genus that already encompasses sage and lavender. Its new botanical name is *Salvia rosemarinus*, leaving behind the previous *Rosemarinus officinalis*.

TECHNICAL
STUFF

Botanists are always refining plants' genealogy themselves. Their changes are often based on microscopic differences in plant structure. They have changed vetiver's botanical name from *Vetiveria zizanioides* to the new *Chrysopogon zizanioides*. This happened after years of speculation that the entire genus called *Vetiveria* should really be merged int *Chrysopogon*.

Chapter **2**

Sniffing the Diff: What to Look for in a Scent

When you get down to the nuts and bolts of essential oils, it's all about scent. After all, that's what makes essential oils smell good and work on the body and mind. An oil's scent tells us many things about its quality and purity. It also dictates how you blend it with other essential oils in your aromatherapy creations. Your nose is your guide on this aromatherapy journey. Don't fret — by using the guidelines in this chapter, the tasks of choosing oils and blending are not as monumental as they may seem. Soon, you'll be able to differentiate between top-of-the-line essential oils and the run-of-the-mill variety, as well as the downright stinky ones.

In this chapter, I tell you how to train your nose to truly understand essential oils. At the same time, you'll be developing your sense of smell so you can judge the quality of essential oils. Knowing what's good and what's not helps you not only when blending oils, but in choosing which ones to buy. This chapter gives you the tricks of the fragrance trade so you can choose the best oils and then make incredible blends with them.

Choosing and Using Oils:
Your Nose Knows Best

To better understand an essential oil, let's dissect scent. We're looking at not just which oils smell good or not so good, but what creates all those interesting layers of different scents. You can use that characteristic scent to identify a certain oil and judge its quality. Also pay attention to the scent when blending an oil with other essential oils to make your final product smell not just great, but fantastic!

The following sections walk you through the tried-and-true sniffing procedure used by perfumers and other smelling experts. Whether you're a beginner or already whipping up your own essential oil concoctions, why not improve your ability to judge essential oils and blending skills like a pro? Both of these talents are important when working with essential oil.

TIP

While you go through this chapter, don't just read about how to understand scent. Put that nose to work. Grab a bottle of essential oil or an aromatic plant and test the techniques for yourself. See what scent categories you can detect with every sniff you take. You'll be amazed at how clever your nose can be! You'll also be delighted at how quickly your brain learns to detect scent.

Sniffing 101

Because you rely on your nose to lead you through the essential oils marketing maze and to become a master blender, you need to teach it the tricks of the trade. First, discover how to smell.

So — nose meet scent. When smelling a finished aromatherapy product, such as shampoo or body oil, you can just sniff away because only a small amount of the essential oil is already mixed into the finished product. However, a bottle of pure essential oil is another story.

Undiluted oils are quite strong when sniffed directly from the bottle. They don't represent how a final product will smell because it's almost always diluted, so that's no help to you as a blender. Even worse, they quickly put your sense of smell and brain on overload. That olfactory overdose while holding the bottle directly under your nose can make you lightheaded, so why suffer?

To sniff essential oils more comfortably and to have a more accurate sense of how they will smell once diluted, try the following:

>> Smell the scent of the oil from the lid rather than the bottle.

>> When sniffing an undiluted essential oil, hold the lid about 6 to 10 inches from your nose.

>> Move the bottle or lid back and forth through the air to dilute the aromatic molecules.

>> After smelling several essential oils, clear your nose palate so that you can keep on sniffing. For tips on how to clear your nose, check out the following section.

Clearing your nose

Your capacity to smell begins to decline after about six or seven good sniffs in succession, especially of the same thing. Along with your ability to smell goes your ability to distinguish an oil's subtle characteristics — an obvious problem when you're trying to determine quality or creating a blend. Keep sniffing, and eventually your nose gives out altogether so that you can't smell a thing.

To regain your sense of smell, simply take a break and stop smelling the oils for 10 minutes or until your sense of smell returns. If you don't want to wait that long, here are simple techniques that the pros use. Granted, they might seem silly, but trust me, they work! You can recover your sense of smell in less than a minute by

>> **Walking outside and deeply breathing fresh air.** Here's a good way to clear your nose of all those scent molecules bouncing around in there. Think of this as an air "wash."

>> **Sniffing coffee beans or hovering over a cup of coffee.** Yes, you read this correctly; I did say coffee. And you thought it was just for a pick-me-up? Exactly how coffee works on your ability to perceive scent is a bit of a mystery, but it does the trick.

>> **Taking several breaths through a wool scarf or cap.** There's something about the smell of wool that changes your smell perception. This trick also works well to filter out the scents that linger in a room when you work with essential oils. Not any cap or scarf will do; make sure that it's a wool one.

>> **Putting a few grains of salt on the tip of your tongue.** This is not only a good way to regain your sense of smell, but it also illustrates the close connection between sense of smell and your taste buds. The salt cuts short the smell information reaching your brain and sets an empty stage that is ready for a new scent experience.

STRENGTHENING YOUR NOSE: WHAT TO DO WHEN YOU FEEL LIKE YOU CAN'T SMELL

I'm often asked, "I have a poor sense of smell, but still would like to work with essential oils. What can I do?" If this is you, try taking a B vitamin supplement. If that works, get more of this vitamin in your diet. You can develop a keener nose by "exercising" it through regular practice sessions. Have smell sessions in which you sniff the same essential oil several times a day for a week. Choose something familiar so even if you can't detect the scent very well, you can imagine it. The only other thing to do is to be patient, especially if your lack of smell is the result of a disease, such as Covid-19, and wait for time to take its course.

How important is your sense of smell? It can affect your life. It influences your sense of taste so much that food only has texture. It also is involved with sexual attraction. Your sense of smell is also a warning system that alerts you to avoid foul smells and rancid food that aren't good for you. While this response becomes so automatic that you may barely notice it, you'll miss it when it's gone. Even though a good nose was important to our ancestors for survival, it's not held in high regard these days. One survey asked individuals which of their five senses they would give up first. The overwhelming response was their sense of smell. I doubt they considered that their sense of taste and a few other things would go with it.

Talking Scents: Language of Fragrance

Although it may seem complex at first sniff, being able to describe different scents is a useful skill for anyone using essential oils, from beginner to professional. I use it all the time when working with all aspects of essential oils.

Aroma language is the terminology that aromatherapists and perfume experts use to describe the components of a smell. It helps you compare one fragrance to another. It helps you clarify what you like in a particular essential oil or in a blend of oils, as well as what you don't like. That's important if you're trying to develop a discriminating nose. It helps you pick out quality products and essential oils or do expert blending. It also helps you figure out when oils get too old to use.

Perfumers are often called *noses*. In the essential oil world, that's a compliment! It means they're good at their trade sniffing out individual compounds in each oil and blending them together. That's also your goal when practicing in aromatherapy! Borrow some tricks of the experts and soon what you create will not only work therapeutically, but it'll smell fantastic!

Perfumers and aromatherapists place essential oils into many categories. These categories give you guidelines for different types of scents to make your blending job easier. For your aromatherapy work, essential oils' scents go into three major categories:

>> **Scent type:** This uses a nature scent to describe what the essential oil smells like. You might say they smell spicy or floral.

>> **Scent quality:** Quality is a description of the essential oil's intensity and richness. Quality discusses whether it smells like a well-rounded "bouquet" or "flat." The scent may also have other characteristics, such as "sharp."

>> Scent notes: This describes the high, middle, or low *notes* that perfumers discuss. It discusses whether a scent is light and airy and is described as a high note or whether the scent carries more of a heaviness to make it a middle or a deep/low note.

Using the three categories, you can judge quality and make good blends. To do so, develop your aroma "language." For example, an essential oil may smell to you like a sharp wood, yet heavy with a low note. Another may seem like a strong, sour citrus but with a hint of a high note. It may be a foreign language now, but after you begin using phrases like these, they come to you automatically with any fragrance. Of course, unless you encounter someone else who works with essential oils, you may be talking to only yourself. It doesn't matter. Mumble away. The point is that by putting a name on it, you better identify what you're smelling.

REMEMBER

A good essential oil blender uses these concepts as guidelines, but not rules. Grasp onto them if you're a beginner but feel free to be experimental as you begin to master the art of smelling. Sometimes creativity is born out of breaking the rules!

Scent type

Identifying the type of scent is the easiest and most familiar way to categorize scents. In fact, you probably already know these scent categories because they are part of everyday life. When aroma geeks talk about different types of scent, they group together scents according to how they smell. This puts them into categories. For example, think of a *floral* scent. It smells like . . . well flowers! Another category that's sure to make you hungry is spice. Think of the aroma of cinnamon buns or pumpkin pie; you'll know mint from the last time you popped a breath mint or enjoyed peppermint tea. You get the idea!

Table 2-1 introduces and explains the basic types of scent produced by nature. This is the typical list of types used by a majority of perfumers and aromatherapists. Feel free to also add your own descriptions, such as "fresh" or "funky." The point is to use whatever you feel best describes a scent. I give you examples of common spices and herbs that fit in each category.

TABLE 2-1   ## Types of Scent

Scent	Description	Oil Example
Floral	Think of the fragrance exuded by a bouquet of flowers.	Rose, lavender
Wood	This is the smell of freshly cut wood.	Cedar, cypress, firs, sandalwood
Citrus	Imagine the fresh scent of an orange, lemon, or lime.	Grapefruit, lemon, orange, petitgrain, tangerine
Herbal	Think of something yummy to eat that contains herbs, like the smell of a pizza, freshly toasted herb bread, or stuffing cooking at Thanksgiving.	Marjoram, rosemary, sage
Spicy	Go to the kitchen for a spicy scent: You can find it in cinnamon-flavored oatmeal or hot cinnamon rolls.	Cinnamon, cloves
Minty	Mint smells of chewing gum and mint breath sweeteners.	Peppermint, spearmint
Camphorous	Imagine the pungent, sharp smell of camphor. Think of the smell of mothballs, although the aromatic wood of the camphor tree itself smells sweeter and much more pleasant. A camphorous smell seems to go directly to the top of your head when you sniff it.	Camphor, pine

Any of these six types of scents can be interesting in small amounts in an essential oil blend but potentially overbearing if it dominates. Take camphor. A camphorous scent can be attractive, as it is in geranium, pine, and rosemary. It's when you sniff it in full force that it becomes unpleasant. Give someone pine oil that smells strongly of camphor to sniff, and the first reaction is to wrinkle their nose and pull their head back. When you see a reaction like that, you know that essential oil is too strong. If you sniff an essential oil and it seems to literally float back and forth between more than one scent type, don't worry. Your nose is doing a great job detecting the complex makeup of an essential oil. That's because most essential oils are not one thing, say a basil or peppermint oil, but a cocktail of different compounds. Each compound contributes its own scent and actions. That actually makes many individual essential oils smell like blends all by themselves. And that's a good thing because the process of blending has already begun before you do anything.

For example, if you detect a floral scent, a citrus fragrance may be lingering beneath it. It may take a discerning and educated nose to detect all that's going on, but the more you can smell, the better you'll be at judging quality and blending. Another example is pine. The scent is decidedly camphor, but can you also detect the woodsy scent? Although lavender is floral, see whether you can pick up the herbal aroma that is mixed in with it. These and many more essential oils fall under more than one category.

Scent quality

Describing a scent's quality is a little more difficult than identifying its type, but not too hard after you get the hang of it. Good essential oils and essential oil blends are described as *full bodied*. This means that the scent carries more intensity and a richer, more rounded "bouquet" of fragrance because it contains more aromatic compounds. On the other hand, you can describe a lower quality oil as smelling "flat," "one-sided," or just plain weak. You could even call it boring.

TIP

Trying to define a term like rounded or flat when you're talking scent isn't exactly easy, but compare it to taste. Imaging biting into a cheese sandwich that is made with a slice of cheese between two pieces of plain bread without butter, mayonnaise, or anything. Your taste buds probably don't get very excited about that lunch! Now envision eating the tastiest sandwich that you can that has all your favorites; perhaps it includes pickles, mustard, and tomatoes. Now, that's a fuller taste experience.

If this scent-describing sounds like wine-tasting, that's because it is so similar — the only difference is that you're smelling rather than tasting. Citrus smells a little sour, but the best oils also have a sweet smell. Contrast the sharp smell of tea tree or eucalyptus compared to more mellow chamomile.

Following are a list of qualities to detect in essential oils. These aren't official terms used in aromatherapy, but they are ones that will aid your descriptions on essential oils. As with the other categories, make up your own terms, if you like. Think about each descriptive pair when smelling an oil. In other words, try to categorize an oil as mellow or sharp and then move on to detecting whether it's smooth or harsh. You won't necessarily find all these qualities in each oil, but many are obvious.

>> Soft or strong (sandalwood versus clary sage)

>> Mellow or sharp (chamomile versus eucalyptus)

>> Smooth or harsh (vanilla versus citronella)

>> Sweet or bitter (jasmine versus angelica)

>> Sour and acidic or sweet (lemon versus jasmine)

>> Full or flat (rose versus orange)

TIP

A trick to familiarize your nose with scent is to choose some common smell — orange or peppermint, for example — and then see whether you can imagine it. It helps to close your eyes and focus on your sense of smell. If this task is too difficult, give your nose a reminder by sniffing an actual orange or a peppermint tea bag and then put it down and let your imagination try again. Then see whether you can identify the quality. Is it well-rounded or flat? If you have an essential oil that you purchased a long time ago and a newer one, compare the two. Chances are that the older bottle will smell flat because it has lost some of its aromatic punch and the newer one will smell more full-bodied.

Scent notes

A third category classifies fragrance as a high, middle, or low *note*. Scent is so analogous to music, that perfumers borrowed the idea of fragrance notes from musicians. They place different scents on a scale, similar to a musical score, and designate them as top, middle, or base notes. A fragrance can just have one note, but more notes in the scent create a richer experience. (You can try to determine the top, middle, and base notes for extra credit.)

It's not easy to pigeonhole an essential oil, especially a complex one, into any scent categories, but perfumers and aromatherapists do it anyway to help them better understand fragrance and blending. If you have a keen nose, you'll pick out many of the oils that have elements of more than one note.

>> A **top (high) note** smells light and is described as airy. A high note is the flirty aspects of smell. It's the first one to greet your nose, but then dissipates quickly. Examples are lemon, grapefruit, lime, and peppermint.

>> A **middle note** is trickier to detect because it falls somewhere in between the high and low notes. A middle note can confuse your nose by seeming to bounce between the high and low note or take on different notes depending upon what other essential oils are mixed with it. Examples are chamomile, fennel, and marjoram.

>> A **base (low) note** is just the opposite of a high note. It smells "heavy" and has staying power. Examples are cedarwood, jasmine, and sandalwood.

TIP

Imagine that you're listening to music. Someone is hitting the same piano key over and over. You have no interest in continuing to listen. In fact, you wish they would stop. It's very *one-sided*. Compare this to hearing a full piano concerto played. Many notes are involved, and it moves all around the scale. There is a much richer sound with a full bouquet of notes that sound musical to your ear. Although lavender is floral, it also smells herbal. Then another note comes carrying just a hint of pine. You can see why lavender and many more essential oils are listed under more than one category.

Blending It All Together

When you understand the language of fragrance, practice identifying individual scents and naming their characteristics. Use the vocabulary in this chapter or make up your own if that's easier. Once your nose is sharp and you've got the fragrance language down, you'll be able to use this information to craft your own concoctions by blending different essential oils that smell good together.

Practice, practice, practice, and your nose will be as keen as a professional perfumer's nose! All your experimentation will automatically settle into the part of your brain responsible for remembering scent. So, practice the language, sniffing, and blending.

Taking baby steps

REMEMBER

When experimenting to see how different essential oils blend, add each oil in small amounts — that's drop by drop. Keep different batches so you can come back and compare. To aid your comparison, be sure to label everything with the exact amounts you used.

When you're learning to create essential oil blends, try starting with a complex essential oil like geranium. Geranium is such a complex oil that it already smells like a blend. This makes it a good starter oil. With all those scents in one oil, whatever you add to it will carry it in a different direction. For example, add rose or another floral, and your blend is decidedly floral. Add any citrus to rose geranium, and your blend moves into that category. In other words, the added scent pulls out the same scent that already naturally occurs in geranium. You can do this same blending trick with other complex oils, such as rose.

Training your nose

Did you know that perfumers go to school to learn their trade? While there, they put their noses through drills. You can try some of these at home. They'll help you better get to know the aromas of a variety of essential oils and how they merge when blended. You need to mix only a few drops of essential oil to complete the drills. This exercise comes in handy. It helps you imagine how your blend will smell before you even start mixing oils. Here are a couple of nose drills in which you compare and contrast aromas.

» **Similar Study:** Mix very similar essential oils together one by one and see how the aroma of the overall blend gradually changes. For example, do a series with citrus. Start with a drop of orange, which is a relatively simple, uncomplex oil. Add another drop of a citrus like lemon. The next drop could be lime or grapefruit. You'll notice the blend becomes more interesting with each drop. Next, try mixing several woods or florals.

» **Contrasting Study:** In this exercise, choose oils that contrast with each other. Select oils from different categories so the blends will smell quite different. That gives you many, many choices. You can mix a drop of a floral essential oil with a woody one or a spicy scent with one of the many citrus essential oils.

SWEET SCENT OF SUCCESS

No doubt about it, fragrance sells. Savvy companies are smelling the sweet scent of success as they jump on the aromatherapy bandwagon. Businesses are looking for "Noses," people who can use fragrance language to create aromatic blends for them. Marketing surveys show that consumers prefer scented products over unscented ones and the better these products smell, the more they like them. The result? Enticing scents waft from the bakery, thanks to strategically placed fans. Cosmetic companies promise to change your mood if you wash your hair with their aromatherapy shampoo. Many stores pump scent through their heating and air-conditioning systems to encourage customers to buy. (And they do.) When Dr. Alan R. Hirsch, Director of the Smell and Taste Treatment and Research Foundation in Chicago circulated pleasant scents through the air-conditioning system of a Las Vegas casino, slot machines sales soared an impressive 40 percent. He also found that just pitching a sale to someone in a scented room made them more likely to buy.

IN THIS CHAPTER

» Finding the best deals on quality oils

» Following the essential oil supply chain

» Recognizing the phonies and identifying the good stuff

» Being eco friendly

Chapter **3**

On the Scented Trail: Shopping

Essential oils are big right now. All types of stores, including mail-order catalogs and websites sell essential oils. The problem is, with such a variety of essential oils and aromatherapy products, how do you decide which ones are actually essential? (You may *need* to use an aromatherapy antistress formula just to get through all the decisions you'll encounter shopping for essential oils.) And when you've made your investment in essential oils and aromatherapy products — and they're not cheap — then you'll want to know how to keep them good for as long as possible. The oils in those little vials have been on quite the adventure before you bring them home, and where they've been might impact your purchase decisions. (And help you sift through all the marketing!)

In this chapter, I show you how to tackle the aromatherapy shopping maze and exactly how to store and keep your precious oils to get the most value and effectiveness from them. Finally, I explain the journey from aromatic plant to that essential oil vial in your hand, so you know where it came from and can decide whether it's right for you.

Searching for Good Scents

Simply put, the kind of oil you're looking for is a quality, completely natural, undiluted essential oil with full potency. To get that, you need to choose oils that come from an aromatic plant that was properly grown and had its essential oil carefully extracted. You also want your oil to be properly stored and shipped.

On your essential oil quest, you need a few tools. You'll want a well-trained nose, a good sense of what to look for in a quality oil, and the ability to choose reliable suppliers. The good news is that you can carry all of these tools with you. (For help training your nose, check out Chapter 2.)

REMEMBER

There's nothing more educational than hands-on, or I should say nose-on, experience. Become familiar with essential oils first-hand and compare the good from the bad. Smell so many essential oils that their scents become etched in your brain. You'll be surprised how quickly that happens. Your sense of smell is connected to your brain's memory areas, so put it to work!

You can sniff the movement of essential oils as they move up an aromatic plant as it matures. Pick an aromatic leaf from your yard or a park. Rub it between your fingers and smell. Visit this plant several times during its growing season and notice how the fragrance increases in its leaves until the plant flowers and then slowly declines.

TIP

It's a good idea to get to know your essential oils by their aromas before you invest in them. Attend an essential oil workshop presented by an aromatherapist, find a store with good samples to sniff, or visit a friend who has a substantial essential oil collection. Better yet, do all three!

Noticing quality

For quality control, teach your nose to know the difference between essential oils that smell full-bodied and complete rather than flat. Use it to sniff out the individual compounds that give the oils their aroma and healing properties. To do this, pick out the aromatic types and notes that it contains. It's helpful to talk this aroma lingo when you're trying to identify what you're smelling. Yes, even if you're just talking to yourself.

TIP

Want to learn how to determine essential oil quality and train your nose, and to pick up aroma lingo along the way? It is all just a few pages away in Chapter 2.

Making the grade

In talking about essential oil grades, the question is whether you always need the best grade and top-of-the-line oils. Is using the highest quality oils practical or even necessary? The answer depends on how you intend to use them. For example, aromatherapy candles and soap require so much essential oil that you can probably turn to a good, but inexpensive essential oil. The quality of oil you put in your facial cream is a different story.

Don't dump out all the essential oils you've already purchased in fear that you didn't choose the best ones. Don't feel that you always need to spend a fortune.

Asking the quality questions

To decide what grade of aromatherapy products and essential oils to use, ask yourself these questions:

>> How am I using the essential oil or finished product?

>> How important is the quality to achieve maximum results?

>> How substantial is the price difference among various qualities?

>> Does the more expensive brand really smell that much better?

>> Do I need to use more of the essential oil to get the desired scent and benefits?

REMEMBER

Using cheaper essential oils doesn't always save money. An aromatherapist I know manufactured a beautiful body cream. One time, she resorted to scenting it with a low-grade essential oil. The oil didn't provide enough fragrance, so she added more and more oil. It took four times the amount of her normal recipe to achieve the right scent. In the long run, it cost her more money, and the cream ended up with far too much essential oil for safety.

Choosing among varieties

Essential oils produce many variations. Different versions of the same essential oil smell different and have slightly different uses. But just because the tea tree oil nicknamed "MQV" is an especially strong antiviral, that doesn't mean common tea tree won't work great to treat infections, acne, or eczema.

In a study, aromatherapist Jane Buckle, R.N., used two different lavender essential oils with patients recovering from heart operations to help them relax during recovery. Lavandin, a hybrid often considered a lesser grade, proved more effective than true lavender.

Also consider your personal preferences. Aromatherapist Mindy Green, co-author of *Aromatherapy, The Complete Guide to the Healing Art*, and I sat down to a selection of rose essential oils from several different species. As we carefully sniffed and compared, we eventually found our favorites. They weren't the same. It wasn't that one was better quality; we each just had a different preference.

Buying Essential Oils

Make your shopping days easier by following these simple tips:

» **Choose your source wisely.** Buy essential oils from companies that have a reputation for quality you can trust. This is not always easy, but look for companies that offer accurate information. It's a good sign if the company is owned by an aromatherapist, or at least has one on staff.

» **Hold back.** Don't buy much with your first order from a new company so that you can sample the oils and check out their quality.

» **Ask about the oils.** Are they undiluted? Ask where they originated. Have the company supply the botanical names and ensure that their essential oils came from those plants.

» **Check for authenticity.** Make sure that the line of essential oils doesn't include any blatantly synthetic essential oils such as carnation, lilac, or strawberry. If so, all their oils may be synthetics, even if they claim otherwise.

» **Check for purity.** See whether the oil stains, has alcohol overtones, or smells weak or not balanced.

» **Check for quality.** Sniff out scents that are fuller, rounder, and more complex. A little essential oil should go a long way.

Sniffing out the best deals

You may think that the higher the price, the better the essential oil. Or, that the grade of an essential oil is reflected in its price. This is often the case but not always your best guide to quality. Lots of factors influence essential oil prices.

Looking at price indicators

If you wonder why you see such a large range of prices for essential oils, consider some of the factors that go into pricing:

>> Cost of harvesting the aromatic plants

>> Ease in producing the essential oil

>> How much oil the plant produces

>> Market demand for the oil

>> Overhead of the company selling the oil

The upcoming "Keep on trucking: Following the supply chain" goes into these factors in more detail.

Adding up the extras

If you run a business, you know it isn't cheap. You need to pay for packaging and brochures and offer information on your website. The same goes for larger companies. Essential oil businesses may offer personalized instruction, a professional aromatherapy formulator, an aromatherapy advisor, as well as customer service representatives. Just keeping a large selection of essential oils on hand gets expensive. You end up paying for these bonuses, but if they enhance your experience as a consumer, they may be worth that higher price tag.

Some companies have their own, expensive lab to analyze their essential oils. They can let you know if an oil is pure and unadulterated. Sophisticated equipment also dissects the oil's composition to see whether it contains the right percentage of compounds. (Small companies may also have this information supplied by their distributors.)

REMEMBER

Essential oil prices might be better on the internet because online companies have less overhead than brick-and-mortar businesses, but you do face a big disadvantage in that you can't smell the oils before purchasing them.

Laboring for oils: You pay for production costs

The cost of an essential oil is based on how much work is involved to get the oil from plant to vial. That can be a lot of work, as you can see in the upcoming "Keep on trucking: Following the supply chain" section.

Growing an aromatic plant can be labor intensive or almost no work at all. The amount of effort depends on whether the plant is grown on a farm or collected from the wild and whether it is a fast-growing annual or a perennial that will be in place for years.

The amount of essential oil yielded by each aromatic plant is an important price influencer. As you can imagine, the better the yield and the less work to harvest, the less expensive the essential oil. Table 3-1 compares eucalyptus and rose oil production.

As the table shows, rose is a real diva that's very high maintenance and is, thus, one of the most expensive essential oils. In comparison, eucalyptus oil sells for just a few dollars an ounce.

TABLE 3-1:   **Comparing Production Methods**

Eucalyptus	Rose
Oil is distilled from the large leaves of very fast-growing trees.	Oil is distilled from bushes that take several years to produce enough oil-producing flowers.
The trees contain natural insecticides and need almost no care while growing.	The bushes require labor-intensive pruning, weeding, and insect control.
The oil is easy to transport and yields a generous amount when distilled.	It takes a pickup truck bed filled with roses to generate a small bottle of precious rose oil.

Clamoring and demanding oils: The impact of supply and demand

Demand for each essential oil in the worldwide market affects its price. High demand lowers costs because farms can grow large crops. They're also assured of having buyers so there's less business risk involved.

You may be surprised to hear that essential oil demand isn't based on aromatherapy needs. For all its popularity, aromatherapy still represents a very small portion of essential oil use. The demand comes from the food, candy, and perfume industries and to scent hand- and dishwashing soaps and cleaning supplies. These commercial uses were in place long before aromatherapists stepped into the picture.

As a result, essential oils made from culinary herbs tend to dominate essential oil lines. That's the oregano, black pepper, sage, rosemary, coriander, and cumin in your spice cabinet. Because these oils are already produced to flavor canned goods and frozen foods, they're relatively inexpensive. The same goes for the clary sage essential oil that flavors some tobaccos. The cost of tea tree essential oil went down as demand increased for it to flavor toothpaste and mouthwash.

Essential oils that don't fit into large markets are comparatively pricey. However, many folks willingly pay the high price of essential oils like helichrysum just to have its skin-care benefits.

Keep on Trucking: Following the Supply Chain

What can go wrong for an essential oil during its journey from the field to your hand? A lot can happen between the time an aromatic plant is growing in the ground and when you lovingly pour its essential oil into your aromatherapy product. You can appreciate the dedication farmers and essential oil suppliers have in bringing their oils into your home. When you consider the effort that goes into each little bottle, prices seem amazingly low.

Producing an essential oil is a journey. Follow the many steps your oil takes to reach you:

1. **Choosing the plant.**

   The grower must choose which aromatic plant species to grow and select the seeds or plant starts from good stock.

2. **Cultivating the crop.**

   Nature's quirks, such as weather and soil type, can alter an aromatic plant's chemistry. Sometimes that's for the better, but sometimes not. Growing conditions for a plant either on the farm or in the wild vary from year to year and from one location to another. As an herb gardener myself, I can tell you that you usually can't do much about most growing conditions.

3. **Maintaining the crop.**

   Depending on the plant, to maintain an aromatic crop, the grower might have to condition the soil, add compost or fertilizer, thin seedlings, control weeds and insects, irrigate, and even prune.

4. **Harvesting the crop.**

   You can harvest most fragrant plants only once a year. To achieve an optimum essential oil, the framer harvests each part of the plant at a different time. With leaves, this is just before they flower. Flowers are ready when they bloom (although you harvest lavender in its bud state). Seeds are ready when they ripen. You dig roots and rhizomes in the fall and spring.

However, sometimes the perfect time to harvest doesn't work out for the farmer. Rain or equipment failure are just a few of the things that can get in the way. When that happens, farmers can't pick plants at their peak, and they don't have prime essential oils.

5. **Drying the plants (maybe) and distilling the oil.**

   You can dry plants for later processing or distill the oil more or less immediately after harvest.

   If you dry the plants before the oil is distilled, the drying process needs to be done with care to retain as much essential oil as possible so the plants don't mold. Even proper drying can result in losing 30–40 percent of the essential oil content. Dry the plant in poor conditions, and oil evaporation rates climb.

   After you harvest and dry an aromatic plant, you need to keep it away from light, moisture, and high heat to retain its essential oils. It takes so much plant material to produce essential oil that you might need a large storage facility.

   Most plants aren't distilled where they are grown. That means someone must transport them from the farm or wild to another town or from one country to another. All sorts of quality concerns come up here. Are they shipped in airtight bags or burlap? Are they moved in open pickups? How good is the storage facility?

   Some aromatic plants are distilled fresh, which means either having a distiller on site or immediately shipping all the heavy, fresh plant material to another location.

   The type of equipment and the temperature used to extract the oil is another consideration. I've encountered essential oils that smelled burnt due to poor production techniques.

6. **Storing the oil.**

   After an essential oil is produced, it still needs to be carefully stored away from heat and light to retain quality. Sure, it's now enclosed in a — hopefully glass — bottle. Yet, it's still susceptible to deterioration.

7. **Getting the oil to the consumer.**

   Your essential oil is on the road again as it travels to you, the consumer. The supply chain from grower to distiller probably involves going to more than one distributor. The oil may detour to a bottling and labeling facility. It finally reaches your online or local brick-and-mortar store, where they may rebottle it one more time.

REMEMBER

Farms and businesses do change hands. Commitment to quality can change along with that.

Navigating the Consumer Jungle

Because the quality of essential oils varies greatly, it can be a jungle out there for consumers. When you begin your essential oil quest, seek out companies you can rely on. It may take some trial and error. Some businesses offer only top-of-the-line essential oils, while other companies are satisfied with pretty-good quality. Then you have companies who stick to the cheapest, let's-make-a-buck ingredients. Those are the ones hoping that you're not reading this book!

TIP

Companies are inclined to use the same grade of essential oil for their entire line, so if you're unhappy with one oil, you probably won't like the rest.

Some companies are inconsistent with the quality of their essential oils. If you go back to buy the same essential oil you purchased and liked a few months ago, you may find the second one lacking. Supply-chain problems lead some companies to stock essential oils below their usual standard so they don't lose sales.

WARNING

Take advice from a company itself with caution. Expect to find, as with other products, a lot of marketing hype. It's just part of the game. Read advertising material with a discriminating eye so that fancy ads and elaborate packages don't sway you.

For example, watch out for declarations that a product line is superior to all others. I can assure you that there's no one essential oil company that's better than the rest. I know through my connections in the industry that many essential oil companies purchase their oils from major distributors, and there's only a few of those. I've seen competitors who claim to have better essential oils than other companies ordering from the same distributor.

When a company says they grow all of the plants to make their essential oils on their own farms, chances are this is true for some of their oils. They probably also contract farms and distilleries around the world, since essential oils-bearing plants need to be grown in so many different climates.

TIP

On your essential oil shopping sprees, come to the store or internet site armed with information and ask questions. Then, weigh everything you hear against what you already know so that you can make well-informed choices.

SHOW THAT ID

Essential oils are identified by many descriptive names that companies use to express the quality of their oils. Some of the terms you may find used to describe an oil include Pure, Aromatic, Quality, 100% Pure, Therapeutic, First, Artisan, Premium, Professional, Aromatherapy Level, Pharmaceutical, Certified, Tested, Grade, Primary, and Guaranteed. What do these terms mean? Well, they mean a lot to the businesses using them but not much beyond the confines of that company. Because these terms are coined and adopted by the company, they don't really tell you about the quality of the essential oils or help you compare one company's oils to another. It's confusing, but you'll have to admit, it's clever marketing.

No official terms for describing essential oil quality are recognized by an aromatherapy association, business group, government agency, or independent standard committee. However, you should look for a couple of designations. Both of these refer to the general safety of that essential oil but not to any particular oil or brand.

- A USP food grade designation from the United States Pharmacopeia indicates that an oil is safe to use as culinary flavoring — extremely diluted, of course.

- Most culinary essential oils also have *GRAS* status, meaning they're Generally Recognized As Safe. Balsam of Peru, bergamot, lavender, and melissa essential oils may also have GRAS status because they are used as flavorings. You can't depend on the GRAS status for all of your essential oils. Many essential oils don't qualify for this status, since they aren't used in food or drinks.

  The GRAS status is also given to some essential oils that are normally toxic. Except in this case, the toxic compound has been taken out in the lab. A good example is wormwood, which has its toxic compounds (thujone) removed. I mention this since at first glance, it may seem safe to use wormwood, but that's only when the toxic compound is pulled out of oil. The safer version of wormwood is created to flavor some alcoholic drinks.

Getting less than the essentials

Sometimes, what is sold as an essential oil isn't essential and may not even be an oil. The essential oils you find for sale may be altered in a number of ways. They may be

>> **Diluted:** A different oil or another substance is added to extend an essential oil.

>> **Enhanced:** An essential oil can be enhanced by adding a compound that the oil already contains. An example is adding extra compounds found in

lavender oil to lavender essential oil. This gives the scent more of the sparkling punch for which lavender is famous.

» **Spiked:** A less expensive essential oil is added that has a very similar aroma but not the exact compounds.

» **Substituted:** One essential oil, usually a less expensive one, is passed off as another oil.

» **Synthetic:** The essential oil or some of its added compounds were synthetically produced.

» **Mislabeled:** An essential oil is improperly packaged. A supplier can accidently mix two different oils or mislabel an oil. Yes, it happens. Trust your gut feeling rather than every label you read.

I explain most of these processes in the following sections.

REMEMBER

Adulteration is making a substance impure by adding an inferior substance. With essential oils, you see adulteration most often with oils that carry a high price tag. Some companies add inferior oils to stretch their dollars, and their ethics, to save a buck. However, with such a long supply chain, it's often difficult to know where to point the finger. It doesn't help that you don't often see additives listed on the label. Alterations change an essential oil's scent and its healing properties. Some adulteration is easier to detect than others with a good nose.

Adulteration is all about altering an essential oil, which creates a new mix of compounds. This can affect the oil's quality and change the scent and therapeutic use. Laboratory analytical equipment can show that the oil contains too few compounds or maybe the wrong mix of them. (For more on essential oil compounds, check out Chapter 15.)

Some popular and essential oils that may be adulterated, substituted, or diluted to save money include the pricey ones in the following list:

» Frankincense

» Jasmine

» Melissa (lemon balm)

» Myrrh

» Neroli (orange blossom)

» Rose

» Sandalwood

The essential oils in the next list are so inexpensive that they are rarely, if ever, adulterated, substituted, or diluted.

>> Citronella

>> Eucalyptus

>> Fennel

>> Orange

Diluting an oil on the sly

Essential oil companies sometimes dilute oils to make a pricey oil like rose more affordable. That's fine, providing they tell you. You should know what you are paying for!

REMEMBER

There's nothing wrong with diluting an essential oil. In fact, you should dilute essential oils before using them. If not, they may burn skin and result in taking toxic amounts. Diluting is only a problem when companies dilute essential oils without telling customers, and then charge for the oil as if it's pure.

The substances that some companies use to dilute essential oils include the following:

>> **Vegetable oil:** Vegetable oil is the easiest type of dilution to detect. Pure essential oils evaporate, leaving no stain. (A few highly pigmented oils like deep blue German chamomile and brown patchouli discolor, but they aren't oily.)

>> **Alcohol:** It's more difficult to detect that an essential oil is diluted with alcohol than with vegetable oil. However, alcohol does have a slight odor. Although alcohol blends well with essential oils, some oils separate from it.

>> **Chemicals:** This is the tricky one. Essential oils diluted with chemicals are difficult to recognize. These solvents are clear, non-oily, do not have an odor, and have a feel similar to essential oil. That's why they're used.

WARNING

>> **Chemical additives:** Chemical additives come with a potential health hazard because they are absorbed into your body when rubbed on your skin or inhaled into your lungs. That's not good, because most of them are suspected of causing health problems.

The problem arises when a company dilutes the oil on the sly to extend it and make more profit from it. One clue to help you detect any type of dilution is that a diluted essential oil smells weaker than the pure oil.

Enhancing an oil

Enhancing is when a company boosts an oil by adding compounds it already contains. You can extract some added compounds from the same plant or from another plant.

Purists object, but not all aromatherapists consider an essential oil that is enhanced with a natural compound as a problem, because the essential oil remains completely natural. What everyone agrees isn't so good is when the added compound has a synthetic source.

A distributor may guarantee that a certain percentage of an important compound is in their essential oil. If a particular oil doesn't contain that compound, a company can cheat by adding the pure compound.

An example is lavender. Some essential oil distributors guarantee that their best quality lavender contains at least 40 percent ester compounds, which provides lavender's characteristic high, almost sparkling aroma. Lavender can contain this much ester naturally, but not always. When it doesn't, the essential oil might be enhanced by adding esters that were extracted from another lavender oil or from another oil that contains the same esters.

As you can imagine, an enhanced essential oil is not easy to detect. It's as if you make lemonade but add natural lemon flavoring because the lemons taste weak. The flavoring you use may be extracted from real lemons or a manmade compound that resembles lemon. If you do this kitchen version of adulteration and add just the right amount, only the lemonade connoisseur will detect your secret.

When rose essential oil is cut with the much cheaper rose geranium oil, both essential oils contain lots of compounds. The blending of all those compounds can make it difficult to sniff out this adulteration. Give it a try anyway. Smell pure rose oil and pure geranium oil individually and then sniff the potentially offending oil. Go back and forth a few times, and you'll begin to detect the aroma of geranium in the rose oil.

Spiking an oil

Spiking mixes a couple of essential oils that have similar aromas together. Most often this means adding a small amount of a less expensive essential oil to an expensive one. The adulterant oil is probably from a close species or may be another essential oil that has a close chemical match.

Examples of spiking are slipping lavandin essential oil into lavender or corn mint into peppermint. Sometimes companies use two parts of the same plant, as in diluting clove bud with the leaf oil.

Substituting an oil

Now we're talking blatant fraud. *Substitution* is when an inexpensive oil masquerades as something else. A common example is when lemongrass, citronella, or lemon eucalyptus essential oil are sold as if they are really the very expensive melissa (lemon balm) oil. Although the substitutes are natural essential oils, they're the wrong one. If you get citronella oil when you thought you bought melissa, not only were you taken to the cleaners, but the oil may not have the therapeutic properties you need. When you're very familiar with the aroma of different essential oils, you'll be able to sniff out some substitutions.

Avoiding sinful synthetics

Aromatherapists won't touch synthetics. That's because aromatherapy is a holistic healing art with the emphasis on natural. As a branch of herbalism, it turns to plants for their healing properties. Aromatherapists agree that nothing does it better than nature. Natural oils — those made from plants — produce far better results than manufactured oils. Your body adapts better to natural medicines than manmade ones. Going natural also results in far fewer allergic reactions and sensitivities such as skin rashes, sneezing, headaches, and puffy eyes.

The safety of many synthetic compounds is questionable. Like natural essential oils, synthetics are composed of molecules that are tiny enough to be absorbed by the skin and inhaled to enter the bloodstream.

TECHNICAL STUFF

Receptors that charge reactions in your brain and the rest of your body are designed to connect to natural substances, including essential oils.

The appeal of synthetic oils isn't hard to realize. Compared to natural essential oils, synthetic oils are

>> Less expensive

>> More stable

>> Have a stronger smell

These are the reasons why many companies — making everything from candles to hair conditioners — sell "aromatherapy" products scented with synthetic oils. The bottom line is that synthetic essential oils save the company money. It's also why some aromatherapy research, with its eye on eventual commercial applications, uses synthetic essential oils. Perfume manufacturers also love the vast array of new and often otherwise unobtainable fragrances offered by synthetics.

Inventing imposters

Whipped up in a laboratory, synthetic essential oils are a brew of chemicals often with a petroleum foundation. Creating new compounds in the lab is much like a puzzle. Imagine that you have a puzzle cut into dozens of intricate shapes. Take out a few pieces and force them to fit into an entirely new puzzle, or in the case of a chemical, a new compound. Because the pieces aren't designed to fit together, you might have to knock off a corner here or there. It's amazing what chemists can do!

Some synthetics need nature's help to even come close to a natural fragrance. Rose is so complicated with its hundred or so aromatic compounds, it's especially difficult to duplicate. Chemists find it easiest to start with a bit of the natural. So, they take rose compounds out of something like geranium oil to mix with synthetics. While the final product mimics it, it never duplicates true rose. When I pass rose oils around in class, all my students spot — or should I say smell — the synthetics.

Sniffing out the disguise

Plenty of synthetics are out there. Next time you go to purchase a fragrant hand lotion or hair rinse, check the label. Even if you plucked your product off a natural food store shelf, it may still contain synthetic oils. The label may not help you at first glance because synthetics are labeled as essential oils. However, body-care companies that go to the trouble of using natural oils like to make a big deal about it on their labels. If you don't see the quality spelled out or the botanical name on the label stating the oils are plant-based, there's a chance what you're holding has synthetics.

TIP

Look for the fragrance industry's code word to distinguish essential oils from synthetic. Essential oils that are called *fragrance oils* are indeed synthetic.

You'll be surprised how easy it can be to detect synthetic essential oils and products containing them, especially after working with the real thing. Smell-wise, some synthetics are better than others, but they're all too sweet, too fruity, overpowering, and something about them just smells blatantly fake. It's difficult to describe, but synthetics can feel like an assault on the senses. One sniff, and I almost instantly feel a headache coming on.

TIP

Smell a synthetic essential oil and then compare it to the same natural essential oil. This little experiment can help you distinguish the difference between the two.

As you sniff your way through a store's rack of essential oils, watch out for the following. Find just one of these, and the other oils in the rack are likely to all be synthetic.

>> **Low prices:** If you find a very expensive oil, such as rose or jasmine, sold at a ridiculously low price — say less than $50 for an eighth of an ounce — you can bet that it isn't a natural essential oil. For true vanilla essential oil, you'll pay $50 for a little vial.

>> **Expensive oils:** Extracting a real essential oil from carnation or violet flowers is so expensive that you'll probably never see the true oil of either one for sale in its real form. That means when you do see these oils, beware. You're probably looking at a synthetic version.

>> **Improbable oils:** Look at other essential oils on the same rack. Popular scents such as lilac, wisteria, and peach can't be produced naturally.

>> **Manufactured scents:** Look at the names on oils. You can guess that an essential oil labeled "Rain" or "Asian Gardens" or "New Mown Hay" isn't real. When you find a brand that carries such obvious pretenders, assume that their entire line is fake.

TECHNICAL STUFF

In the 1950s, chemists were excited about new developments of manmade synthetics, my dad among them. It was the wave of the future, and it was theirs. The new chemistry expanded their field greatly, offering the hope of all sorts of new compounds, including drugs. Back then, chemists felt confident that they could duplicate nature's compounds — or at least they thought so. The modern, state-of-the-art equipment now available to analyze essential oils shows us a different story. What once looked like matches now display different traits, so they have different characteristics and reactions.

Shopping with the Environment in Mind

People are very concerned these days about the environment, and for good reason. Aromatherapists work with plants to make us all healthier. It's no surprise they also want the plants they use, as well as the environment, to be healthy. Aromatic plants need to be in abundance for us and for future generations.

Particularly worrisome are plants harvested in the wild. Unlike cultivated plants, they often have no backup because they're not always replanted. The limited native habitat of many plants is rapidly changing.

All sorts of conditions hurt the environment where wild aromatic plants grow including drought, fire, today's ever-changing weather patterns, livestock overgrazing, housing or factory development, pollinator loss, pest attacks on weakened trees, and, of course, overharvesting.

The greatest environmental problem is with trees and roots because trees take so long to grow. Trees are cut down for their roots or bark or damaged when their bark is stripped. Harvesting wild roots or rhizomes means first waiting a few years so they are large enough to harvest. Then, the entire plant needs to be dug up.

A solution to losing wild medicine sources is to propagate and grow plants sustainably on farms or use a new practice called *wild farming*, which cultivates plants in the wild. Wild farming uses less labor to potentially have stronger, wild-grown medicine. Meanwhile, environmental researchers are searching for ways to completely stop wild harvesting. They hope to leave the land where these plants live wild, giving the plants a chance to flourish again.

Protecting the endangered

Sustainability issues are in constant flux between conservation issues and companies invested in wild harvesting. CITES is an international organization with a Medicinal Plant branch that monitors wild harvesting. It lists wild plants as vulnerable, threatened, or endangered. United Plant Savers is made up of herbalists concerned about the non-sustainable harvest of wild medicinal plants. You can support organizations working to save medicinal and aromatic plants in the wild. See the Appendix for more on these and other environmental organizations and their work.

Some of the popular aromatic plants currently in trouble include the following:

>> **Atlas Cedarwood *(Cedrus atlantica)*:** Weakened by drought and overgrazing, these magnificent trees are on the decline, so they're considered threatened. Himalayan Cedarwood *(Cedrus deodora),* which is harvested for timber, is not threatened, but is still a concern.

>> **Sandalwood *(Santalum album)*:** It takes sandalwood trees 20 to 50 years to reach maturity. Fussy about where it grows, it's a parasitic tree that needs host trees growing nearby. India was the primary source, and the government controlled Madras and Mysore sandalwood. However, an active black market exists. Other species growing in Indonesia and Polynesia are now being distilled. Currently, Australia's plantation-grown sandalwood seems the most ecofriendly choice.

» **Rosewood or Bois de Rose (*Aniba rosaeodora*):** This South American tree has been cut down without being replanted for so many years, I don't even use its essential oil. The Brazilian Institute of Environmental and Renewable Natural Resources has begun certifying wild tree harvests when conservation methods are in place and the trees replanted. Rosewood's main linalool compound is abundant in essential oil plants. Its rosy spice scent is often replaced with coriander essential oil. (Just to be clear, this isn't the rosewood tree used in making furniture.)

» **Spikenard or Jatamansi (*Nardostachys grandiflora*):** Spikenard only grows wild in high-elevation alpine forests. It has become so rare that harvesting the rhizomes (roots) is banned even in its native Uttar Pradesh region of India. It is harvested wild but now also cultivated in Pakistan and Nepal, where the Fairwild Standard is promoting a sustainable international trade.

Buying mindfully

Money talks. You as a consumer have the ability to sway companies through what you buy. If a company's salesperson doesn't know the answers to questions about sustainability, ask them to find out. Even if you don't get answers, it doesn't hurt to remind companies that many consumers are eco-conscious and appreciate transparency about their products' origins. This encourages companies to pay more attention to where they source their oils.

Some questions you might ask when purchasing essential oils include the following:

» Are these oils from plants that were sustainably grown?

» Where were these plants grown?

» Are these fair-trade essential oils?

» Do you know the work conditions where the plants are harvested?

TECHNICAL STUFF

Unfortunately, the aromatic plant farmers producing essential oil crops tend to be in the poorer areas of the world. Like most farmers, they get only a very small percentage of what's made on the finished product, but rely heavily on this income. If consumers shift away from essential oil production, these farmers would need an alternative to make a living.

One environmental question that you'll likely encounter is whether essential oils should be avoided, because it takes so much cropland to grow them, and that may not be environmentally sound. I always consider environmental concerns but don't see a problem here. It does require more land to cultivate a pound of essential oil compared to a pound of herbs, but it takes more land to grow plants for essential oil production than for an aromatic herb drop. Or does it? When you consider that a quarter cup of dried herb is roughly equal to only one drop of essential oil, the amount of land needed comes out to about the same, especially when you consider how much essential oils are diluted before being used. So, while it may take more farmland to produce one ounce of essential oil than one ounce of herb, whether you turn to the oil or the herb, there's not that much difference.

Thinking organically

Organically grown essential oils are becoming more available. They come from plants that aren't grown with chemical pesticides (or chemical fertilizers) or treated with herbicides.

Organic farmers are typically on a mission to grow aromatic plants that produce high quality essential oils. This says a lot for their oils. Supporting these farmers and the companies that buy from them encourages less chemical pollution in our environment. This is true, even though essential oil chemists find that the compounds in pesticides are generally too heavy to go through the distiller that separates out the oil, so they don't end up in the finished product.

WARNING

Essential oils that are pressed from fruit rinds, such as citrus, are a different story. Pesticides are often used on citrus, and they cling to the surface of the fruits' rind.

Not all plants need to be protected with the use of pesticides. Some essential oils are natural pesticides. Wild plants harvested for their essential oils aren't eligible for organic certification because they aren't cultivated.

REMEMBER

Organically grown certification varies from state to state in the United States, but it is well regulated, and the organic farms are inspected. Essential oils are produced all over the world, so the requirements for certification aren't consistent. Some countries still don't have the designation; other countries have it, but they are unable to completely regulate it.

IN THIS CHAPTER

» **Using and storing oils correctly**

» **Noting the side effects and sensitivities**

» **Proceeding with caution during pregnancy**

» **Steering clear of toxic oils**

» **Checking measurements**

» **Keeping pets oil-free**

Chapter **4**

Safety First

You know the power of essential oils. You see how effectively they work to ease and heal many physical and emotional conditions. This makes them potent medicine for both physical and emotional problems, but it also means that you need to use them responsibly. Along with their powerful actions come some potential side effects that you want to avoid.

REMEMBER

All essential oils aren't created alike. They have different properties and aromas, and they also have different levels of toxicity. Some oils are safe if well diluted, but you need to think twice about using other ones.

If just the thought of toxicity makes you ready to abandon the aromatherapy ship, don't worry. This chapter helps you play it safe. I explain the problems that can occur when you use too much essential oil, apply the oil incorrectly, or use oils that are toxic. This chapter helps you choose which essential oils and aromatherapy products to use and which ones to avoid.

Playing It Safe

Everyone can agree that aromatherapy should heal, not harm. The best way to achieve that is to use small amounts of any essential oil and avoid the potentially toxic ones.

Applying a product that contains essential oils to your skin exposes you to much more of that oil than sniffing it out of a vial or hanging out in a scented room. My rule is to limit your personal exposure to essential oils to a couple drops a day for all the oil you use.

REMEMBER

Don't forget to consider the amount of essential oils in the aromatherapy products you rub on your skin, such as your hand lotion and toothpaste, and that scented candle or room freshener.

Don't confuse limiting your use of essential oils with limiting your use of the herbs themselves. Certainly, you can enjoy cinnamon buns and oregano on your pizza, no problem! Essential oils are much more concentrated than herbs. On the one hand, that's why you love them. They work so well and quickly because they're concentrated. On the other hand, their concentration gives them the potential to cause harm — burn your skin or worse, impact your kidneys.

TIP

Every time you consider using an essential oil, think about this: Just one drop of oil easily equals several cups of tea made from the herb. No one would think of downing 24 cups of tea in one sitting, although I've heard of people slathering themselves with the equivalent amount of essential oil.

Seeking treatment: DIY or going professional

Use essential oils for healing conditions that you already treat yourself anyway. You know, those times when you become your own doctor. You diagnose yourself and figure out the best way to treat a simple cold, headache, or other minor ailment.

When you have a health problem that normally sends you to a doctor — either conventional or holistic — then by all means make an appointment with your health-care provider. Don't wait for a medical situation to get out of hand.

REMEMBER

When treating yourself with essential oils, consider this your golden rule: Use essential oils therapeutically only when you're certain you know what's wrong and only if you feel confident treating it on your own. When you take care of injuries and conditions on your own, there's always a chance that you'll use the wrong remedy or treat the wrong condition.

WARNING

If you have any doubts about what you're doing when your health is at stake, don't take chances by using essential oils alone. Seek advice from a health-care professional.

When you're dealing with minor first aid — say a burn or a sprain that isn't bad enough to send you to your doctor — use your aromatherapy treatment to help relieve your pain and start the healing process right away. Your condition should show signs of healing within a day. The same is true if you come down with a cold or flu.

A seemingly minor infection can spread and rapidly worsen if not properly treated, so if you get sicker, re-evaluate that trip to your physician, acupuncturist, aromatherapist, herbalist, or somebody! How long you wait depends upon how much of an emergency you're facing, so listen to your common sense.

Following safety guidelines

Use these general guidelines to ensure you use essential oils safely and effectively:

» Dilute essential oils even when using them on your skin. Putting an undiluted essential oil directly on your body generally isn't wise. They're just too concentrated.

I admit at times it's quick and convenient to dab a half drop of lavender essential oil on each temple to ease your headache. Maybe you place a drop of tea tree essential oil directly on an insect bite or a herpes outbreak. When you're dabbing, make sure it's with the gentlest essential oils.

» Keep essential oils away from your eyes and ears and other sensitive areas.

» Don't take essential oils internally except under the supervision of a health-care professional.

» Don't use products containing *photosensitizing* essential oils — oils that, when applied to the skin, make that area of skin more sensitive to light — such as citrus oils and especially bergamot, before spending time in the sun or in a tanning booth with that area exposed.

See "Shining a Light on Sun-Shy Oils" later in this chapter.

» Use only the very safest and gentlest oils during pregnancy and for babies and young children.

» Do a patch test if you suspect that you're sensitive to an essential oil. (See "Testing for Scentsitivities" for instructions.)

SWALLOWING WITH CARE

Most aromatherapists prefer to stay on the safe side by using essential oils only on the outside, not their insides. Ingesting essential oils is not a good idea because they're so concentrated.

The safest and most effective method when ingesting essential oils is to take low doses. More is not better when it comes to aromatherapy.

Say you throw a few drops into a smoothie or a cup of tea; you may not be prepared for the way the oil moves through your body. Because essential oils are — no surprise — oil based, they quickly migrate out of whatever you eat to a more friendly surface like the roof of your mouth or your cheek. Some reaches your throat, and a little bit might make it to your stomach, but mostly the oil ends up treating your mouth. If your intended destination is your intestines, say to get rid of bowel problems, be aware that essential oil never makes it that far.

Special enteric capsules that stay intact and don't dissolve until they reach your lower gut help oils actually made it to your intestines. *Enteric capsules* contain only tiny amounts of essential oil in a carrier oil. For example, an enteric capsule of peppermint essential oil can reach the colon to treat problems such as irritable bowel syndrome. Follow the directions on the package to use them safely.

>> Keep essential oils out of the reach of children.

>> Use tiny amounts of essential oil on your pooch and avoid using oils on your cat.

Combining drugs and essential oils

Very few studies address the interactions of essential oils with drugs, but in most instances using essential oils while taking prescription medication is no big deal. Be aware of potential problems when combining essential oils and certain medications:

>> Don't use blood-thinning essential oils such as birch, wintergreen, clove, or garlic, while taking aspirin, warfarin, heparin, and other anticoagulant drugs.

>> Some researchers worry that relaxing essential oils like melissa (lemon balm) and chamomile may boost sleep aid and sedative barbiturate drugs like Pentobarbital and increase your sleeping time.

>> Because cinnamon bark energizes the mind, it may counter the sedative action of acetaminophen drugs.

Considering Oil the Effects

Essential oils help with all sorts of physical and emotional healing. So, why am I so concerned about safety? Because even the gentlest essential oil can be a problem to process if you have certain health conditions.

REMEMBER

Effects from many essential oils can be cumulative. Sometimes the resulting problems don't show up until years later.

Although I've heard some people say that burns and headaches from essential oil are a sign that the body is healing, I'm quite sure these effects aren't healthy. As a clinical herbalist and aromatherapist, I've dealt with people suffering from essential oil overdose, so I have reason for concern. Of course, I'm a big fan of using essential oils, but I like to see careful, well-educated use.

Considering your health conditions: Preventing toxicity

Do you have liver or kidney problems? Do you have any other chronic illness or condition that impacts your overall health? If so, you may be more susceptible to illness from essential oils.

To sum up who should be extra careful with essential oils and use very small amounts of essential oils, or use none, check this list:

>> Use essential oils cautiously if you're elderly, convalescing, or have a serious health problem.

>> If you have possible liver or kidney problems or these organs may be weak from previous disease or toxic exposure, you should avoid essential oils.

>> If you have a nervous system condition, stay away from the essential oils classified as neurotoxins (See "Your nervous system" later in this chapter.) If you have epilepsy or other seizure-related disorders, don't even sniff essential oils that promote the problem.

>> Although it may not be a problem, to be on the safe side, avoid essential oils that promote the hormone estrogen if you have an estrogen-related cancer or other disorders like endometriosis. The most estrogenic essential oils include anise, basil, clary sage, fennel, and myrtle.

Cut down the amount of oil you use or avoid essential oils altogether.

If you and your health-care provider decide that limited use of essential oils is safe for you, you can cut down the amount of oil you use. Several ways to create a lighter dose are

>> Choose only the safest essential oils, such as those recommended for use during pregnancy. (See "Exploring Essential Oils for Mother and Child" later in this chapter.)

>> Cut the recommended amount of oil in half.

>> Use essential oils as sprays or potpourri, or to scent a room rather than applying them on your skin.

>> Use the aromatic herb itself in tea, pills, or an extract rather than the essential oil.

>> Use a hydrosol instead of an essential oil. A by-product of distillation, hydrosols are water-based and contain only a small quantity of essential oils. (For more about hydrosols, see Chapter 14.)

Feel free to enjoy aromatic spices in your food or inhale the fragrance in a spray.

Taking care of your physical body

You may wonder exactly how essential oils act on your body and what happens if you use too much or use an oil that's toxic. In the next sections, I break down the effects on five areas of your body: your liver, kidneys, nervous system, brain, and skin.

Your liver

Your liver breaks down toxins as well as any essential oils that enter your body. Otherwise, the oils remain in your system and keep on cycling through it. Having large amounts of essential oils hanging around can slow down your liver as it tries to process them. That can be a problem because the liver already has a lot of work to do.

Unfortunately, your liver can be sick for years without letting you know it's in trouble. It's your body's manufacturing plant. Initially, it often causes digestive problems, but then leads to your body not being able to function. With all the pollution in the modern world, many people have livers that are quietly struggling to keep up.

If your liver is healthy and you follow the guidelines in this book for properly diluting essential oils, you should have no problems. (See Chapter 5 for more on diluting oils.)

WARNING

Rather than make a tired organ work harder and risk a toxic buildup, stick to using the mildest essential oils, especially if you suspect that you have poor liver health. Having an active case of hepatitis or cirrhosis of the liver are two good reasons to avoid essential oils altogether.

You only need to look at your spice shelf to find examples of aromatic herbs that can overwork your liver when they're in essential oils form — anise, cinnamon, clove bud and leaf, and fennel seed.

Your kidneys

Like your liver, your kidneys deal with essential oils once they hit your bloodstream. It's up to your kidneys to clear essential oils out of your body, generally in just a few hours. If you use a lot of essential oils, it taxes your kidneys.

Even healthy kidneys are susceptible to damage from excessive essential oils. Weak, injured, or sick kidneys can't keep up with even small amounts of essential oil.

WARNING

If you have weak kidneys, some of the essential oils to avoid are *anticoagulants* that hinder blood clotting. These include birch, wintergreen, clove, and garlic oils, as well as angelica, bergamot, and the citrus oils. Don't use essential oils at all if you have kidney disease.

Your nervous system

Essential oils that aggravate the nervous system aren't your friend if you have MS (multiple sclerosis), Parkinson's disease, or any physical problem that causes shaking, tremors, or physical instability. Anxiety, nervousness, and some mental conditions can worsen with certain essential oils.

WARNING

Using essential oils that are toxic to the nervous system demands caution. Be wary of using camphor, hyssop, wormwood, tansy, thuja, and even common culinary sage if you have nervous system problems. Simply inhaling neurotoxin oils like thuja and hyssop can bring on seizures in epileptics and others who are prone to them. For some folks, sage, "spike" lavender, and even rosemary can be a problem.

If you have liver or kidney problems, oils that are toxic to the nervous system compound the problem because these oils keep recirculating in your body rather than being broken down and eliminated.

What determines an oil's potential toxicity are the compounds it contains and how much is in that oil. *Ketones* are compounds that are particularly concerning. They make essential oils like wormwood and hyssop toxic. However, a few ketones aren't toxic. For example, a compound called fenchone in fennel is safe. Go to Chapter 15 to learn more about essential oil chemistry. Here are some problems ketones can cause.

>> Hurt the liver

>> Build up toxicity in the body

>> Not be metabolized, so they pass through your body unchanged, which can be rough on the kidneys

>> Overstimulate the nervous system

>> Be toxic to the nerves

Your brain

I've had aromatherapy students complain about slight headaches or feeling a little dizzy when working with essential oils at an all-day seminar. You may encounter these symptoms as well, but they're not a good sign. This sensory overload is your body's red flag warning that enough is enough. It also means your sense of smell's not working accurately, so you might as well quit.

To clear your head when you find your world is too aromatic, try these tips:

>> Take breaks so you don't work with essential oils for long periods of time. The amount of time depends upon how sensitive you are to the essential oils you're using. I generally stop after twenty minutes and take a fifteen-minute break.

>> Stop sniffing oils until your headache or dizziness is gone.

>> Go get some fresh air.

>> Take a lot of deep breaths — away from the essential oil aromas, of course.

>> Smell coffee beans to clear your nose.

Sometimes, in the excitement of making essential oil blends, I forget to monitor my time. At the first sign of an emerging headache, dizziness, or more likely for me, feeling less focused, I stop. I also reach for an herb extract that I keep on hand in case of an aromatic overload or an accidental essential oil spill. I down it several times throughout that day. My blend contains herbs like burdock root, turmeric, milk thistle seed, and dandelion root, but there are plenty of herb combinations to keep your liver and kidneys happy. Follow the dosage directions on the label.

Your skin

Skin reactions are common when you use essential oils topically, but usually, they are not severe.

REMEMBER

Any oil that burns your skin will burn sensitive areas like mucous membranes even more. Your mouth, for example.

Everyone's skin reacts to essential oils that are irritating, but if you already tend to get skin reactions, be extra careful with any essential oil.

Some essential oils that can irritate, redden, and even burn your skin are

>> Cinnamon

>> Cinnamon

>> Citronella

>> Clove

>> Oregano

>> Thyme

>> Wintergreen or birch

>> Citrus-peel oils, such as lemon and lime, with orange oil especially notorious

>> Lemon-scented essential oils that can produce reddening but aren't as troublesome are lemongrass, lemon verbena, and litsea.

TECHNICAL STUFF

Essential oils made from citrus peels can irritate and burn the skin due to a couple of different compounds they contain —aldehydes and phenols. If someone shows me a new essential oil and mentions it's high in either one of these compounds, my initial thought is to use that oil cautiously. To read about different oil compounds see Chapter 15.

Testing for Scentsitivities

Different people have different body types and constitutions and deal with different types of health issues and sensitivities. Your reactions to essential oils are different from mine. Sensitivity to essential oils or full-on allergic reactions can happen with any essential oil, but some oils are more inclined to produce adverse effects than others.

The side effects of essential oils can vary. A reaction might make your eyes puffy or cause you to start sneezing. It depends on how your body reacts to allergens and to anything that causes a sensitivity.

REMEMBER

If you find yourself sensitive to most fragrances, you're likely reacting to the synthetic ingredients in the fragrances — not to the essential oils in them. The problem almost always goes away when you switch to natural essential oils. I can't count the number of folks who told me they're allergic to rose scents and then had no reaction at all to rose essential oil. Chances are that you'll have fewer problems when you make sure you're sniffing the real thing.

You may hear that lavender and tea tree are the two gentlest essential oils you can use. Yet I've met plenty of folks who have sensitivity and allergic reactions to lavender. The same is true for tea tree, which contains some strong compounds.

They don't react to the oil itself, but to particular compounds in it. If you're sensitive to a particular oil, you probably react to other oils that contain the same compound.

TIP

If you find an essential oil product burns or irritates your skin, or you accidentally spill essential oil on yourself, wash it off with warm, soapy water. Soap plus warm water pulls off essential oils. Rubbing alcohol also works. Just reach into the liquor cabinet or use the rubbing alcohol in your first aid kit. Whatever you choose, work fast because the essential oil quickly absorbs into your skin. If you accidentally rub your eyes with essential oils on your hand, use eye drops or an eye cup with warm water to wash out your eye.

TIP

When you work with essential oils, it's a good idea to keep an eye cup and rubbing alcohol on hand so you're ready for an irritation or allergic reaction.

If you have a tendency toward allergies or sensitivities to plants, try a patch test before you use an essential oil:

1. **Set aside a bowl of warm, soapy water or have rubbing alcohol nearby.**

   If you have an allergic reaction, you need to wipe the oil off quickly.

2. **Dilute a drop of essential oil in ½ teaspoon of vegetable oil.**

   If you're testing an aromatherapy product, no need to dilute it.

3. **Rub a little oil or aromatherapy product in the crook of your arm.**

4. **Check your reaction.**

   If your skin reddens even slightly, you're having a mild reaction. You still may be able to use the oil or product if you dilute it more. If the spot you dabbed on the oil burns, itches, or turns your skin seriously red, this essential oil or product is not for you. Wash off the oil immediately with warm, soapy water or alcohol, and choose an alternative oil.

Shining a Light on Sun-Shy Oils

A few essential oils can cause a skin reaction in sensitive people when they go out in the sun after using the oil. This *photosensitization* reaction most often is uneven pigmentation that may look like a rash. The discoloration occurs where you applied the oil or a product containing it. Distilling the essential oil instead of pressing it removes the offending compound.

Citrus has a reputation for causing skin reactions. Generally, citrus essential oil is pressed from the peel, but it won't have the photosensitizing action if it's distilled. Bergamot is the most notorious of the photosensitizing citrus due to a compound called *bergapten*. Check the label for bergapten-free oil.

The following is a handy list of photosensitizing oils. Aromatherapists often recommend diluting these essential oils more than other oils (usually 2 percent in 98 percent of a carrier). I've included those dilutions below.

>> Angelica root (0.8 percent)

>> Bergamot (0.4 percent)

>> Cumin (0.4 percent)

>> Grapefruit

>> Lemon

>> Lime (0.8 percent)

>> Orange, bitter (1 percent)

I recommend that you don't use the photosensitizing essential oils of rue and marigold because they are very strong oils.

Compounds called *coumarins* are found in some essential oils. You may have heard your doctor mention this compound as a blood thinner. Herbs with coumarins are popular because they have a calming and uplifting effect when you inhale them. However, they're also the main culprit in sun sensitivity. The photosensitizing property isn't a huge concern with small amounts of essential oil, although you can stay on the safe side by avoiding the use of these oils if you've been instructed to avoid blood thinners.

WARNING

Be wary about applying essential oils and aromatherapy products that contain coumarins (or any photosensitizing essential oils) on your skin and then exposing that skin to the sun or sun tanning lights.

Exploring Essential Oils for Mother and Child

Aromatherapy can greatly enhance pregnancy; you just need to proceed with caution. Even the gentlest essential oils may be too stimulating for women prone to miscarriage. When in doubt, don't use essential oils while pregnant.

Instead of using essential oils, pregnant women can choose a safer route and drink gentle herb teas. Use aromatherapy mostly for sniffing to keep your emotions balanced.

REMEMBER

Be very cautious in using aromatherapy, especially during the first trimester when so much early development occurs.

Not everyone agrees on which essential oils to use during pregnancy or whether it's safe to use any at all. The truth is no one knows for sure, so everyone's taking an educated guess. I say play it safe and stick to light use of the mildest essential oils. Be especially careful about any essential oils that I say are potentially toxic.

Choose products designed for pregnancy or babies. If you're making aromatherapy products, follow these guidelines:

>> For pregnant women and young children, use half the usual amount of essential oils and keep to the gentle ones.

>> For babies, use one-quarter of the adult dose of only the gentlest essential oils, such as lavender and chamomile.

WARNING

Don't use citrus oils on babies.

Most children love citrus such as lemon, tangerine, mandarin, grapefruit, and orange. When they sniff them, kids (and adults) feel happier and more content. Citrus oils are fine for kids but be sure to dilute them properly and use them as a spray or just to sniff. Concentrated citrus oils can burn delicate skin, so never apply them directly to anyone's skin.

Essential oils considered okay to use during pregnancy and on young children include

>> German chamomile

>> Frankincense

>> Geranium

>> English Lavender

>> Neroli

>> Rose

>> Sandalwood

>> Spearmint

Avoiding Toxic Oils

Natural doesn't always mean safe. Some essential oils are simply too toxic to use. Other oils you need to use with care — in small amounts and always diluted properly. I divide the essential oils that you need to use with care into three categories:

>> Oils that can cause some minor issues, but are fine to use

>> Oils that can be toxic and shouldn't be used

Okay oils to use sparingly and carefully

These essential oils are fine to use, but can all cause skin irritations, and even burn your skin if used undiluted, so use them carefully.

>> Allspice (*Pimenta dioica*)

>> Camphor (*Cinnamomum camphora*)

>> Cinnamon

>> Clove (especially clove leaf)

>> Oregano (*Oregano vulgare*)

>> Thuja (*Thuja occidentalis*)

>> Thyme (except the gentler linalool chemotype)

>> Wintergreen/birch

Potentially toxic oils to run away from

Some essential oils are so strong, your best bet is not to use them at all. In fact, you won't even find these oils described or used in this book. I include the botanical name of the plant so that there's no confusion about which oil it is.

These oils all contain one or more compounds that adversely affect the nervous system, liver, and/or kidneys. However, all of these can be used for culinary and medicinal use in their herb form; just don't overdo it. And it's a good idea for you to read about the herb's potential toxicity first. Still, please feel free to slather your sandwich with mustard! You can eat that parsley garnishing a meal and go for horseradish wasabi that gives your sushi some zing. Just promise to not use the essential oils of any of these because they're so concentrated.

>> Bitter almond (*Prunus amygdalus var. amara*)

>> Calamus (*Acorus calamus*)

>> French tarragon (*Artemisia dracunculus*)

>> Horseradish (*Armoracia rusticana*)

>> Hyssop (*Hyssopus officinalis*)

>> Mugwort (*Artemesia vulgaris*)

>> Mustard (*Brassica nigra*)

>> Parsley (*Petroselinum sativum*)

>> Pennyroyal (*Mentha pulegium*)

>> Rue (*Ruta graveolens*)

>> Sassafras (*Sassafras albidum*)

Storing Oils Properly to Minimize Safety Risks

Store your essential oils with care. You can turn them toxic by contaminating them with how you store them.

Using the right container

Storing pure essential oils in plastic can lead to disaster. For one thing, molecules from the dissolving plastic contaminate the essential oil, so you end up with a lot more than you bargained for in your oil. Also, essential oils are so strong that they may completely dissolve a plastic container. I've heard some funny and not-so-funny stories about this happening.

As tempting as it is to keep your essential oils in dropper bottles for handy dispensing, essential oils eventually break down the rubber. Just the fumes coming off the essential oil does this even if the oil itself never touches the rubber. (Don't ask how I discovered this!) For the same reason, think twice about using those handy plastic inserts that fit inside the top of a vial to dispense your oils drop by drop. Guess where this rubber and plastic end up over time — you got it, in the oil. At the very least, keep the vials and bottles upright during storage. Glass is also best to store aromatherapy products containing essential oils.

I know it's convenient to keep your aromatherapy hair rinse, massage oil, or travel lotion in an unbreakable plastic bottle. If so, look for hard plastic containers, preferably ones designed to resist essential oil. The softer the plastic, the easier it migrates into liquid, even water-based hydrosols.

Preventing oxidation

To keep your essential oils fresh and potent you want to avoid *oxidation,* a reaction that occurs when oxygen combines with the aromatic compounds in an essential oil.

Oxidation breaks down the compounds in the oils causing

>> Scent to diminish, causing the oil to smell flat and not as lively. You can notice this in citrus aromas that don't have their whole spectrum of smells.

>> Loss of some therapeutic properties

>> A shorter shelf life.

WARNING

Oxidized oils are not good for your skin. Citrus essential oils are already harsh on the skin, and oxidation increases their irritating quality.

Considering that the air is filled with oxygen that causes oxidation, the obvious solution is to expose your essential oils to as little air as possible. Ways to curb air exposure include the following:

>> Keep oils in dark glass containers with tightly sealed lids away from sunlight and heat, the culprits that encourage oxidation.

>> Have as little air in the container as possible. Rebottle small amounts into smaller containers.

>> Make sure containers are super clean so you don't introduce bacteria into the oil. Run the containers through the dishwasher or boil them. Dry the containers thoroughly before filling them.

Examples of essential oils likely to suffer most from oxidation include

>> German chamomile

>> Ginger

>> Grapefruit

>> Fir

>> Juniper

>> Lemon

>> Orange

>> Pine

>> Tea tree

Avoiding Oiling Your Pets

Let's not forget your furry friends. The American Society for the Prevention of Cruelty to Animals, Animal Poison Control Center database says to watch out when using essential oils around your pets, especially cats. Pets experience depression, weakness, and muscle tremors and become uncoordinated when exposed to essential oils.

When your cat has been exposed to too much essential oil, it is typically agitated and drooling. Cats that ingest or are exposed to essential oils can even die. Dogs are inclined to lethargy and vomiting.

When exposed to natural flea preventatives, 92 percent of cats had adverse effects within 24 hours. These lasted from 30 minutes to 6 days. In these documented cases, about three-quarters of the owners applied the products correctly according to the label. Half of the animals recovered after a bath while others received intravenous fluids, muscle relaxants, and anticonvulsive medications. Of the cats treated with products applied to their skin that contained essential oils like tea tree, peppermint, cinnamon, lemongrass, and clove, 5–9 percent experienced symptoms of poisoning.

IN THIS CHAPTER

» **Converting your kitchen into a laboratory**

» **Diluting essential oils to make an aromatherapy product**

» **Making your first blends**

» **Extracting fragrant herbs into vegetable oil**

» **Figuring out proportions**

Chapter 5

Essential Oil Alchemy: Making Your Own Scents

P laying mad scientist in your kitchen is one of the benefits of your interest in aromatherapy. I warn you, though, that it's a fascinating hobby that can take over your life. That's what happened to me. And, it has not only taken over my life, but my kitchen. I devote vast stretches of kitchen cupboards and even a section of my refrigerator to aromatherapy supplies and projects. In fact, I don't cook as much as I'd like to because I'm too busy concocting my newest aromatherapy brainstorm. Instead of creating a carrot cake or soufflé, my kitchen's more likely to feature a neroli-rose facial cream or a lemon-oatmeal skin scrub.

When I began using aromatherapy products made with essential oils and other natural ingredients, I couldn't get anything commercially, period. I know that seems hard to believe considering the abundance of products you can buy nowadays, but it's true. There was only one thing for me to do: Make them myself. One thing led to another and pretty soon I started sharing my creations with friends and then selling them.

In this chapter, I tell you all you need to know to get started creating your own blends and products with essential oils — and to make sure that they smell good. (Aromatherapy's never going to work if you don't like the smell!) I also tell you what to do with your fabulous blend after you make it. Okay, are you ready to roll up your sleeves and get to work?

Getting in Touch with Your Inner Mad Scientist

Consider yourself lucky. Nowadays, you can find a wonderful selection of essential oils and aromatherapy products in a variety of places. If you're busy (and who isn't?), you can purchase anything you want. But why not dabble in making your own custom creations? It's as easy as it is fun.

Some concoctions are so simple, there's no reason not to make them yourself. They involve no more than adding drops of essential oil to vegetable oil or water. You can find many examples of these simple recipes in the Symptom Guide at the back of this book.

Making your aromatherapy creations is as simple as one, two, three:

1. **Turn your kitchen into a lab.**

2. **Choose the essential oil or oils you want to use.**

3. **Decide how to dilute them.**

TIP

Before you get started, read the basics on essential oils in Chapter 2 along with safety tips from Chapter 4. They give you a good foundation to stand on. The sections in this chapter delve into how to choose the oils and the material to dilute them with.

Converting your kitchen into a lab

No, you don't need fancy beakers or expensive microscopes. Except for the essential oils, you probably already have all the equipment and most of the supplies you need to turn your kitchen into an essential oil laboratory. The next sections talk specifics about what you need.

Gathering the right equipment

Before you go into production, make sure you have

» A glass measuring cup

» Stainless steel measuring spoons

» Small glass, stainless steel, or ceramic funnels to fit your bottles

» Vegetable oil

» Distilled water

» Rubbing alcohol

» Unflavored vodka

» Glass vials and bottles with tight-fitting lids (for storing your finished concoctions)

» Labels for your vials

» A notebook to document your recipes

Most of your fluid supplies are readily available from local stores or online retailers. You can buy or order fancier vegetable oils such as almond, apricot, and grapeseed at natural-food stores.

TIP

You'll probably want to gather some paper towels or rags and rubbing alcohol to help with spills and cleanup.

REMEMBER

Make sure to label everything so that you always know what's what and keep notes so that you can duplicate a winning success or avoid repeating a complete flop! I've had a few recipes that could have made a fortune . . . if only I'd remembered to write down the ingredients.

Managing the oils

You need a way to measure small amounts of the essential oils and transfer them from the vial to your project. Some essential oils are sold in bottles that have an insert called a *reducer* that has a small hole in the middle to let out only a drop of oil at a time. Allow yourself a few tries to get the technique. (If you shake the bottle, several drops slide out at once, so don't shake it.) Some essential oils are sold in dropper bottles that have special oil-resistant droppers. (Droppers are convenient, although they add to the cost of the oils.)

If your essential oil doesn't come in a bottle with either a reducer or a glass dropper, measure small amounts of essential oils with separate droppers (sold by drugstores, natural-food stores, and essential oil suppliers). You can also use a *pipette* (sold by essential oil suppliers). This long, narrow, plastic tube has a bulb at the top. You squeeze the bulb and then release. This makes the oil go into the tube and then drop out. Be sure to not let essential oil residue stay in the pipette because the oil dissolves plastic.

TIP

If you use a dropper or a pipette, practice first with water to get the hang of it before you start transferring your precious essential oils.

WARNING

Don't contaminate your essential oils by putting a dropper or pipette directly from one oil into another. If you don't have a separate dropper for each oil, rinse out all the essential oil with rubbing alcohol. In only a minute or so, the alcohol will completely evaporate so that you can put that dropper into another oil. Having two or three droppers allows you time to let one dry while you're using another one.

Deciding to blend scents

Why blend essential oils? Imagine sniffing lemon peel, or a sprig of lavender, or a single rose. Very nice, of course, but then imagine rose and lavender mixed with a hint of lemon. The result? A scent so spectacular that you can't get enough of it!

A blend holds the advantage of combining attributes offered by different fragrances. For example, you can use an aromatherapy blend to scent your bedroom that helps reverse your insomnia or an energizing blend to scent your office that keeps you awake and alert.

THE CASE OF MISTAKEN IDENTITY: A TRUE STORY

Mishaps can happen when you turn your kitchen into an aromatherapy lab. One time I put a facial cream I made into a clean mayonnaise jar and popped it into the refrigerator. Unfortunately, I didn't remove the original mayonnaise label. The next day at lunch time, I was writing in my office when I heard screams from the kitchen as my family bit into sandwiches that had been spread with some very expensive neroli-rose cream.

All I could do is joke that at least the natural ingredients I use are pure and quite edible! Rather than revealing any more embarrassing stories, I'll say that it's important to do as I say instead of as I do. Label everything appropriately!

Your first step is to decide which scents and which emotional qualities you want to combine. You have a whole lifetime of deciding which fragrances you do and do not like, and the Essential Oil Guide at the back of the book can help you choose what to combine. You can start out simply: Try combining just two scents.

TIP

You may think putting opposites together is counterproductive, but that's not the case in aromatherapy. Don't be afraid to combine a scent that increases energy with one with relaxation properties. After all, isn't that everyone's ideal state: Being perfectly relaxed yet having boundless energy?

There are many possibilities for using your blended scents. You can keep them in a glass vial to sniff whenever you want. That's all you need to affect a mood. Your blend can go into an essential oil diffuser to scent a room. (See Chapter 6 for diffusing ideas.)

REMEMBER

The important part of blending essential oils is that the final result smells good and is effective.

Talking Intensity

Essential oils vary in the intensity of their odor. To make a formula smell good, add small amounts of strong essential oils and larger quantities of the subtle ones. Otherwise, the strong ones will completely overpower the weaker ones.

It is far too easy for an especially potent oil such as rosemary to completely overpower the soft scent of sandalwood or cedar. When mixing small experimental quantities, even one drop of a high-intensity oil like cinnamon can be way too much. Try adding just a smidgen of oil with the end of a toothpick.

You can easily figure out which essential oils are subtle. I use more of these subtle oils than other oils:

>> Cedar

>> Orange

>> Sandalwood

Sniff any of the following very strong essential oils right from the vial and chances are you'll turn away because they're so strong. I generally use only one drop of these oils for every five drops of other oils:

>> Chamomile

>> Cinnamon

>> Clary sage

>> Patchouli

>> Rosemary

>> Ylang ylang

Some powerful essential oils aren't pungent, just intense. With the following, use only one drop for every ten drops of other oils:

>> Jasmine

>> Neroli

>> Rose

Tricks of the Trade: Blending Essential Oils

To make the best blends, rely on a few tricks of the trade:

>> **Choose one essential oil as the main scent.** You can then add small amounts of other essential oils to enhance the blend so that what you smell is the primary scent with the others in the background.

Start with an oil with a complicated aroma that already smells like a blend. Rose geranium, lavender, jasmine, and bergamot are good examples. Make it easy on yourself by starting with one of these and then layering. Add small amounts of additional essential oils to produce an interesting blend. Each choice sends your creation in a different direction.

TIP

>> **Add small amounts of strong scents.** Sharp smelling scents, such as fir, eucalyptus, peppermint, and cinnamon can overpower the other scents in your blend.

Use ylang ylang sparingly. The fragrance is intense, and most people find its fragrance overly sweet.

WARNING

>> **Be aware of how concentrated the oils are.** Rose and jasmine are expensive essential oils, but fortunately they are also extra-concentrated so that a little goes a long way. In fact, the scent is so powerful that you can substitute one drop of rose, jasmine, or neroli (orange blossom) essential oil in a recipe that calls for ten drops of another oil.

An interesting way to expand a blend is to choose oils that have similar characteristics. This performs a delightful trick on the nose as the scents play off one another. It makes your blend seem more complicated and mysterious because no one can pinpoint exactly what the aroma is. Try combining peppermint and spearmint, lemon and bergamot, or cinnamon and ginger.

A First Formula

With info on all these oils, you already have the makings of a formula. Sniff this blend when you need a quick pick-me-up.

>> Preparation time: 3 minutes

>> Yield: 13 drops

>> Ingredients:

8 drops orange oil

4 drops lavender oil

1 drop clary sage oil

1. Mix these essential oils together.

2. You're done. Didn't I tell you blending is easy?

Vary It! Known for promoting a dreamy relaxation, clary sage has a heady smell. If you prefer something more stimulating, replace the clary sage with one drop of cinnamon oil. For a sensual and sedating blend, use ylang ylang instead. A drop of cedar oil turns the blend more woodsy. It's your choice, and the options are almost endless.

Concocting the Simple Stuff

You make aromatherapy products by diluting the essential oils into a *carrier* (the substance, such as olive oil, that you use to dilute the oil). The oil may be just one essential oil or a blend of several different oils.

REMEMBER

Typically, you add 10 to 12 drops of an essential oil or a blend of oils to one ounce of the carrier.

The following sections describe both parts of the process.

Diluting into a carrier

Essential oils are so concentrated, you almost always dilute them into the carrier.

REMEMBER

A typical dilution ratio is 8 to 12 drops of essential oil per ounce of the carrier. Sometimes you use a little more or less depending upon the strength of the essential oil and what you're making.

Common carriers include

>> **Alcohol:** Essential oils mix well into alcohol much better than into water. Alcohol is a mild astringent with drying properties and is often used in oily skin products. It is also useful in your essential-oil skin products when the greasiness of vegetable oil is a problem — say for those times when you want to apply a pain reliever to your shoulder but don't want an oily shirt.

Unflavored vodka is the preferred alcohol because it's pure alcohol and water and has almost no smell.

Some other forms of alcohol include

- *Witch hazel distillate* is witch hazel bark and leaves extracted into alcohol.

- Rubbing alcohol is an ingredient in some commercial liniments but it's poisonous to drink and has a strong smell. (See Chapter 11 for liniment recipes.)

- An herbal tincture is medicinal herbs extracted into alcohol. For example, you can start with a St. John's wort tincture as your carrier (for nerve pain and inflammation) and then add essential oils.

>> **Salve or lotion:** If you want a thicker product than oil or alcohol offers, buy unscented lotion, cream, lip balm, salve, or hair rinse and stir in your choice of essential oils.

You may have to slightly heat a salve so that it turns semi-liquid before you add the oils. The easiest way is to place the jar in a hot water bath on the stove. Make sure the water level is below the top of the jar.

TECHNICAL STUFF

You can make salves, lotions, and other carriers from scratch. Get a book with recipes for making aromatherapy salves and creams such as my book *Aromatherapy* (Crossing Press). To find out more about herbs themselves, check out *Herbal Remedies For Dummies* by Christopher Hobbs, L.Ac. (Wiley).

- » **Vegetable oil:** Vegetable oil's molecules are too large to penetrate the skin. Instead, they smoothly slide over your skin, holding in moisture and protecting dry skin. This makes it ideal for body care. For advice in choosing a vegetable oil, check out the upcoming section "A slick question: Choosing a vegetable oil."

- » You can make your own infused oil to use as a carrier instead of plain vegetable oil. For example, you can start with a vegetable oil infused with calendula to soothe irritated skin and add essential oils to it. I explain the infusion process in "Making your own infused oil" later in the chapter.

- » **Vinegar:** Only a few aromatherapy products call for vinegar because it's difficult to mask its strong smell even with essential oils. With all the newfangled products available, vinegar has lost the popularity it held for centuries. That's too bad, considering that it improves your complexion and hair. Apple cider vinegar contains more minerals than distilled vinegar, which makes apple cider vinegar the preferred choice. You'll find that essential oils don't mix into vinegar as rapidly as they do into alcohol so you may need to shake the final product before use.

- » **Water:** Even though oil and water don't mix — even essential oil — the two form a good partnership in a facial spritzer, a household air freshener, or an aromatherapy compress. Use distilled water, which doesn't contain the bacteria that's in well water or the chlorine found in tap water.

  You can use other water-based liquids such as aloe vera juice, which is excellent for skin care and helps to heal burns.

The carrier you choose depends on how you intend to use your concoction. For example, opt for a vegetable oil such as olive oil for a body, complexion, or massage oil. Alcohol is very drying to the skin, but is useful to treat some skin conditions, such as oily skin with acne. Either one can be used as a carrier for essential oils that treat internal conditions, such as pain. You'll find that alcohol and vinegar aren't as easy to apply as vegetable oil, but both of these evaporate quickly, so they won't leave a residue on clothing. Water as a carrier is mostly restricted to a spray for a complexion moisturizer, foot or hand bath, or sprayed in the air as a mood changer.

A slick question: Choosing a vegetable oil

Vegetable oil slides smoothly over your skin without penetrating it, so it's ideal to use in body-care products.

TECHNICAL STUFF

Not all vegetable oils come from vegetables. In fact, they're far more likely to come from fruits, seeds or nuts. The word *vegetable* just means the oil is plant based.

Some people (including me) refer to vegetable oils as *fixed oils* because the oil is fixed in the plant and not easily released compared to an essential oil that moves into the air or on to your hand without any hesitation.

If you choose *cold pressed*, unrefined vegetable oils for your kitchen, you're making a good decision for your health. The best-quality oils are pressed when cold, which means they are processed under 110 degrees Fahrenheit (about 43 degrees Celsius). Quality oils are also good for your skin, although be aware they often come with a strong aroma.

Some oils smell so strongly they overpower the aroma of the essential oils. Olive and sesame oils are good examples. Another oil you want to avoid is peanut oil. No matter how much essential oil you add, it still smells like peanut butter sandwiches.

WARNING

Another reason to avoid peanut oil is that many people have serious peanut allergies.

What distinguishes one vegetable oil from the other isn't as well-defined as marketing literature suggests. The basic difference is the degree of thickness and texture and how much glide it produces when you rub over your skin.

The more solid the oil is at room temperature, the more preservative action it tends to have. That places olive oil, and especially coconut oil, right up there as long-lasting oils.

The following sections go through a whole selection of common fixed oils and their uses in aromatherapy.

Common vegetable/fixed oils

The following oils are the ones most commonly used in essential oil blends:

>> **Apricot kernel oil is similar in price, color, and texture to almond oil,** with a slightly lighter scent and texture.

>> **Avocado oil is deep green, rich, and heavy.** It's loaded with skin-nourishing nutrients and is recommended for dry skin. It's a little pricey, so you usually blend it with other vegetable oils.

>> **Castor oil is helpful in treating skin problems such as eczema.** It's so thick that you typically blend it with thinner vegetable oils to make cosmetics. Castor oil helps break down fibrous tissue and enhances immunity where it's applied. It is often used in *castor oil packs,* which are a special type of compress that help with these types of problems.

» **Coconut oil has a wonderful scent and a creamy texture.** Containing twice as heavy a fat as lard, coconut oil is solid at room temperature. Its thickness gives products that contain it a creamy consistency that seems to melt into the skin. You usually mix it with other oils because by itself your concoction would melt in a warm place. (If you're ever in a large southern Mexico market, be sure to visit a coconut oil factory where you can see them pressing the delicious-smelling oil with a hand crank.)

» **Grapeseed oil is odorless, mildly astringent, and has a light texture and scent, so is favored in aromatherapy cosmetics.** Use it for dry or acned skin treatments that don't tolerate a thicker oil.

» **Olive oil is often preferred for medicinal uses because it's rich in healing chlorophyll.** It can be cold pressed without solvents and keeps longer without refrigeration than other vegetable oils — for more than a year. The strong smell of the dark green virgin oil overpowers other aromas, so choose lighter versions for aromatherapy.

» **Sesame oil is a favorite in *Ayurvedic medicine* (a traditional medicine from India).** It contains a natural preservative and provides some sun protection (equivalent to SPF 4 or 5). You rarely find the unrefined oil used in aromatherapy because it smells so strongly of sesame.

» **Sweet almond oil has a light, sweet scent with a good glide for skin care.** It's a little more expensive than most vegetable oils.

Fancy vegetable/fixed oils

The following fancy (and more expensive) vegetable oils are popular in aromatherapy skin care. Due to their expense, you often use small amounts and combine them with an oil from the list in the preceding section.

» **Hazelnut oil has a mild fragrance and is light in texture.** It's often used in products for oily skin.

» **Jojoba oil joins this list, although it is actually a vegetable wax rather than an oil.** Use it like vegetable oil, anyway. It has the advantage of not turning rancid, which means your aromatherapy project won't spoil. It's expensive, so you may want to save it for products you intend to keep for a year.

» **Kukui nut oil is the thinnest, lightest of these oils and the least greasy — suitable even for oily skin.** It has its own distinct odor but usually blends nicely with the aroma of essential oils. In its native Hawaii, the nut is used to recondition sun-exposed skin, although it isn't a sunscreen.

>> **Macadamia nut oil has a very light texture but is still quite rich. It is slightly heavier than kukui.**

>> **Rice bran oil has a smooth, nongreasy texture.** It's especially high in vitamin E, so it doesn't spoil rapidly.

>> **Tamanu oil hails from tropical regions of Asia and is popular in Polynesia.** Anti-inflammatory and pain-relieving properties make it useful for treating sciatica, arthritis, rheumatism, and shingles, along with skin problems like acne, chapped skin, and burns.

>> **Wheat germ oil is so thick that you need to dilute it with another vegetable oil.** It contains high amounts of vitamins A and E so it nourishes and heals the skin, but it does spoil easily.

Herb seed oils

Oils derived from herbs are expensive, a fact usually reflected in the price of products that contain them. All of the oils listed here are high in *GLA (gamma linoleic acid)*, an important fatty acid that maintains healthy skin and is often used for mature skin. GLA helps repair and regenerate skin damaged by sun or burns and can mitigate stretch marks and scars.

TIP

All the benefits are great, but GLA oils are also expensive with a relatively short shelf life. Keep them refrigerated and store the final product in a cool place.

Generally, you use these GLA oils to make up only 5 to 10 percent of your essential-oil formula:

>> **Borage seed oil is derived from the seeds of this popular garden herb.**

>> **Black cumin seed oil is from a Middle Eastern plant that destroys bacterial and fungal infections and is used for respiratory problems.** It's also a pain reliever.

>> **Black currant seed and red and black raspberry seed oils come from these fruits.**

>> **Evening primrose oil is from the seeds of this herb that is found growing wild in the United States.**

>> **Rosehip seed oil comes from the hip that forms after a rose flowers and contains the seeds.** It can have a strong fragrance. This, along with the expense, usually dictates that you use it in small amounts.

> » **Sea buckthorn seed oil is often recommended to promote skin repair and for mature skin.** It reduces redness and dermatitis.

Oil butters

Oil butters are thick and creamy, so they feel great on the skin. You need just a small amount to thicken a skin lotion or cream. The resulting product seems to melt into your warm skin.

Because an oil butter can make your aromatherapy product melt, you usually mix them with other oils rather than use them by themselves.

> » Cocoa butter is derived from cocoa beans so it has a distinctive yet light chocolaty aroma that can contribute or detract from the scent of your blend.

> » Shea butter is an oil from an African tree. Its texture is especially buttery. It's light scent usually adds to a product's aroma. Its best to use products containing it right away because it does go bad easily and becomes quite stinky.

Making your own infused oil

Extracting essential oils from aromatic plants into a vegetable oil base is a fairly simple process. You use a very early form of extracting essential oils that predates steam distillation, the method used to extract most essential oils today.

You can make infused oils from plants not available as natural essential oils such as wisteria, gardenia, and lilac, and from plants such as rose and jasmine whose essential oils are quite expensive.

The scent of infused oil tends to be light because a relatively small amount of essential oil is extracted.

To make infused oil, you soak aromatic herbs in warm vegetable oil so that the scent and properties of the herb are drawn into the oil, thereby infusing the herb's fragrance and properties into the oil.

When you use these oils instead of plain carrier oils in your preparations, you add the healing benefits provided by the herbs and the essential oils they contain. Two very popular choices of infused oil are St. John's wort and calendula.

Infused Oil Recipe

Use this herbal oil as a base and add essential oils to it.

>> Preparation time: 15 minutes

>> Yield: About 1¼ cups of herb oil

>> Ingredients:

  1 cup dried herbs

  Approximately 1½ cups vegetable oil to cover

1. Coarsely chop the dried herbs in a blender or with a knife.

2. Place the chopped herbs in a wide-mouth jar with a lid.

3. Add enough oil to cover the herbs and completely submerge them (see Figure 5-1).

  Make sure all the herbs are submerged in the oil. If some are floating, give them a few hours to absorb the oil and sink down.

4. Stir the oil with a chopstick or table knife to release any air bubbles.

5. Put the lid on the jar and place it in a warm location, such as outside in the sun or near a heater or wood stove in the winter.

6. Check the jar every day to make sure that all the herbs remain submerged in the oil.

  Some herbs absorb a lot of the oil, so you may need to add more.

7. After about three days in the sun or one to two days with continuous heat, strain out the herbs using a metal strainer or cheesecloth.

This recipe uses dried herbs, but you can also do this same process with fresh herbs from your garden. Using fresh herbs is a little tricky because you need to make sure the jar and lid are very clean and be extra careful stirring out any air bubbles. You also need to keep the plant material completely submerged so it doesn't get moldy.

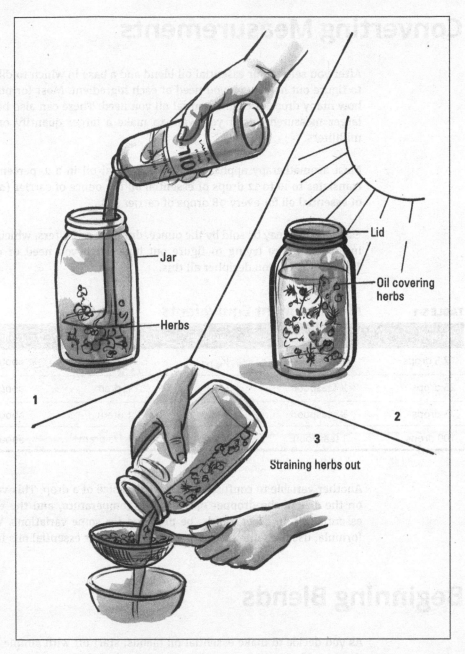

Lid

Jar

Oil covering
herbs

Herbs

1

2

3

Straining herbs out

FIGURE 5-1:
Making your own
herbal oils.

Converting Measurements

After you select your essential oil blend and a base in which to dilute it, you need to figure out how much you need of each ingredient. Most formulas will tell you how many drops of each essential oil you need. These can also be converted into larger measurements if you want to make a larger quantity or into drams or milliliters.

Most aromatherapy applications add essential oil in a 2-percent dilution. That translates to 10 to 12 drops of essential oil per ounce of carrier (or that's 2 drops of essential oil for every 98 drops of carrier oil).

Essential oils may be sold by the ounce, dram, or milliliters, which can be confusing when you're trying to figure out how much you need or compare prices. Table 5-1 helps you decipher all this.

TABLE 5-1   ## Measurement Equivalents

Drops	Teaspoons	Ounces	Drams	Milliliters
12.5 drops	⅛ teaspoon	$\frac{1}{48}$ oz.	⅙ dram	about ⅝ ml.
25 drops	¼ teaspoon	$\frac{1}{24}$ oz.	⅓ dram	about 1 ¼ ml.
75 drops	¾ teaspoon	⅛ oz.	1 dram	about 3.7 ml.
100 drops	1 teaspoon	⅙ oz.	1 1/3 dram	about 5 ml.

Another variable to confuse the issue is the size of a drop. This varies depending on the size of the dropper opening, the temperature, and the thickness of the essential oil. In other words, be prepared for some variations. When making a formula, use the same size droppers for all of your essential oils for consistency.

Beginning Blends

As you decide to make essential oil blends, start off with simple blends, such as the examples in this section. To use any of these blends, sniff them as is or place a few drops into a diffuser to scent a room. (Chapter 6 helps you choose a diffusing method.) This book is filled with lots and lots of ideas along with lists of potential essential oils that you can include in your recipes as you gain confidence and get more creative.

The following blend formulas ask for the standard 10 to 12 drops of essential oil in a carrier, but if you want to make more product, just double the amount of drops and the amount of the carrier. Do the math and make even more.

Squeaky Clean: Lemon and Eucalyptus

In the kitchen or bathroom, this scent enhances a feeling of cleanliness.

» Preparation time: 3 minutes

» Yield: 10 drops

» Ingredients:

8 drops lemon oil

2 drops eucalyptus oil

1. Combine all ingredients in a glass bottle.

2. Seal the bottle tightly.

Pop-up Plus: Orange, Cinnamon, and Mint

This combination of spice and mint increases energy, makes you more alert, and relieves anxiety. Cheerful orange relieves stress, and cinnamon and the mints are perky scents that increase mental awareness and make you feel energized. Use it when you need energy or to think faster — as a physical or mental uplift. While entertaining company, studying, or simply trying to get the housework done, you can appreciate its energizing effects.

» Preparation time: 3 minutes

» Yield: 12 drops

» Ingredients:

8 drops orange oil

1 drop cinnamon oil

1 drop peppermint oil

2 drops spearmint oil

1. Combine all ingredients.

2. Seal the bottle tightly.

Relax Away: Chamomile, Lavender, and Ylang Ylang

This blend produces a great way to relax with fragrance — and it works! Use this combination to relax your children (and yourself!) in the evening. Plus, both chamomile and lavender lift your spirits if you're feeling blue.

» Preparation time: 3 minutes

» Yield: 12 drops

» Ingredients:

10 drops lavender oil

1 drop chamomile oil

1 drop ylang ylang oil

1. Combine all ingredients.
2. Seal the bottle tightly.

Meditative Mood: Sandalwood and Rose

This is a favorite combination in India where both scents are used to increase a meditative focus and to inspire prayer and contemplation. These oils may be expensive, but I bet you'll agree with me that the end result is worth the price.

» Preparation time: 3 minutes

» Yield: 10 drops

» Ingredients:

9 drops sandalwood oil

1 drop rose oil

1. Combine all ingredients.
2. Seal the bottle tightly.

Bouffant Bouquet: Rose Geranium, Lavender, and Bergamot

These floral scents blend well together. The combination produces an uplifting, relaxing, floral bouquet that makes a good scent for a general living area or for a working space. These scents create a sense of relaxation and emotional balance.

They are equally good for company or just for keeping the family happy. These three scents are also antidepressants — in case anyone is feeling down and needs an emotional boost.

» Preparation time: 3 minutes

» Yield: 10 drops

» Ingredients:

6 drops lavender oil

2 drops bergamot oil

2 drops rose geranium oil

1. Combine all ingredients.
2. Seal the bottle tightly.

2

Inscentives for Living: Essential Oils in Your Life

Fill your home with feel-good scents.

Feed your skin and hair with beneficial essential oils.

Try out fragrances that enhance romance.

Ease stress and focus your mind with aromatherapy.

Aid your digestive and immune systems.

Use essential oils to live pain-free.

Up your energy while enhancing your workout regimen.

Get bugs out of your home and garden and off your pets.

Chapter 6

Surrounding Yourself with Scents

Fragrance makes any environment more enjoyable and inviting, and it creates a comfortable place to work and play. So why not bring aromatherapy into your home and workplace? Mood lighting dims lights for relaxation or mimics sunlight to keep you alert and happy. How about trying mood scents that enhance the "feeling" of your personal space? Go for therapeutic aromas that can cheer you up or make you feel more energized.

In this chapter, I show you how to select the best scents for a variety of moods. Then I explain quick ways — all simple and practical — to fill a room with the fragrance you choose. Read on to discover how to make your home smell great and provide benefits to everyone who enters.

Setting the Mood by Choosing a Scent

When aroma researchers in the United States and Japan put people in scented rooms and observed their behavior, a variety of different fragrances were tried. All the scents that the room's occupants found pleasing put them in a feel-good mood. Simply put, smells that you enjoy make you feel great.

Good scents also tend to make people feel more sociable and inclined to get along better. It really is all in your head, say the researchers. That's because aromatherapy influences the way you think. Fragrance leaves you feeling more positive about yourself and your environment. A room containing a light, pleasing scent even makes people more friendly and improves their dispositions. Aromas can also inspire confidence and self-motivation and improve thinking.

Scent can make you feel more alert, or relaxed. It can ease depression or create a romantic atmosphere. Say that someone in your household feels down in the dumps. Then turn to one or more of the scents suggested for depression to provide an emotional lift. Having a party or working on an important project? How about something to pick up everyone's energy? Counter insomnia with an aromatic bedroom. Or maybe it is romance you have in mind. And imagine, all of this is just a sniff away! To fill your environment with fragrance, first choose your scent. There are very few rules. You can find many suitable fragrances to scent your abode. Use the information in this chapter to select a particular mood that you'd like to enhance. Also follow your nose to go with what you like best. If you just can't decide on just one, it's okay to mix and match different scents into an aromatic blend. So, your first assignment is to sniff a selection of essential oils and discover your favorites.

You can start your scented journey by referring to Table 6-1. This table shows you which scents help alleviate which emotional conditions. Decide what mood you'd like to create or cure, and then choose one of the suggested scents. Easy-peasy!

TABLE 6-1   **Emotions You Want to Positively Impact**

Scent	Stress/ Depression	Mood Imbalance	Lack of Energy	Romantic Blahs	Insomnia
Bergamot	X	X			
Chamomile	X	X			X
Cinnamon			X	X	
Eucalyptus			X		
Fir		X	X		
Jasmine			X	X	
Lavender	X	X			X
Lemon	X		X		
Orange	X				X

Scent	Stress/Depression	Mood Imbalance	Lack of Energy	Romantic Blahs	Insomnia
Peppermint			X		
Rose	X	X		X	X
Rose Geranium	X	X			X
Ylang Ylang				X	X

REMEMBER

Even if this is your first plunge into using essential oils, it's hard to go wrong. Choose the emotional quality you want from this chart. Then, select your favorite scent. If you're wondering which oils to purchase, here is your perfect starter kit.

If you just can't decide on just one, it's okay to mix and match different scents into an aromatic blend.

TIP

Find out even more about each of the selected oils by turning to the Essential Oil Guide. When you're ready to move beyond these starter scents, then look through the other scents the guide covers to select something new and different.

Scenting Your Home Sweet Home

You may already know what scents you enjoy and which scents put you in which mood. When you've got your chosen oils ready for use, the next step is to decide the best way to get those scents spread around the room. Here are eight easy tools and methods you can use to disperse whatever scent (and mood) you choose throughout your home.

>> Aromatherapy diffuser

>> Spray bottle

>> Scented candles

>> Incense

>> Steam

>> Potpourri

The following sections give you the scoop on each of these tools and methods.

Lighting aromatherapy candles

There are scented candles, and then there are aromatherapy candles made with good quality essential oils. Once you smell a quality aromatherapy candle, you'll have a difficult time going back to the overly sweet, fruity scented synthetics. (If you're unsure how to sniff the difference between good and poor-quality essential oils, then turn to Chapter 2.)

If you have a favorite style of candle, but alas, it comes without a scent, no problem. Scent it yourself. Give that tired box of unscented candles a makeover. Unlike candles that are already scented, you need to re-scent them every time you use them. However, that also gives you the opportunity to change the scent with every use! Here's a quick method to transform your tapers and wide candles.

Instant Aromatic Candles

Use this quick method to transform your tapers and wide candles into aromatherapy treats.

» Preparation time: About three minutes

» Ingredients:

Candle

10 drops essential oil or a blend of oils of your choice

1. Trim the wick of an unburned candle to ½ inch.

2. Place 10 drops of an essential oil (or a blend) directly on the wick and around its base.

That way, the liquid wax that puddles around the wick will mix with the oil. The wick is very absorbent and will "pull" the scent down into the center of the candle. If you aren't sure which oil to use, choose an oil from Table 6-1.

3. Wait at least 30 minutes before lighting the candle and enjoy.

If you want to scent a candle that has already been burned, trim off the burnt wick because this part is no longer able to absorb the essential oil. Then dig down into the wax to expose ½ inch of the unburned, white wick. Scent this wick the same way you do an unburned wick.

TIP

When not using any scented candles, keep them sealed in an airtight container so that they retain their fragrance.

Diffusing your mood changers

An excellent way to fill a room with a mood-changing scent is with an essential oil *diffuser* that sits on a table or shelf. These units are called *diffusers* because the scent that it emits is *diffused* throughout the air.

REMEMBER

Diffusers run on electricity, so you do need to have a nearby outlet.

A diffuser provides a continuous scent for several hours, making it a good choice for times when you need a longer lasting scent, say when entertaining guests. It is also ideal for a professional office. If your work includes seeing clients or massage therapy, you can diffuse a light, natural scent into the air to produce a calming, relaxed atmosphere.

Using a diffuser is pretty simple, although check the directions for the model you have. Typically, you place a few drops of essential oil in or on the diffuser and then switch it on. After it warms for a few minutes, you can begin to smell the scent of the essential oil.

Search for a diffuser, and you'll find lots of models. They've become a very popular way to scent a room. Whether you're interested in a fancy or plain model, plenty are available.

The following list describes different types of diffusers. Figure 6-1 shows you what a simple diffuser looks like.

TECHNICAL STUFF

TIP

>> **Glass diffusers:** These models resemble tiny laboratory glass equipment. They use a small pump, which is usually a modified fish-tank pump, to continually puff light scent into a room. An advantage of this type of diffuser is that it does not heat the essential oil, producing a purer aroma.

The tubing needs to be periodically cleaned out to keep it from becoming clogged. Unless you don't mind the scent combining with the last one that was in the diffuser, clean it every time you switch from one scent to another. Do a clean out by running rubbing alcohol through the tubing. Let the alcohol completely evaporate, which happens quickly, before using the diffuser. Don't even try using thick essential oils (such as patchouli, myrrh, benzoin, or vanilla) or essential oils mixed with vegetable oil or glycerin. These oils are sure to clog the works and make a mess inside that may be difficult to clean.

If you buy a "fish pump" diffuser, be sure to get a quiet one. Some pumps are so loud that they can ruin the relaxing mood you want to create.

>> **Ceramic diffusers:** Some models rely on very low electric heat instead of a pump, which makes them quiet, but that means that they do heat the essential oil to disperse it into the air. Too high a heat will alter the pure scent.

TIP

>> **Clay diffusers:** These diffusers, made of porous clay, are often made into a figurine or miniature pot or formed into a design. All you do is add a few drops of essential oil. The clay absorbs the oil, which then slowly dissipates it into the air. A light aroma will linger for several hours. Clay diffusers scent the immediate area, although usually not a whole room, so it's good for small spaces or somewhere your nose will be close by. As I'm writing this, a clay flower disk is fastened on the edge of my computer screen, scented with a fragrance that helps me keep alert.

If you want to go the simple route, a low-fired red clay flowerpot works similarly. Place a clay diffuser where essential oils won't injure wood finishing or fabric.

>> **Wall plug-ins:** These inexpensive, little models have absorbent pad inserts. You place a few drops of the essential oil on the pad, which slips into the unit. When plugged into an electric outlet, the pad heats and releases the scent. An innovative version of this type of diffuser plugs into your car's USB port to make your journeys more pleasant and relaxing.

>> **Decorative diffusers:** These tend to be fancy and often attractive units that are designed to go with your room's decor. Some of these send out the aroma in puffs of vapor while others coordinate the release with lights and even music. I have one on a turntable that changes the scent every hour. Various aromatic alarm clocks are available to wake you up to a good aroma, putting you in a good mood. Some of these can also be programmed to send you to sleep with relaxing scents.

MAKE A DIY DIFFUSER WITH YOUR FAN OR HEATER

This quick method adds scent to your house. While you're cooling down with a fan on a hot summer day, take advantage of all that air flow to scent the room. Place about six drops of essential oil on a small strip of fabric or paper and tie or tape this on the grill in front of a fan. When you turn on the fan, air rushes past the scented cloth or paper to sweep the aroma into the room. This same technique works with an air-conditioner, a swamp cooler, or an air-flow heater. You can even use it with the air-flow control in your car. Absorbent pads to scent and fit in your house's heater vents are even available.

All of that air flow means the scent blows off within half an hour and then it lingers in the room for another half hour. However, it's a simple matter to keep reapplying essential oil — either the same or something different to change moods.

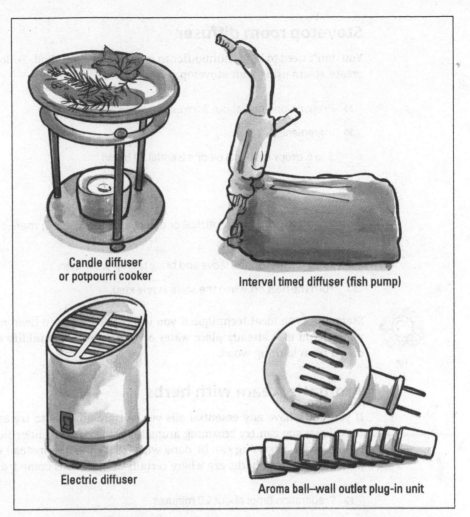

FIGURE 6-1: Various types of aromatherapy diffusers.

Candle diffuser or potpourri cooker

Interval timed diffuser (fish pump)

Electric diffuser

Aroma ball—wall outlet plug-in unit

Creating a steamy atmosphere

One of the easiest methods to scent a room is with steam. The rising steam carries the fragrance into the air. The essential oils quickly go out of the steaming water into the surrounding air, but the lingering scent fills the room. It won't last forever, but you'll have a delightful hour of scent.

The idea here is to release aromatic steam into the room without having to buy a diffuser. This is the same technique you would use to do a facial sauna. By all means, take advantage of that, if you like. You can multitask by treating yourself to a facial steam while scenting the room at the same time. (You can find instructions on giving yourself a facial in Chapter 7.)

Stovetop room diffuser

You don't need to buy a humidifier to use the steam method. Follow these steps to create steam using your stovetop.

>> Preparation time: about 3 minutes

>> Ingredients:

3 to 6 drops essential oil or essential oil blend

2 cups or more water

1. Place 3 to 6 drops essential oil or essential oil blend in 2 or more cups of water in a pan.

2. Place the pan on the stove and bring to a light simmer.

3. Turn the heat off when the scent is released.

TIP

Steaming is an ideal technique if you use a wood stove to heat your home in the winter. You may already place water on your stove to humidify the dry air produced from burning wood.

Aromatic steam with herbs

If you don't have any essential oils yet, but are anxious to try an aromatherapy technique, you can try steaming aromatic herbs, like lavender flowers or cinnamon powder. Steaming can be done with fragrant herbs instead of the pure oils. (After all, fragrant herbs are where certain essential oils come from.)

>> Preparation time: about 20 minutes

>> Ingredients:

1 to 2 heaping tablespoons fragrant herb

1 quart water

1. Place 1 to 2 heaping tablespoons of a fragrant herb into a quart or more of water in a pan.

2. Place the pan on the stove and bring to a light simmer.

3. Turn the heat off when the scent is released.

TIP

Want a good wintertime suggestion? A combination of equal amounts of cinnamon and orange peel thrown into simmering water will warm your spirit. Use either essential oils or the herbs. Or, simply toss in a mulled cider mix instead of making cider. Yet another good idea for winter is to fill your room with the scent of fir essential oil.

Spraying it up

An aromatic room freshener spray instantly transforms your room with fragrance. Basically, it's scented water and possibly a few other ingredients in a pump-style spray bottle. Essential oil is added to water and placed in a spray bottle. Spritz away, and a scented mist floats on the air to bedding, carpeting, and furnishings.

Oil and water separate so some room freshener sprays that you purchase need shaking before they're used; others do not. It depends upon what other ingredients they contain besides water and essential oil to stabilize and mix the oil and water. You can buy these, or it's simple to make your own. (The following section explains how to do this.)

You can also use a hydrosol to spray around a room. This is an aromatic water and essential oil combination that comes from producing essential oils by distillation. (See Chapter 14 for an explanation of hydrosols.)

WARNING

Room freshener in hand, keep your distance from fabrics such as silk and satin and wood furniture because water droplets can stain them.

Spraying a room freshener does not last long, often less than an hour, but you'll find it is a quick way to freshen or disinfect the air, get rid of unpleasant odors, set a particular mood, or simply make your house smell wonderful. Freshener sprays are versatile and come in handy for a variety of uses. I use them everywhere. Be sure to let the water dry before the item you spray is used. It only takes a few minutes. Following are some ideas to get you started:

>> A sparkling citrus on the towels in your bathroom

>> Lavender on your bed sheets to assure peaceful sleep

   One mom says that she sprays her kids' bedrooms every evening with a relaxing mix of chamomile and lavender — and it works to get them to sleep quickly!

>> Eucalyptus or peppermint on the kitchen counter to ward off pesky ants

>> Cedar on your dog's bed as a flea repellent (Allow it to dry before pup lays down.)

>> Bay rum in the stinky locker room and certainly on athletic socks

On trips, a room freshener spray is a must so that you can scent your home away from home. You can choose one essential oil, or if you're feeling that creative bug, then design your own blend using several different oils. Make up your own themes. Here are some ideas to pique your imagination:

>> A wake-up-and-keep-sightseeing spray like peppermint

>> A calm-down-and-sleep-now scent like chamomile

>> An enough-bugs (or mold) eucalyptus spray

>> A something's-a-little-fishy lavender spritz for your boat

>> An all-purpose, home-on-wheels rose geranium freshener for the kitchen and bathroom of your motor home

TIP

If you're a schoolteacher or a caregiver at a nursing home or work any place where air fresheners are already acceptable, you can spray your aromatherapy room fresheners on the job to provide a therapeutic fragrance.

Mixing your own sprays

Make your own aromatic room freshener spray to create a custom-designed fragrance. All you need is essential oil, distilled water, and a spray bottle for your final creation. Glass bottles are preferred because essential oils eventually erode plastic, but the oils are so diluted in this spray, you can get by using a plastic spray bottle to dispense the spray when out and about. For long-term storage, use glass containers.

Because water and oil do not mix, most essential oils float on the water's surface. Solve this problem by shaking your aromatic room freshener before spraying to better distribute the essential oils in the water. Fortunately, the tube in spray bottles goes down close to the bottom of the bottle and that helps them release a good mix of water and oil. Store-bought sprays solve the problem by adding emulsifiers that keep the essential oil distributed. However, I don't mind a little shaking before use, so I make my sprays without added ingredients. The essential oils will merge a little into the water after a few days.

Some essential oils mix with water better than others. For example, rose goes into water fairly easily, while citrus oils such as orange and lemon do not. Resinous essential oils such as patchouli, benzoin, and myrrh are especially stubborn mixing with water and may require more shaking than it's worth. They also tend to clog up the little tube inside the sprayer. When using resinous essential oils, make them only a small fraction of your recipe. The following sections include some easy recipes to get you started.

Aromatic spray

Here's an all-purpose spray you can use for all sorts of occasions. This five-minute recipe yields four ounces of spray. It uses lavender, which has an uplifting and fresh scent, but feel free to replace it with another essential oil.

» Preparation time: 5 minutes

» Yield: 4 ounces of spray

» Ingredients:

   4 ounces distilled water

   20 drops lavender oil

1. Put the water in a 2-ounce spray bottle.

2. Add the lavender oil to the bottle.

3. Shake before using.

Disinfectant room spray

If you are looking for a fresh-smelling spray that also cleans the air, I have a recipe for you. This recipe takes five minutes to make and yields four ounces of spray. Spray it in the bathroom, kitchen, or sickroom.

» Preparation time: 5 minutes

» Yield: 4 ounces of spray

» Ingredients:

   12 drops lavender oil

   12 drops eucalyptus oil

   12 drops orange oil

   5 drops white thyme oil

   4 ounces distilled water

1. Add the essential oils to the water in the spray bottle.

2. Keep the mixture in a spray bottle.

3. Shake before using.

AROMATIC FASHION STATEMENTS: WEARING YOUR SCENTS

One way to scent the immediate environment around you is to scent yourself. Of course, you can wear a drop of essential oil for perfume, but you can carry a scent in other innovative ways. Aromatherapy jewelry is specially designed to emit fragrance while making a fashion statement. You can purchase anything from elegant stones or tiny vials with a small depression for a drop of your favorite essential oil to small clay figurines to filigree hearts and globes that open with small pads to scent inside. My own favorite is a silver-engraved heart container with a stopper on top. The scent of rose emanates from it when I pop open the top.

Some unusual aromatic items include scented pantyhose imbedded with time-release capsules and men's ties in your choice of spice, leather, or — I kid you not — tobacco scent.

Cruising with scents

There's a good chance that whatever you do, you spend a lot of time in your car. You may commute a long way to work or travel in your job, or perhaps you chalk up a pile of miles just driving the kids back and forth to all their activities. Considering all the time people spend in them, they deserve to be scented as much as houses.

Cars are the perfect vehicle to infuse with scent because they are such a small space. I first got the idea when I started using essential oils. I broke a vial of oil in my car door. Now, that was more than overwhelming for the first days, but after that, my car smelled great.

Scent can keep you calm when you're stuck in traffic or late for an appointment. It comes in handy to cover up musty car smells or fume-filled air from traffic. The best part is that a perk-up scent like peppermint or eucalyptus will keep you alert on those long drives or those late-night runs to the store.

You've probably seen the tree-shaped car air freshener at auto parts stores, car washes, and gas stations. It's supposed to smell like a "new car." So, go natural. Toss out that cardboard car scenter that's loaded with synthetic berry smell. Replace it with a good aroma that gives you an aromatherapy boost.

The aroma dissipates into the air rapidly. If your car is wide open and you're flying down the expressway, then your car may need an additional spray every 15 minutes or so. Techniques that you can use in your car include:

>> **Aromatherapy spray:** I carry a selection of several mood-changing and refreshing sprays in my car and keep them between the driver's and the front passenger seat.

>> **Plug-in diffuser:** Yes! These are available. These small, plastic models fit in your cigarette lighter. Add the essential oil of your choice to the pad, and the lighter's low heat will emit the aroma into your car.

>> **Potpourri:** Tuck a porous bag filled with an aromatic somewhere in your car to scent the space.

>> **Solid perfume:** I keep a small box of a solid perfume from India that's sold as "amber" in my ash tray because it keeps a light scent in the car.

>> **Car jewelry:** "What?" you may ask, but jewelry is the best description to describe the scented objects that hang from your car's rearview mirror. Several types of jewelry are sold for cars. Or, how about making your own? Simply dab a couple drops of essential oil on a small piece of absorbent cardboard. Feeling crafty? Make it decorative by gluing a favorite photo or a picture cut from a magazine or greeting card on the cardboard.

>> **Clay stick-ons:** Small, arty objects made from absorbent clay can dissipate scent into your car. The ones that have a sticky back come ready to place wherever you like.

Burning incense

Incense is made from a blend of essential oils mixed with charcoal and a little *saltpeter* — a combustible compound that ignites to keep it burning. Most incense also contains some adhesive plant material to help it stick together. All of this is mixed together and wrapped around a slender stick or formed into a roll, coil, or cone and baked, traditionally in the sun, to a hard consistency. When lit, the incense releases the scent of the essential oils as it burns. Be forewarned; it's messy working with powdered charcoal. You and your workspace will not be pretty sights afterward!

The smoke from burning incense is strongly fragrant and lingers in a room for hours. All you do is light the tip and find a landing spot for a little ash that falls off as the stick burns. The downside is that the smoke itself bothers some people.

TECHNICAL
STUFF

Anthropologists guess that incense was the earliest form of aromatherapy. Its use goes back long before recorded civilization, when fragrant barks, leaves, and saps of plants containing essential oils were tossed into the fire to release their scent and for purification rituals. Buddhists, Hindus, and the Catholic and Greek Orthodox churches still use incense to inspire prayer and meditation. In Japan, making incense is a highly refined art that is part of the celebrated Japanese tea ceremony.

Quick Incense Recipe

To make your own incense, buy premade unscented incense sticks, called *incense blanks,* from a craft store or off the internet. You can also recycle old incense sticks that have lost their scent and re-scent them.

» Preparation time: 5 minutes

» Yield: one incense stick

» Ingredients:

1 incense blank

24 drops essential oil for an 8-inch incense blank

1. Place the incense blanks on a pie pan or cookie sheet.

2. Partly fill a glass dropper (like the ones sold at a drugstore) with the essential oil of your choice.

3. Apply 3 drops for every inch of the stick.

Apply the oil slowly, giving it time to absorb into the stick.

4. Let the stick dry for one hour and then put it in a tall glass jar.

Your incense will be ready to use the next day.

 TIP Whether you make or buy your incense, be sure it retains its scent for a long time by keeping it in an airtight container. Although incense is usually sold in a plastic or cellophane bag, glass is best. Always store homemade incense in glass, because it gums up plastic bags.

Bringing potpourri back

Just the name *potpourri* may ring of another era, but this attractive mix of scented dried herbs, flowers, and foliage is making a comeback. Placed in a glass container, a basket, or in a bowl and set in a room, it offers twofold charm as both an eye-catching and pleasingly fragrant center of attention. In an open container, potpourri scents the air around it. In a closed container, it invites the visitor to open it and experience the burst of fragrance.

Potpourri is a great project to do with kids. Give each child a plastic, sealable baggy and have them partially fill it with a selection of dried plant material, perhaps some things that they collected themselves. Most children love selecting the ingredients. Then, you drip in the essential oil they choose.

You can buy potpourri or be creative and make your own. The following sections guide you through the entire potpourri producing process, from gathering supplies to preserving scents for months to come.

The benefits of DIY potpourri

Your homemade potpourri that is made with essential oils from plants is sure to be more therapeutic compared to many commercial versions that are made with synthetic oils. With homemade potpourri, you can be creative and have fun. Here's a few ideas to get you started:

>> Use natural essential oils that have therapeutic effects.

>> Bring the colors and fragrances of the garden indoors — if you have your own garden or have access to colorful fresh or dried plant materials.

>> Choose your own scents, colors, and textures.

>> Match the scent to the mood you want.

>> Coordinate the colors of your room for added visual appeal.

>> Stuff potpourri in a pillow or stuffed animal scented with a pick-me-up essential oil to help a child or a bedridden individual.

>> Keep enjoying cut flowers from a special occasion, such as weddings, birthdays, or anniversaries. You'll have jars filled with special memories!

TIP

Place potpourri where people can notice it, like by an entrance, close to the couch, or next to a bathroom sink, and your guests will be welcomed with beautiful, great smelling décor.

How to prepare your materials

To preserve cut flowers from your garden or a special occasion, cut them right before the fresh flowers and greens begin to wilt or lose their colors. Flowers and greenery for your potpourri dry best at room temperature or warmer. Keep them out of direct sunlight while they dry because the sun will blacken the various colors and destroy the scent. Spread the plants thinly on a piece of newspaper, cookie sheet, or cutting board to dry them. Or tie them at their base with either string or a rubber band around the stems and hang them upside down — a good way to decorate your kitchen or pantry. Any of these methods provides enough air circulation to allow the plants to dry. When the plant material feels very dry — brittle enough so that the pieces snap in your hands — they're ready for an attractive container.

Steps for making potpourri

When you're ready to make potpourri, use dried plants from the garden, a floral bouquet, and/or bulk herb section of your local natural-food store. Look for interesting colors and textures. One way to do this is to mix dark colors with light colors to create visual contrasts. For example, yellow and white chamomile flowers contrast with dark green rosemary leaves or brown cinnamon sticks. You will be amazed at the beauty that dried cut flowers give to a potpourri.

The scent of your dried plant collection doesn't have to match the essential oils that you choose to scent the potpourri. In fact, because you're adding scent, they don't have to smell at all. Ready to make your own? Follow these steps:

>> Preparation time: 10 minutes to combine ingredients once they are collected

>> Yield: 1 cup

>> Ingredients:

1 cup dried plant material

1/8 teaspoon essential oil or a blend of essential oils

1. Mix several types of dried plant material together in a bowl. You'll want the ingredients to look good together. Don't worry about the smell yet; that comes later.

2. Drop by drop, add essential oil to the herbs. Select one or more essential oils. (The amount called for in this step is for all the essential oils combined, not for each oil you add.)

3. Place your newly made potpourri in a sealed plastic bag or in a jar with a tight lid for at least five days. This gives the essential oils a chance to penetrate all the herbs and the various fragrances time to blend, so that the scent "matures."

4. After five days, put your potpourri in an attractive container — basket, fancy glass jar, or handmade bowl — and display. You'll want to try all sorts of gorgeous containers to show off your potpourri.

TIP

If you want to get more serious about your potpourri making, consider using a potpourri cooker. Simmering potpourri cookers have a small bowl set over a candle or electric heat source. When the candle is lit or the electricity turned on, it heats the water and releases the fragrance into the room. In a cooker, potpourri acts mostly as a carrier for the essential oils that scent it. In fact, often the essential oils are responsible for all the scent.

Make your creation last

The scent of potpourri lasts for months in a closed container and for several weeks in an open container. When the scent eventually grows faint, revive it by placing a few drops of essential oil directly on the dried plants.

If you want to make your potpourri scent last longer, add ½ teaspoon of dried, finely chopped orris root to every cup of dried plants. Few potpourri makers use it these days, but it does make the scent last longer. Called a *fixative*, this fragrant root comes from the root (technically a *rhizome*) of a white-flowered iris. It is available in some herb and craft stores and on the internet. (Avoid powdered root. It will put a powdery coating on your potpourri.)

WARNING

Just be aware that some people are allergic to orris root. Craft stores also sell an alternative cellulose fixative.

Chapter **7**

Mirror, Mirror on the Wall: Skin and Hair Care for Us All

Body-care products containing essential oils are big sellers these days. You find essential oils in creams, hair conditioners, complexion soaps, body and massage oils, bath salts, shower gels, and all sorts of items specially designed for skin and hair.

Of course, you can always grab the product that smells the best. But why not seek essential oils and products that improve the health and beauty of your skin and hair? Plus, they have scents appeal.

Aroma plays a big role in choosing what you use and contributes to your enjoyment as you use body-care products. Watch your initial reaction the next time you buy a skin lotion or hair rinse. I bet that the first thing you do is open the lid to discover how it smells. So, I'm going to not only consider each product's effectiveness, but how good it smells.

In this chapter, I concentrate on how aromatherapy benefits your skin and hair. I put the types of products available into a few categories. Then I help you figure out your own skin and hair type. I take the stress out by making your task less overwhelming and, I hope, even make it fun!

Reaping All the Benefits for Your Hair and Skin

For a truly special product, consider not only how an essential oil benefits your skin and hair, but its other properties. For example, you can choose an essential oil that's good for your skin, relaxes your muscles, and is an antidepressant. (Stumped? Some examples are lavender, chamomile, ylang ylang, and rose.)

Despite all the hoopla over new and improved body-care products, they all boil down to three basic ingredients:

>> Vegetable oil or wax to protect the skin

>> Water to moisturize it

>> Herbs and essential oils to add medicinal and beauty properties

I talk a lot about buying your own body-care products in this chapter. But you can also go the simple route and dilute essential oils directly into an oil or water base and use that on your skin.

To give your skin the beneficial effects of using both oil and water, you can adapt a two-part program:

1. **Use a spray with essential oils added to it on your skin.**

2. **Apply a protective vegetable oil that also contains essential oils.**

Chapter 5 provides recipes for making your own essential oil products.

No matter what you put on the outside of your skin and hair, it's what's inside that really counts. Having healthy skin and hair depends on your general health — and even more on what you put in your body rather than what you put on your skin.

Healthy skin and scalp need oxygen and nutrients to bring the skin nourishment, and young skin cells are especially heavy feeders.

REMEMBER

I hate to be the one to break it you, but your hair's dead. Please don't take this personally because it's true for everyone. Being dead, your hair has no resources to recover from mistreatment. So, you need to be good to your hair from the jump. The best thing you can do besides use natural hair-care products is to treat it right.

Thinking about dying your hair? Consider this: Chemicals that change hair color first must enter your hair's inner structure and strip away the original color. This breaks down your hair's natural protective armor. In short, it can partially destroy your hair. That's why so many bleached blondes eventually end up with frizzy hair.

TIP

To color your hair, try a henna blend made with natural herbs, which coats and protects your hair. *Henna* is a plant-based dye, so it's natural and free of chemicals. Henna eventually fades, so the next best thing is a partially natural dye sold in natural-food stores.

Here are some things that essential oils can do for your skin:

>> Penetrate lower skin layers to work on moisturizing and healing. (See Figure 7-1 for a diagram of skin layers.)

>> Stimulate and regenerate skin cells to heal skin damaged by sun, burns, wrinkles, or injury.

>> Destroy infectious bacteria, viruses, and fungi, such as those associated with acne and other skin problems.

>> Reduce inflammation and puffiness.

>> Soothe sensitive or injured skin.

>> Regulate over- or underactive oil glands.

>> Encourage removal of waste products.

>> Contain plant "hormones" (for hormonally related skin problems).

>> Treat stress-related skin problems.

Choosing Products for Hair and Skin

Choosing aromatherapy body- and hair-care products can be complicated, much more so than simply sniffing an aroma to influence an emotion or putting a scented cloth on your forehead to relieve your headache. If you feel confused as you gaze over shelf after shelf of aromatherapy bottles and jars and essential oil vials, you're not alone.

How to choose the proper skin and hair preparations is a question I often get from my students, customers, and even people who follow me down the aisle in the natural-food store! You may find yourself reaching for a calming essential oil to inhale to help you through your decision making!

The reason selecting body-care items can be difficult is because they contain an amazing number of ingredients. One list I saw had more than 400 substances! This means that you, as a consumer, not only have to consider the quality and the uses of the essential oils in each formula, but also the numerous other ingredients that may or may not be suited for your skin and hair.

When you look at the wide assortment of products offered for sale, you may not realize that there are only a few types of body-care preparations but many, many variations. You see all the variations when you shop for them. Look for those that contain the essential oils recommended in this book for your own skin type or condition.

Ideally, ingredients such as vegetable oils, glycerin, lanolin, alcohol, and herbs work with essential oils to enrich your skin and hair. However, that's not all you find in the bottle. Body-care products contain waxes and other stabilizers to prevent all the ingredients from separating. Preservatives slow spoilage, and additional ingredients provide a desirable color and texture.

You don't need these fancy chemical ingredients in your homemade essential oil products. Most items you find on a store shelf go through all the shipping, shaking, and long-term shelf-sitting a commercial product experiences, so they need to combat those conditions. The same is true of products you buy online.

If you're feeling ambitious and have the time, you can try your hand at making body- and skin-care products from scratch. That's one way to ensure that what you put on your skin contains only the best quality ingredients. Chapter 5 can help you realize that ambition.

Looking at body-care options

Popular aromatherapy body-care products are scented with essential oils. Of course, those oils also provide them with beneficial properties for the health of your skin. Some common aromatherapy products are

>> **Body or complexion oil that** is vegetable oil-based. It's rubbed on the skin as a massage, body, or bath oil. While not a moisturizer itself, it provides a barrier to keep moisture in the skin. It also makes a good baby oil.

» **Cream** combines oil with water, so it's an ideal moisturizer, especially if you have dry or mature skin. You can find night creams, cleansing creams to remove makeup, and first-aid creams for damaged skin.

» **Emulsions** are moisturizers that have a milky or gel-like consistency. They are water-based, so they're non-greasy. Think of them as lighter versions of moisturizing creams.

» **Lotion** contains more water (50 to 90 percent) than oil, so it's thinner and less oily than cream and is better suited than cream for normal to oily skin. Unlike cream, it doesn't leave an oily coating and spreads easily over your skin.

» **Powders** are just that, powder that is infused with essential oil to scent them. They are used for conditions that need a drying treatment, such as deodorant or skin fungus and as baby powder.

» **Skin toner** is usually a non-oily base, often aloe or witch hazel, making it ideal for oily skin. It improves circulation and skin tone to give your skin a healthful glow. It sometimes contains vinegar, although the smell makes this a less popular ingredient.

» **Salves and lip balms** are made from oil that has been thickened with beeswax (rather than petroleum products) to make them semi-solid. They keep lips from drying out and help repair skin injuries and irritation.

» **Scrubs** cleanse your skin. They can be made with course material, such as the abrasive ground almond shells, or the gentler cornmeal or ground oatmeal.

Sudsing up: Shampoo and soap

It used to be easy: You washed everything with plain soap — skin, face, hair, floors, and even clothes. Times have changed and so has soap.

Skin and hair cleansers come in all sorts of fun shapes and consistencies, and most of them aren't even soap. This list gives you the dirt on when and how to use common cleansing products for your skin and hair:

» **Bar soap** is very alkaline, which helps it remove dirt, but this also makes it harsh, especially on delicate skin and dry skin. I have nothing against soap, but unless you have oily skin, use it on your face only when you need to remove makeup, dirt, grime, or grease.

If you're dealing with a skin condition, try switching to washing that area with something other than soap until it clears up.

TIP

After you use bar soap, quickly restore your skin back to its natural acidity with a product that contains vinegar. See the sidebar about vinegar on your skin and hair.

» **Glycerin** is produced during the soap-making process and then removed. Without the glycerin, soap is more concentrated and cleans better but also becomes harsher on skin. But many people prefer the gentle action of soap with glycerin included. It's translucent and easily molded, so it often comes in bright colors and interesting shapes.

» **Liquid skin soap** is popular because it's dispensed in a convenient pump. It usually has a balanced pH so that it isn't overly alkaline.

Liquid soap isn't overly alkaline like regular soap and convenient to use in a push-top dispenser.

Shampoo and bath and body gel are made with liquid shower soap. They are very similar, except the gel is thickened. Shampoo washes your hair, and gel is to clean your body.

» **Facial sauna** See the sidebar "Giving your face a sauna." You can also purchase a facial steamer at a large drugstore, facial steamers plug in to produce steam that contains a few drops of essential oil. A soft padding on top of a large tube cradles your face so that you can experience the gentle aromatic steam.

TECHNICAL STUFF

There's controversy over the use of sodium lauryl sulfate, which, until recently, was *the* cleansing agent in shampoo, body gels, and liquid hand soap. Labels say sodium lauryl sulfate is derived from nut oils like coconut, so it sounds natural — but is it? It takes an elaborate laboratory process to produce it. It produces super suds that everyone loves in a cleanser, but you may have noticed that, recently, there's been an increase in sodium lauryl sulfate-free products on the market. That's because sodium lauryl sulfate dries out your skin and hair. It also easily irritates skin and eyes, especially with frequent use.

Diluting with essentials

If making your own products isn't in the cards, you can add your own essential oils to high-quality, unscented products to customize them for your personal needs. You can try this with all sorts of body-and hair-care products, such as hand or body lotion, shampoo, hair conditioner, body washes, and liquid soap.

When you're adding essential oils to existing products, the rule of thumb is to add about 6 drops of essential oil total (not each individual oil) for every ounce of the product. I know that's not much, but it shows the concentration and strength of these oils.

Add the oil drop by drop. Then, using a chopstick, toothpick, or narrow knife, stir the oil thoroughly into the product. If the product is liquid, add the drops of essential oil, cap it off, and shake. Just like that, your job is done!

TIP

Before you go altering a whole bottle of shampoo or jar of face cream, my advice from experience is to try out a small batch first. After you get the hang of it, you'll find it easier to enhance a product without making a test sample. And start small; you can always add a few extra drops if the product doesn't smell strong enough.

The amount of essential oils you need can vary depending upon the oils you select and the type of product you're enhancing. You need to be light-handed with strong-smelling essential oils like clary sage and ylang ylang. Fortunately, the same goes for the very concentrated and expensive essential oils such as rose, neroli, and jasmine.

TIP

If you're adding essential oil to a large bottle of liquid, you use a lot of drops. Save time by adding your essential oil by the teaspoon instead of going drop by drop. Generally, you get 25 drops of essential oil in a ¼ teaspoon. If you're adding about 6 drops per ounce, that's 48 drops for one cup, or close enough to half a teaspoon.

Salves and balms hardened with beeswax are a bit more work. You need to gently heat them or set them out in the sun on a hot day before stirring essential oils into them.

Most commercial face and body creams are air whipped and contain some natural stabilizers, so it's possible to stir in essential oils. You won't be able to stir a homemade cream, because that can cause the water and oil to separate.

WARNING

It's important to dilute essential oils rather than use them straight, or what's referred to as *neat*. If you're buying your skin-care products, they contain only tiny amounts of essential oils and are ready to use. If you're adding essential oils to existing body-care products, be sure to follow the guidelines and add only a few drops.

The same thing goes if you're making your products from scratch. Appling essential oils directly on the skin can easily lead to an overdose for your kidneys and liver — not what you want when you're trying to do something good for yourself. In some cases, an essential oil can burn your skin. Essential oils are so concentrated, they work just fine when diluted without damaging your skin or organs. Chapter 4 explains safety issues in detail.

Typing Your Skin

You don't need to put lots of stuff on your skin to maintain a beautiful complexion. Choose products that contain simple ingredients and are suitable for your skin type. If you have dry or oily skin or problems with acne, what you use can correct these imbalances. Even if you're blessed with normal skin that's not too oily or too dry, you still can benefit from complexion products to keep it that way.

To figure out which essential oils and products you need, you need to first determine your skin type. If your complexion is oily, you want essential oils and other ingredients that differ from somebody who has dry skin. Take everything into consideration. Do you tend to get acne and have overly sensitive skin? Are you dealing with a skin problem such as eczema or trying to prevent premature wrinkles? Also consider where you go and what you do. If you're often in the sun or wind, maybe sailing or skiing, you need extra protection so that your skin doesn't dry out or burn.

See which categories best describe your complexion. If some places are dry and others oily, you have combination skin — for example, your forehead and around your nose are oily, and the other areas are dry. If so, use two different skin-care products or one specially designed for combination skin.

>> **Dry skin** doesn't produce enough oil, so it tends to be flaky and look dull.

>> **Oily skin** produces too much oil, making it shiny. It may even feel greasy to the touch.

>> **Normal skin** is just right. It isn't too dry or too oily.

If you're wondering what kind of complexion you have, try this experiment.

1. Go to bed without putting anything on your face — no creams, no lotions.

2. When you wake up, cut three small strips of paper, say two inches by half an inch, from a clean brown paper bag.

3. Before you wash or do anything to your face, press one strip of paper on your chin, one on your nose, and the third on your forehead.

4. After at least five seconds, peel the strips off.

If you have oily skin, you see a definite oil stain on the paper strip. Dry skin leaves no oil on the paper at all. Normal skin shows only a slight stain caused by a small amount of oil. Figure 7-1 shows skin layers.

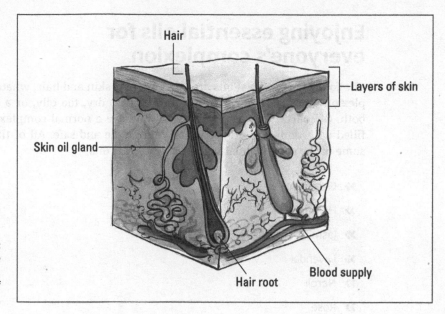

Hair

Layers of skin

Skin oil gland

Hair root

Blood supply

FIGURE 7-1: A close-up of the skin layers, hair, and oil glands of your skin.

The more you can define your skin, the easier it is to pick out the perfect products for it.

You may find that more than one condition describes your skin. For example, your dry skin may be mature skin with acne that's also sensitive. If you fall into more than one category, you have combination skin. If this describes you, turn to the essential oils for all skin types.

You can apply *spot therapy* in which you use different products on different areas of your skin. For example, use a general product for dry skin and apply an acne treatment to those problem spots.

REMEMBER

Just like your skin, your hair can be too dry or too oily. It's not actually the hair itself that produces oil; it's your scalp, which is skin, so it's usually the same type as your complexion. If you have dry skin, you probably have a dry scalp. If your skin is oily, then your scalp is likely also oily. So, your skin and your scalp benefit from the same remedies.

When thinking about what you need for healthy skin, consider where you take your skin. Wind, icy-cold air, dry air, sun exposure, and air pollution all take a toll on your complexion. So do some less obvious conditions, such as the recycled air in an office, car, or airplane. This is especially true if you sit directly in the line of the air stream, which is as drying to your skin as spending the day skiing or sailing in a heavy wind.

Enjoying essential oils for everyone's complexion

The following essential oils are good for your skin and hair, whatever your complexion type. Use them if your hair or skin is dry, too oily, or a combination of both. Of course, they're also great if you have a normal complexion. Each oil is filled with skin-care properties and are gentle and safe. All of this makes them some of the most popular body-care essential oils.

>> Geranium

>> Helichrysum

>> Jasmine

>> Lavender

>> Neroli

>> Rose

>> Ylang ylang

Focusing on special skin conditions

In addition to thinking about how dry or oily your skin is, you may also need to take a special condition into consideration:

>> **Acne:** Your skin breaks out easily in pimples. In severe cases, this can leave scarring. Use skin-care products designed to counter the inflammation and infection that often accompanies pimples and blackheads.

>> **Mature skin** tends to have wrinkles and is thinner and not as plump as younger skin. Use products that keep down irritation and help to rejuvenate skin cells.

>> **Enlarged blood vessels** are called a *couperose complexion*. Avoid heat and essential oils that encourage blood near the surface.

>> **Sensitive skin** may be sun-damaged or easily flare up with an allergic reaction. Treat it gently with products that reduce sensitivity and inflammation and contain skin-healing ingredients.

GIVING YOUR FACE A SAUNA

Steam is a great way to carry the cosmetic and healing properties of essential oils directly to your face. Use whatever essential oils are most appropriate for your skin concerns. As an added benefit, steam moisturizes your face. The heat helps to clean the pores in your skin and also relaxes facial muscles.

1. Add about 4 drops essential oil to a pan of water that contains at least two cups. Then, heat the water until it steams.

   An alternative method is to pour boiling water over a handful of fragrant herbs to release their essential oils.

2. Take the pan off the heat and set it where you can comfortably sit next to it.

3. Lay a towel over the back of your head, put your face over the steam, and secure the ends of the towel around the pan to capture the steam.

4. Hold your face about 12 inches from the water with your eyes closed (so that the essential oil doesn't irritate them).

   Steam for a minute or so and then back away and take several breaths of fresh air.

5. Go back under the towel and repeat a few times.

   Altogether, steam for five or ten minutes at the most.

You can also purchase a facial steamer. These appliances plug in to produce steam. You just need to add a few drops of essential oil. A soft padding on top of a large tube cradles your face so that you can experience the gentle aromatic steam.

Sensitive skin reddens or becomes irritated and inflamed easily. Essential oils that reduce that redness, irritation, and inflammation include

>> Chamomile

>> Helichrysum

>> Lavender

Skin problems such as psoriasis or eczema or a constant infection like ringworm need extra care. Look up these conditions in the Symptom Guide at the back of the book to find out more about how to care for them.

Caring for your acned skin

Acne may not present a hazard to your health, but it has the unfortunate habit of impairing your looks. It always strikes at a most untimely moment. Just when you least want your complexion to look like a geological survey map, that's when your skin pores become clogged with oil and infected. A hormonal imbalance takes most of the blame for causing acne. However, holistic practitioners suspect that stress, diet, and toxins in the blood (not effectively filtered out by the liver) contribute to the breakouts.

Essential oils come to your skin's rescue, balancing hormones, reducing inflammation, and regulating your skin's oil production. This makes aromatherapy the ideal treatment for blemishes, pimples, and other skin eruptions. Shop for something that you can apply directly on the acne.

Dermatologists say not to pop pimples, but if you do, wash the spot and use a compress on it before and afterward. A *compress* is a few layers of soft, absorbent material that is soaked with a medicinal solution. (See the upcoming "Simple Pimple Compress" recipe.)

The following essential oils work well for any type of acne:

>> Chamomile

>> Geranium

>> Lavender

>> Sandalwood

>> Tea tree

The following essential oils work well for acne with oily skin:

>> Cedarwood

>> Eucalyptus

>> Lavender (or Spanish) sage

>> Lemon

>> Tea tree

The following essential oils work well for acne with dry skin:

>> Clary sage

>> Fennel

>> Frankincense

>> Juniper berry

>> Patchouli

>> Rosemary

Simple Pimple Compress

Making a compress for your skin is simple. You can reheat the water and re-apply the compress several times. This recipe calls for tea tree oil, but you can replace it with another essential oil of your choice. Cotton is the suggested material for compresses because it's absorbent.

>> Preparation time: 3 minutes

>> Yield: Several compress applications

>> Ingredients:

   1/4 cup hot water

   2 drops tea tree essential oil

   cotton ball or cotton cloth square about 3 inches square

1. Heat the water so that it's hot to the touch.

2. Pour the hot water into a container.

3. Add the essential oil.

4. Slosh the cotton ball or cloth in the mixture and gently squeeze out.

5. Lay the cotton ball or cloth (fold it first) on your skin, applying a little pressure for at least a couple minutes.

6. Reapply several times.

Discovering Secrets of Ageless Mature Skin

As your skin matures, it loses elasticity and the ability to retain water. The dryness and the thinness gradually increase, especially after you turn 40, and mature skin is almost always dry. (To keep water from evaporating, young skin contains natural moisturizing factors that attract and hold in water and oil glands that keep it and your scalp lightly coated.)

Not to worry: As you age, you can gradually adjust the way you care for your complexion. If you're relatively young with dry skin, you may be prone to developing wrinkles early. You can think ahead and treat your skin now with products designed to use on a dry complexion.

The essential oils suggested for mature skin all help skin cells regenerate and rejuvenate. These oils help to heal the slight skin abrasions that dry, mature skin tends to develop. Following is a list of anti-aging essential oils:

>> Carrot seed

>> Frankincense

>> Geranium

>> Helichrysum

>> Lavender

>> Neroli

>> Rose

>> Rosemary

Slicking Back Your Oily Skin and Hair

Oily skin has a lot of luster. The oil reflects light to give it a smooth, silky texture and a healthy glow. It protects your skin from drying so that it takes longer to develop wrinkles. However, having oily skin is not always as slick as it looks. Excess oil creates coarse skin texture that can be prone to enlarged pores and acne. The real downfall is excess oil clogs your pores and then acts like a sponge to collect dirt and dead skin cells, and that leads to pimples, blackheads, and sometimes infection.

TIP

If you have oily skin, wash daily with an aromatherapy soap to remove the excess oil. Use a skin lotion rather than cream because it contains more water and less oil.

Witch hazel and grain alcohol in a skin toner help dry your skin, but don't overdo it; too much drying works against you by encouraging your skin to produce more oil. Vinegar is good for oily skin. A hydrosol made from any of the herbs in the following list is also a good choice. *Hydrosols* are the scented water produced when an essential oil is extracted from the plant via distillation. (See Chapter 14 for a description of distillation and hydrosols.)

Just like oily skin, oily hair has an attractive shine, but too much makes it look dull, lifeless, and heavy. You need to get to the root of the problem: roots of your hair where the oil is produced and where it concentrates. Brushing your oily hair from the roots to the tips helps to distribute the oils. Wash it frequently and brush beforehand to make it easier to remove the excess oil. Don't use protein or balsam shampoos because they attract oil.

The best essential oils for your oily skin and hair include

>> Basil

>> Cedarwood

>> Clary sage

>> Cypress

>> Eucalyptus

>> Helichrysum

>> Juniper berry

>> Lemon

>> Lemongrass

>> Myrtle

>> Palmarosa

>> Patchouli

>> Sage

>> Sandalwood

>> Tea tree

>> Vetiver

VINEGAR — OLD AND NEW AGAIN

Vinegar is an example of a new idea that's as old as the hills. After a glorious history as a facial toner and hair rinse, vinegar fell from fashion in the 19th century due to its smell. (If you're concerned about smelling like pickles after using it, don't worry — the odor quickly dissipates.) Herbalists who know its reputation still produce facial products that contain vinegar.

A component of vinegar is a modern rage in skin care. AHAs, or alpha-hydroxy acids, maintain your skin's natural acidity and, along the way, moisturize and soften your skin, temporarily smooth out fine lines and enlarged pores and improve texture and discoloration. Suitable for all types of skin and hair, AHAs quickly restore natural acidity when used as a rinse after using soap. As if that's not enough, AHAs also help to heal skin infections, psoriasis, eczema, and blemishes.

AHAs are so common you can find them lurking in your kitchen. Yogurt, sour milk, wine, apples, and some fruit juices are loaded with these acids. It's no wonder legendary beauties such as Cleopatra bathed in sour milk or wine! The purified form of AHAs used in cosmetics is most often derived from sugar.

Keeping a Dry Wit: Caring for Your Dry Skin and Hair

Dry skin has its advantages because it tends to develop less acne. However, to stay soft and supple skin normally contains 50 to 75 percent water. Look under a strong magnifier at dry skin, and you see a resemblance to a dry lake bottom in the Sahara Desert: A rough, flaky, cracked surface layer of skin with dry areas that slightly curl up on the edges. (Refer to Figure 7-1 for a diagram of skin layers.) The lack of oil in dry skin and hair also makes them look rough and dull because they don't reflect light.

Underlying skin cells rapidly reproduce into a tightly packed layer that gradually moves upward to replace surface skin as it flakes off. Dry skin has a tendency to shed too quickly, and the underlying skin and scalp are too immature and tender to take on the job of keeping moisture in. Thus, your skin or scalp easily become irritated and inflamed.

Hormones determine the amount of oil produced by your skin and scalp, and women tend to have drier skin than men.

TIP

If you have dry skin, use cream and lotion to retain and add water to your skin. Stay away from skin products with water-based ingredients, which pull water out of your skin and make it dry out even more. Also avoid skin-care products containing alcohol, which is very drying. Choose a gentle oatmeal scrub (see the Scrub-A-Dub Oatmeal Scrub recipe in this chapter) over bar or liquid soaps, which irritate dry skin.

The following essential oils are good for your dry skin and hair. They encourage production of your own natural oils in your skin and scalp. Many of these also increase the ability of your skin and scalp to hold in water. Quite a few are anti-inflammatory oils, which are good for dry skin because they reduce skin irritation and puffiness that so often accompany the dryness.

>> Carrot seed

>> Cedarwood

>> Frankincense

>> Myrrh

>> Palmarosa

>> Peppermint (small amounts increase oil production)

>> Rosemary

>> Sandalwood

>> Thyme (the variety called linalool)

>> Vetiver

The source of your dry hair is too little oil on your scalp. When hair emerges from your scalp, it's dead, and it depends upon oil from your scalp to coat it and make it look alive.

Dry hair is dull and flat, often with that flyaway look. At its worse, it can be unmanageable and brittle and easily develop split ends and dandruff — all because there isn't enough oil in your scalp to coat your hair and hold in moisture.

Protein-rich and balsam shampoos coat your hair to smooth down individual frayed hairs and make your hair look thicker, at least until the protein coat wears off. (High-protein herbs include comfrey and henna.)

TIP

For a quick dry-hair treatment, rub a couple drops of an essential oil — rosemary or cedarwood are good choices — on your brush or comb before brushing or combing your hair.

Scrub-A-Dub Oatmeal Scrub

This scrub washes your skin when you're not dirty enough to need soap to cut through the grime. It's also a great soap alternative if you have dry skin. An ingredient list doesn't get much simpler than this one. You may already have everything you need waiting for you in your kitchen.

» Preparation time: 5 minutes

» Yield: About ½ cup scrub

» Ingredients:

2 tablespoons oatmeal

1 teaspoon cornmeal (optional)

¼ cup distilled water

5 drops lavender oil

1. Grind the oatmeal in an electric coffee grinder (clean out the coffee grounds first!) or blender.

2. Drop in the essential oils.

3. Add enough water to make a paste.

4. Gently massage your face for two minutes. Use the rest in two days or keep it in the refrigerator where it will last about a week.

Vary It! Use rose water or aloe vera juice, both of which are excellent for your complexion, instead of water. You can also leave out the water and store the dry scrub in a jar or decorative bowl. Dampen fingers with water and dip into the dry mixture, then scrub damp face and rinse. Or you can make a "soap" bag by tying the corners of a piece of loose-weave cotton fabric (about 8 inches square) into a pouch to hold about a 1/4 cup of the dry scrub. Add water, and then use this scrub bag in place of a bar of soap.

Chapter **8**

Essential Oils in the Bedroom

I f there's one place that fragrance steps into the limelight, it's the bedroom — or anyplace you have sex. Scent is the ultimate sex appeal and has been for at least 3,000 years. Perfume, cologne, aftershave, diluted essential oil — however you choose to scent your body becomes a personal statement about you.

And what a statement it makes! There's no denying that scent is a downright sexy language complete with allure and mystery. The fragrance you choose and exude says that you're appealing, attractive, alluring, and worth being near, yet mysterious enough to be intriguing. Just how sexy you seem depends upon the fragrance you choose.

In this chapter I show you essential oils that have earned the name *aphrodisiac* (an agent that arouses sexual desire) and help you select your favorite essential oils in this category. I introduce you to sexy essential oil scents from around the world and offer ideas on how to use them. Remember that fragrance can be captivating, sensual, and even downright erotic, but the rest is up to you!

Relating Sex and Smell

You may take your sense of smell for granted. The truth is that it's connected to more than just your ability to detect odor. The value of your sense of smell doesn't stop there. A keen nose detects all the subtleties in food and makes everything you eat taste better. Chances are you experience the complete opposite when a stuffy nose prevents you from detecting much, if any, flavor in your food.

A good nose lets you feel more enjoyment from the aromas as well as the sights around you. Smell makes the world more enjoyable.

Plus, a good nose makes for good sex. Your ability to smell is tied to sexual enjoyment in several ways. In fact, your sense of smell is one of the most scents-ual things about you. A smell researcher from Duke University, Dr. Susan Shiffman, sums it up nicely, "People who don't like each other's smell don't make it as a couple."

Our ability to perceive smell decreases as we age. By the time we reach 65, about half the population has lost some of our sense of smell. For women, this is especially true of musky scents.

The decrease in your sense of smell doesn't have to be a dramatic decline. It turns out your sense of smell is one of those things in the "use it or lose it" category. Working with essential oils improves your sense of smell and keeps it going. To explore the sense of smell and how to improve it even more, go to Chapters 1 and 2.

Harnessing pheromones and hormones

Whenever you get excited, *adrenaline* rushes through your body. Adrenaline fuels your excitement and makes you hyper-alert. This hormone also activates your scent glands to release strongly aromatic *pheromones* (a Greek word for "excitement").

TECHNICAL STUFF

Pheromones go into action when you reach puberty, triggered partly by the pheromones of the opposite sex. Certainly, you can recall when your own teenage hormones accelerated into hyperdrive!

Sex hormones (substances that spark actions in your body including influencing moods and behavior) definitely play a role in your sense of smell. During ovulation, when women are most fertile, their sense of smell greatly heightens, and their noses become a high-functioning pheromone detector, helped along by their own hormones, including estrogen. An ovulating woman can detect essential oils, sexy scents, and other aromas more clearly than when they're not ovulating.

SEXY PERCEPTION OF FRAGRANCE

History has left an unabashed scent trail concerning fragrance. Those who could afford it in ancient cultures may not have had vials of essential oils, but they still made extravagant use of fragrance.

This fragrance wasn't just room fresheners to override foul odor or sacred incense to appease the gods. The aromas they chose are legendary aphrodisiacs. And they perfumed everything — their skin and hair, their clothes, their bedding, the wall hangings — you name it, it was fragranced.

One look at the seductive role of scent as portrayed in the world's great literature, and you'll have no doubt of aromatherapy's lurid past. You might even take a few scentful hints from history. The *Kama Sutra*, a famous Indian tell-it-like-it-is treatise on love and sex, refers repeatedly to aromatherapy. Here it sets the stage:

> "... the outer room, balmy with rich perfumes, should contain a bed ... having garlands and bunches of flowers upon it.... There should also be ... fragrant ointments for the night, as well as flowers and other fragrant substances."

Just to show how sexy fragrance is, the stuffy religious Puritans hated it. During the era when they held power in England, they passed a law forbidding women from wearing perfume and any scented accessories. A 1770 parliamentary bill declared that a woman who seduces someone with scent can be charged with witchcraft. Ginger, long known as an aphrodisiac, was out and banned lest someone get a whiff of it and lose control.

TIP

If you ovulate, practice training your nose to judge the quality aromatherapy products when you're ovulating or right after, when you're better at discovering the source of each aroma. You can detect what's being whipped up in a restaurant or your own kitchen, especially if it's fried and fatty foods!

Spreading your scent

The close relationship of your skin's chemistry with essential oil occurs because you have your own unique, personal odor. Yes, it's yours alone and as individual as your fingerprint. And guess what? It's more important for lovemaking than that sexy outfit you just bought.

It's not just about how well you can smell, but how you smell! You may already know that fragrance changes depending upon who wears it.

TIP

Test whatever you wear as perfume or cologne on your skin before you buy it. When you find a scent that really works for you, your smell preferences encourage you to stick to that fragrance.

As much as people try to subdue their personal odor with deodorants and hide it with cologne, perfume, and aftershave, your biological smell holds the key to your sexual allure. It attracts sexual partners, or at least flirts with them.

When famed sex therapists and researchers William Masters and Virginia Johnson suggested that odors influence sexual arousal in the 1960s, they weren't exactly coming up with something new. The word for "kiss" is the same word as "smell" in several languages.

Your body makes its very own essential oils. I'm not referring here to body odor but to the musty, subtle, warm, personal smell unique to every person. You become finely attuned to the scent of a lover's skin — or more accurately, their armpit. I often hear this personal smell called *that* scent. Students at my aromatherapy seminars shyly comment that they know what I'm talking about. It's *that* scent that swept them off their feet when they first encountered *that* person. Many describe it as intoxicating.

Hankies have quite an aromatic history and are excellent carriers for essential oils. Just a couple drops on it will do. Whipping the cloth through the air is a perfect way to distribute the scent. No respectable Edwardian or Victorian would have blown their nose in public, but their embroidered, and certainly scented, handkerchief served to politely protect the nose from the city's smells, to fend off impolite people with a flick of the wrist, or serve as a come-hither gesture to one's beloved.

TIP

Scent a handkerchief, or any square of cloth, with a couple drops of essential oil or wrap an aromatic plant like lavender or sage in cloth. Stick it in a drawer or bag for a couple days so the cloth can absorb the aroma.

Buying essential sexiness

Sometimes you use essential oils to cover up your own personal scent, but they're far sexier when you use them to enhance your personal scent.

Banking on the irresistible mix of sex, essential oils, and imagination, perfume companies devise provocative names such as Obsession, Poison, Tabu, and Touch. To add a little heat to the equation, there's Fahrenheit for Women. A lot of masculine scents have names that exude power: Brut, Tsar, Boss, and Musk, with few secrets about what they're trying to sell. With that in mind, I can't help smirking at the name of a fragrance line called Contradiction.

Body powder, cologne, aftershave, and other products accompany perfume lines. Even shampoo and hair rinse are advertised for their sex appeal. Body and massage oils follow suit, not to mention the slew of sexual enhancement products.

To create your own sexy products from scratch, see the instructions for making body and massage oils in Chapter 5. And sexy scents aren't just for your body. You can give your environment – a room, a pillow — a sexy vibe by following the advice in Chapter 6.

REMEMBER

One key thing to note about sexual attraction and choosing your essential oil: Not everyone likes the same scent. Everyone has their own preferences when it comes to what they love to smell.

Patchouli's fragrance may be a potent aphrodisiac, but there are patchouli lovers, and there are patchouli haters, although even this strong-smelling oil can dive into a well-constructed blend and not be detected. But try a blend in which patchouli dominates, and you're in for a disappointing experience if your partner hates it and flees the room. Be prepared with either an alternative or be willing to go scentless until you discover the offending essential oil so you can avoid that one in the future.

WARNING

Use essential oil carefully and responsibly. Essential oils can enhance an intimate moment, but use too much, and they can also ruin one. They are highly concentrated and some of them can burn or irritate skin even if you're not allergic to that oil. Be aware that people do have allergies to certain essential oils or have a sensitivity to them. There's nothing like having your perfect aromatic romance turn into a sneezing fest or an allergic rash. Not that you should shy away from using essential oils in romantic settings. Just be safe and remember that light fragrance does the trick. Be especially mindful about using even diluted products on sensitive skin areas. Just the friction of applying a warming oil increases the heat.

Scenting Up Your Sex Life

Essential oils as aphrodisiacs can be a spicy subject in more ways than one, especially musky and woodsy aromas along with vanilla. All these scents are incorporated in your own unique blend of personal body scent. The musky ones are usually the easiest to detect, although personal scent can be subtle to the nose. No matter, you can still enhance it using essential oils.

TIP

While you're sniffing out what you desire in an aphrodisiac essential oil, consider bringing in other attributes for your sexy blend. For example, fall into a more romantic mood by taking the edge off of a hectic day with an essential oil like lavender. The relaxing aroma of lavender still lets you maintain focus, so you don't just roll over and fall asleep. Try the do-it-right-this-time essential oil of rose that opens the heart and brings love and receptivity into the mix. Think of other combinations that suit the time and space. You don't need much of these adjunct oils; just a hint will do.

Aphrodisiac themes for essential oils

Look at a selection of some of the world's most famous aphrodisiacs. Use these scents at your own risk — they work:

TIP

>> **Musky** scents like myrrh are reminiscent of personal scents. They resemble the human pheromone androsterone secreted in male sweat.

Use musklike scents in small amounts so your blend doesn't become over-powering and smell animal-like, conveying a message of being unwashed rather than in the mood.

>> **Spicy** scents are hidden in personal scent. This explains why pumpkin pie spice is such a sexy aroma. Sometimes there's also just a hint of sour or citrus scent hidden underneath all that spiciness.

>> **Vanilla** is considered one of the most comforting scents there is, perhaps because it's the closest scent to mother's milk. At the same time, it's an aphrodisiac that combines well with different types of scents. Sweet scents like benzoin that have vanilla-like aromas have the same effect.

>> **Woodsy** describes another aspect of the human smell. Hormonelike odors are often described as smelling like incense or wood. Like musky aromas, woodsy scents like sandalwood resemble masculine pheromones.

Love potion number 9 (through 17)

The spicy, musky, woodsy, and vanilla scent themes are well represented in the following list of aphrodisiac essential oils. Some of these essential oils carry more than one of these themes. Go ahead: Pick your "poison."

>> **Anise** smells like licorice and incites sex, at least according to the ancient Greek herbalist Dioscorides. The Chicago Smell and Taste Treatment and Research Foundation says anise is a favorite sexy scent for both men and women.

>> **Cardamom** blended with cinnamon, cloves, nutmeg, black pepper, and clove-scented carnations creates a classic Indian and Arab aphrodisiac. Medieval and Renaissance Europeans gave cardamom the nickname of "Fire of Venus" after the sensual goddess of love. Since Victorian England, Europeans have nibbled on cardamon seeds to freshen their breath after dinner and to spice up their evenings.

>> **Cinnamon** entered Western Europe with the Crusaders returning from the East. Along with it came its reputation as an aphrodisiac. Today, it's ranked as one of the most popular spices worldwide and rated high in the studies as a sexy scent.

>> **Clove bud** is regarded as a sexual stimulant. The Egyptians, Persians, Arabians, and Europeans all agree on this one. Sudanese women wear a fertility blend of clove, sandalwood, and musk to wedding parties so that its scent floats through the air as they dance.

>> **Coriander** is *the* aphrodisiac of the Middle East, Egypt, and Palestine. You can read about it in the classic tale, *The Arabian Nights*. Brought to Europe during the Crusades as a love potion, it flavored a popular drink called *Hippocras* that was drunk at weddings to inspire love and sex.

>> **Ginger** was for "burning desire," according to the Persian physician Avicenna. His recipe mixed it with honey for use during lovemaking. Ginger's hot stuff, so it's sure to at least get a rise from the guy emotionally! Women in Senegal entice lovers by wearing ginger in their belts. In New Guinea, men scent their face, arms, and chest with ginger to make them smell irresistible. They also tuck the fragrant flowers, along with other aromatic herbs, into their armbands.

>> **Jasmine** is called "Queen of the Night" because it releases its fragrance at night. As a symbol of both sex and love, it's also associated with passions unleashed at night. In India, jasmine is used to anoint the body and is placed in bridal wreaths. It's one of the five fragrant flowers the Indian god of love, Kama, puts on his arrows to penetrate the five senses. The fragrance is also said to rekindle fading romance. The Arabian *Medical Formulary of Al-Kindi* suggests jasmine massage oil for "strong lust."

>> **Myrrh's** musky scent is used in the Middle East to inspire both spiritual and sexual awareness. The Old Testament's *Song of Solomon* reads, "Delicate is the fragrance of your perfume, your name is an oil poured out . . . . My beloved is a sachet of myrrh lying between my breasts."

>> **Myrtle** was a major ingredient in the 16th-century "Angel Water" used as skin toner, but also drunk by women to increase their sexual attractiveness. It's a potent aphrodisiac in the Middle East. In ancient Greece, it was strewn beside the bridal bed and worn by brides.

>> **Nutmeg** is favored by the Chinese as an aphrodisiac. Although it smells spicy, this relaxing scent creates a euphoric feeling. In 18th century North America, it was popular in nightcaps; I wonder if they ever considered why.

>> **Orange blossom (neroli)** scents the popular perfume Poison. Long before this perfume's creation, prostitutes in Madrid, Spain, seduced their customers with it. Mediterranean brides also wear the flowers.

>> **Patchouli's** deep, earthy scent is said to overcome inhibitions. It has a similar association with the counterculture of the 1960s, when it was the *only* fragrance to wear.

>> **Peppermint** helps overcome frigidity. Arab men drink it to ensure virility. On New Guinea, a mint-coconut scented love charm is slipped into the bed of one's beloved to inspire passionate dreams of the two lovers together.

>> **Rose** inspires love as well as sex. Cleopatra scented the sails of her barge with rose water to entice Mark Anthony to her bed. (It worked!)

>> **Sandalwood** is close to human personal scent and is considered an aphrodisiac throughout the Eastern world. The famous tenth-century Arabian physician Avicenna recommended it to "exhilarate" and "heal passions" of the heart. India's ancient erotic text, the *Kama Sutra,* suggests that a man "give her your jasmine garland, lie her back gently, and massage her body with sweet sandalwood oil."

>> **Vanilla** is often mixed with chocolate (which causes a release of a stimulant related to amphetamine in the brain when people fall in love). Tonga Islanders rub vanilla in coconut oil on their bodies to smell sexier. The tribe Kellaway in Bolivia rub vanilla-like balsam of Peru under their arms. Jivaro women in Peru and Ecuador wear vanilla bean bead necklaces for their intoxicating fragrance. In the early 20th century, sex researcher Havelock Ellis found workers in a vanilla factory were sexually aroused from the scent.

>> **Ylang ylang,** sometimes described as intoxicating, is used to treat impotency and frigidity. Indonesians take the flowers along on their honeymoon.

Maybe not aphrodisiacs, but close

These essential oils are classified as mild aphrodisiacs. They're usually mixed with one or more of the more erotic scents.

>> **Basil** is used to attract a lover by Italian women who place the potted plant on their doorstep.

>> **Black pepper** has a reputation of perking up waning sexual desire.

>> **Clary sage** produces euphoria and, thus, releases inhibitions. Not a bad idea when you're using an aphrodisiac.

>> **Vetivert** smells like dirt to most people — that is, until small amounts are blended with richer fragrances; then it more closely resembles human scent. It's long been a popular scent in men's cologne and aftershave and is an important ingredient in Asian-style fragrances.

Sniffing out sexy scents for the sexes

Sex is always a hot topic that perks everyone's interest, including scientists. As a result, you can find plenty of research data on sex and scent.

The studies say that the scent that especially turns men on is the aroma of pumpkin pie spice, which has prompted many jokes over the years, but the food theme doesn't stop there. Add to that cola drinks, licorice candy, cinnamon buns. Not just any food will do, though. The aroma of cranberry and chocolate definitely don't captivate men's fancy.

Going back to ancient Rome and Greece, men favored heavy, clinging floral scents and wouldn't think of going to bed or to war without their fragrant ointments. According to surveys, most modern men say they'd rather not smell like flowers.

Women are also foodies when it comes to scent, just not as much. They tend to like the aroma of anise and also go for pumpkin pie spice. Cucumber's also on the list, although it's only available as a synthetic. And the favored herby scent of women? Lavender, of course. On the second-best list are the scents of chocolate and bananas — not a bad combination!

Planning Some Enchanted Evening: "Scentsual" Seduction

Placing a dab of perfume or cologne on the pulse point behind each ear and on the inside of your wrists is a good start to your scentual adventure. Because the blood vessels are close to the surface of your skin in these areas, they heat the scent and help diffuse it. However, you have other great hot spots. Just don't overdo it — you don't want to cover up your natural pheromones.

Scenting yourself

Throughout the world, from the jungles of the Amazon to the high-rises of New York and neighborhoods of Paris, scent captures people's imagination. African Bushmen say that the sweet scent of rain is the most seductive scent of all. You can draw on the world's aromatic traditions to come up with innovative ideas for yourself and your love life.

>> **Your body:** Take a hint from Arabic women: They first wash and then anoint their whole body with a scented paste made of musk, rose, and saffron. Their hair is perfumed with jasmine in sesame or walnut oil. On their ears, they place a red-colored blend of fragrant plants that includes saffron, rose, musk, and a very aromatic wood called oud. On their neck is rose, narcissus, oud, ambergris, or musk. Armpits are perfect for sandalwood or ambergris. Arabic men wear rose and oud behind their ears, on nostrils and beard, and on the palms of their hands. India's ancient Vedic texts also describe using different fragrances on different areas of the body.

Go ahead and try a little scent in your armpit where it can mix with your own personal scent.

>> **Your breath:** For perfumed kisses, chew on an aphrodisiac — a clove bud or cinnamon stick — as do people seeking passion throughout the Middle East. Or use a mint- or cinnamon-flavored breath lozenge. Most everyone likes the scent of mint on another's breath, although some people are repelled by it.

>> **Your hair:** Your hair — anywhere on your body — holds scent even better than your skin. Take advantage of this with shampoos and hair rinses that contain essential oils with aphrodisiac scents. After all, they are often advertised with this implication.

Polynesian women treat their hair with ylang-ylang scented coconut oil while Japanese women scent their hair and garments by holding them over incense. Geishas unpin their scented hair, so that a cascade of fragrance fills the space around them.

>> **Your loins:** Women of Nauruan stand over scented steam that comes from fragrant plants placed on a hot rock inside a miniature oven. In the Columbian Amazon, men stick sweet-smelling herbs under their loin cloths.

These days, you can buy almost anything scented. How about scented underwear? Scent them yourself by tucking a sachet that smells strongly of your favorite aphrodisiac in your underwear drawer. Or spritz your underwear or lingerie before your romantic evening.

>> **Your very being:** South Pacific Islanders of Nauru say that sipping an aromatic coconut oil drink makes the breath and skin irresistible. (I'd share their method, but it's a closely guarded secret.) The Desana people of Colombia down strong cups of aromatic herbal tea so they exude fragrance. See my suggestions in the section "Sharing a sumptuous scentual supper," later in this chapter.

TIP

Spritz your clothes so that a light scent lingers on them. This technique works best done with clothing that floats, such as scarves and loose shirts and blouses. That way, an aura of scent surrounds you and draws the loved one in closer.

>> **Your lover:** You don't have to look very far to find cultures that use scents-ual massage with aphrodisiac fragrances. You can buy a blend specially designed for this purpose. You can also choose your favorite scent from the list in this chapter.

>> **Your surroundings:** Cleopatra probably needs no introduction. This Egyptian queen enveloped herself, her barge, and its sails in scent to entice Mark Anthony to her bed. Granted, you may not find yourself sailing to your prospective lover drenched in perfume but look around. You can scent a lot of things in your surroundings — the curtains, couch, towels. A sprayer filled with scented water does the job quickly.

Make a trail of scent that leads your partner to new frontiers by applying a unique scent to each spot. You can keep your lover guessing, as well as wanting more. For more ideas on scenting rooms, see Chapter 6.

>> **Your bed:** In ancient Greece, men sprinkled their beds with fragrant powder so that their entire body was scented as the smell was released throughout the night. Louis XIV scented his sheets with jasmine. Greeks and Egyptians would literally cover the bed in rose petals.

You, too, can scent your sheets, and don't forget the pillows, too. (You can forget the blankets; you won't need them with all the hot passion.) You can either scent your entire linen closet with aromatic sachets or spritz just the sheets.

>> **Your food:** King Solomon's Garden was said to be filled with fragrant and edible aphrodisiacs, such as almonds and pomegranates. Two of life's greatest pleasures are eating and making love, so why not combine them? Because taste and smell are so intimately linked — you can't taste without smelling — food scents are definitely "in" when it comes to sex. See the section "Sharing a sumptuous scentual supper" and have a romantic, sensual meal.

Sharing a sumptuous, scentual supper

When it comes to fine, erotic dining, pass on the musk and jasmine and go for the yummy, edible foods. Many of the scents considered the sexiest are those that remind us of food. That makes it an easy task to choose what's on the menu for your sumptuous scentual supper.

You may find a box of licorice and a pumpkin pie more appropriate than candy and roses on your next Valentine's Day, next hot date, or romantic pursuit. Rather than wine, ply your lover with the licorice-flavored liqueur Ouzo. Because the smell of mint and sometimes chocolate is a favorite to scent your breath, the choice for dessert is obvious: a delicious chocolate mint mousse. Or, while you're at it, how about a rose water rice pudding with cardamom, pomegranate syrup over vanilla ice cream, or neroli ice cream over chocolate cake?

After dinner, going to the movies may be your best choice for a date. This is not to a movie with a sexy or romantic theme, but to make sure that they get a box of Good 'n Plenty licorice candy or buttered popcorn and orange cola. And, guys, play it safe and skip the cologne — many women consider it a turn-off.

The following seasonings are aphrodisiacs and can turn any meal into an erotic adventure.

>> Black pepper

>> Cardamom

>> Cinnamon

>> Coriander

>> Ginger

>> Nutmeg

>> Orange blossom (neroli) water

>> Rose

>> Vanilla

The first five on the list are hot spices used as mental, physical, and sexual stimulants. The last three — the orange, rose, and vanilla — are calming. You may want to use them all in one meal. That way, your lover will be relaxed, but not too relaxed. You certainly don't want them falling asleep.

Making Sexy Recipes

Let me put all of this scent-ous talk into action in these sure-to-please recipes. I generally don't recommend the internal use of essential oils, but these are the exceptions. You'll see why! Just promise to use a steady hand when adding the essential oil and stick to the small amounts called for in each recipe. One drop more, and you may ruin the batch.

Scents-ual Touch Massage Oil

This massage oil can also be a body or anointing oil. Only use this sensuous blend if you're intending the experience to go beyond a massage.

>> Preparation time: 5 minutes

>> Yield: 2 ounces massage oil

>> Ingredients:

8 drops ginger

5 drops myrrh

2 drops jasmine

1 drop cardamom

2 ounces vegetable oil

1. Add the essential oils to the vegetable oil.

2. Store in a closed container and enjoy!

A-romantic Whipping Cream

This sensual delight was invented by herbalist Diana DeLuca, author of *Botanica Erotica, Arousing Body, Mind, and Spirit* (Healing Arts Press) for your lover to eat on a rich cake, hot chocolate, or anywhere else that you can imagine.

>> Preparation time: 6 minutes

>> Yield: 1 cup cream

>> Ingredients:

   1/2 pint whipping cream

   1 drop essential oil

1. Whip cream to desired consistency.

2. Add the essential oil and mix well.

3. Add a touch of honey or sugar, if desired.

4. Refrigerate it if you don't use your whipping cream right away. Although it may lose a little of its airiness, the cream will last in the refrigerator at least a couple days, but why wait?

Midnight at the Oasis Balls

This dynamite blend created by herbalist and aromatherapist Mindy Green who co-wrote *Aromatherapy: The Complete Guide to the Healing Art*, (Penguin Random House) is something you can make days ahead of time and keep in the refrigerator until the mood strikes you — or your lover.

>> Preparation time: 15 minutes

>> Yield: 12 to 24 balls

>> Ingredients:

   1 cup hulled sesame seeds

   1 drop rose essential oil

   1/2 teaspoon vanilla extract

   2 tablespoons almond butter

   2 tablespoons honey

1 tablespoon finely chopped dates

1 teaspoon cardamom powder

1 teaspoon bee pollen

1 teaspoon ginseng powder

2 tablespoons shredded coconut

2 tablespoons cocoa or carob powder

1. Grind the seeds in an electric coffee grinder or blender.
2. Add the rose oil to the vanilla to dilute it.
3. Combine all ingredients, except the coconut and cocoa or carob powder, and mix thoroughly.
4. Form the mixture into balls.
5. Roll the balls in a combination of the shredded coconut and cocoa or carob powder.
6. Keep refrigerated.

Chapter 9

Essential Oils to Ease Stress and Brain Fog

The good news is that aromatherapy can help. Essential oils offer you many ways to deal with the stress and strain of everyday life. They help keep you sharp, alert, and on your toes, ready to deal with each new challenge. They also prevent you from lagging and keep your efficiency from dropping.

In this chapter, I talk about how essential oils help prevent stress and put a smile on your face. I throw in some fragrant techniques to reduce tension and improve your memory, and basically, make life a little better. You also get some advice on bringing aromatherapy wherever life takes you. Finally, I help you use essential oils to catch some Zs at the end of your busy day.

Seeking a Balanced Approach

Researchers studying aromatherapy's effects on emotions find that it eases feelings of apprehension, loneliness, and rejection. Some scents even help you feel less embarrassed and happier.

One study asked participants, "What kind of person makes you angry?" After getting everyone riled up by describing infuriating people, participants exposed to pleasant scents calmed down faster than the folks who didn't have anything to sniff.

The New York City subway doesn't usually exemplify great etiquette. It's push and shove all the way to your destination. However, researchers discovered that when cars are scented with pleasant food aromas, passengers push each other less and act more considerately than usual.

One study described the scent of lavender as creating "an inner sense of peace."

Adapting to your needs

Geranium, and to a lesser extent lavender, have both a stimulating and sedative effect on your brain. Called *adaptagens* because they "adapt" to your personal needs, these herbs also teach your body to "adapt" well in different physical surroundings and emotional circumstances. Likewise, some essential oils have adaptagenic scents useful in easing a variety of emotional problems.

The roselike fragrance of geranium creates a harmonious space and makes you feel better about yourself and others when you sniff it. I like to call it the "living room space." I highly recommend spritzing your living room, or any room, with geranium before bringing up a touchy subject.

TIP

An apple a day may keep more than the doctor away — it can fend off nervousness. Apple is one of the scents that make people less anxious, especially when mixed with cinnamon and clove. Apple scent is available only as a synthetic, but the next time you're going to speak before a group, try eating an apple beforehand and inhale its sweet smell. And, if you have a chance, sprinkle a little cinnamon on it as well!

Recognizing the possibilities of essential oils

Don't expect essential oils to push you into super-drive and enable you to get twice as much done as ever before. You won't experience that head-snapping alertness that comes from caffeine pills and other eyepopping drugs.

You can expect essential oils to assist you in plenty of ways, mostly through scent alone:

- » Provide a boost when you need to wake up
- » Keep you relaxed enough to ride through tension and tight deadlines
- » Power up your brain and memory
- » Eliminate brain fog
- » Maintain your attention and energy levels through a long day, whether you have yet another meeting or a fussy baby
- » Help you bounce back from jet lag

In fact, whenever you find life challenging, essential oils help you literally change the atmosphere. Not too bad from smell alone. And you won't be riding on the roller coaster of highs and lows experienced when you rely on coffee or drugs to sustain your energy. (For more on the way your brain comprehends aroma, see Chapter 1.)

Soothing Stress

Life is stressful; that's just a fact. Another sad fact is that stress doesn't improve your memory or level of efficiency one bit. On the contrary, it contributes to their slowdown. The problem with stress is that if you endure enough of it for long enough it short-circuits your brain so that you can't think as quickly or as clearly as you should. If you're already under stress at work, having brain fog, or even a brain meltdown, is the last thing you need.

Hanging out in any stressful environment, straining to get a project done, being bored by monotonous tasks, or being always on the go increases your body's workload by pushing your adrenal glands into overdrive. You end up working overtime in more ways than you realize: While you're working hard at your job, your body is working hard to deal with the physical and emotional effects of stress. No surprise that you feel worn out!

You may become drowsy and irritable and develop headaches. If you think that's enough reason to slow down at work, listen to this: Researchers find that the more stress you experience, the more likely you are to get sick. You get sick and then you really fall behind at work (not to mention use up your sick days).

The following list lays out stress-related problems and symptoms. Answer the questions for a quick check on how well you're dealing with stress:

>> **Circulation problems:** Do you ever have heart palpitations, an irregular heartbeat, high blood pressure, or get out of breath easily?

>> **Digestive upsets:** Do you experience heartburn, a loss of appetite, indigestion, constipation, or diarrhea?

>> **Emotional responses:** Do you sometimes feel nervous, hostile, overreact emotionally, or frequently want to cry? Do you feel an increasing amount of depression?

>> **Fatigue:** Do you ever feel endlessly tired?

>> **Headaches:** Do you get migraines or tension headaches?

>> **Insomnia:** Do you have sleep disturbances? For example, do you wake up often and can't get back to sleep? Do you have vivid dreams accompanied by restless sleep?

>> **Teeth clenching:** Do you find yourself clenching your jaw, or is your jaw or neck extra tight or sore?

>> **Sexual problems:** Do you have a lack of sexual desire?

>> **Sweating:** Do you sweat when it's not even hot, have a very dry mouth, or feel exceptionally thirsty?

If you answer yes to even one of these questions, you may already have a stress problem. If you answer yes to several of these questions, you're probably over-stressed. Keep reading for ways to cope with the tension.

WARNING

The listed symptoms are symptoms of stress, but they are also associated with other — sometimes more serious — illnesses. If you experience several of the listed symptoms or they severely affect your life, consult a doctor.

TIP

If you're dealing with chronic exhaustion, try to determine its cause and go to the source of your problem. Refer to the Symptom Guide under "Fatigue" for more energy hints when you're burning the candle at both ends.

STOP AND INHALE

The big breaths you automatically take when you sniff an essential oil have an added benefit. Taking deep breaths slows your breathing down, and that makes you feel less anxious and stressed. Breathing sends oxygen to your brain and also to your muscles to help them function properly and relax.

Watch out for those midday yawns. They're your body's attempt to convince you to breathe more deeply, and they signal that your brain is longing for more oxygen. Working at a desk, especially on a computer, puts extra strain on your neck and can interfere with your need for oxygen. The tight muscles that result constrict your blood vessels and all of the oxygen-rich blood traveling to your brain. In a vicious cycle, the neck tension impairs your brain activity. That slows down your work pace and makes you stressed. To top it off, the longer work hours increase your neck tension.

Taking a breathing break every so often is good for your productivity and for your health.

Dealing with adrenal exhaustion

Stress affects your adrenal glands. Your adrenals keep you alert when you're stressed so you feel ready to deal with anything. However, if you push your adrenal glands to the limit, they stop functioning properly. You then enter the wearying cycle of stress impairing the ability of your adrenal glands to operate and making you more easily stressed.

In the early stages of overload, your adrenal glands go overboard when responding to even small amounts of stress. Eventually, they hit the hammock in exhaustion, and you end up with "tired" glands. They can't rouse enough energy, leaving you feeling drained and unable to get excited about much of anything: work, family, sex, vacation . . . it all becomes blah.

The adrenal glands respond well to certain scents. Sniff the following essential oils and use them in a massage oil — along with a massage, if possible! (Massage is one of the best stress-reducing techniques in aromatherapy — and probably in life.) Look for aromatherapy blends that combine these essential oils with other antistress oils:

>> Clary sage

>> Pine (especially the species called *Pinus syvestris*)

>> Spruce

Lessening stress: Mind over matter

Your body's responses to stress are linked to your brain's hypothalamus, which controls many functions in your body. Because the hypothalamus is part of your limbic system that processes smell, aromatherapy directly eases stress.

TECHNICAL STUFF

Relaxing fragrances — the ones that help you deal with stress — tend to produce slower frequency brain waves (delta waves), and they also prompt some relaxing theta waves. Both delta and theta waves bring out your quiet and meditative side. Many relaxing aromas increase another type of brain waves — alpha waves. Alpha waves make you feel centered and focused.

REMEMBER

The aromas of lavender, bergamot, marjoram, sandalwood, lemon, chamomile, and valerian produce sedating brain wave patterns.

Check out this list of the most important essential oils for decreasing your stress:

>> Bergamot

>> Chamomile

>> Lavender

>> Lemon

>> Melissa (lemon balm)

>> Marjoram

>> Neroli (orange blossom)

>> Petitgrain

>> Rose

>> Sandalwood

>> Valerian

Choose any aromatherapy method, such as an aromatherapy diffuser, to dispense scents that relieve anxiety into the air. If you're on the go a lot, carry them with you in an aromatherapy inhaler (easy to buy) or as smelling salts that you make yourself (easy to make). (See Chapter 6 for diffusion tips and the "Smelling Salts" recipe in this chapter.)

REMEMBER

Essential oils are safe to use even if you're taking anti-depression or anti-anxiety medication. Scents that ease stress also have anti-depressant properties.

Stress-Less Massage Oil

This massage oil reduces stress and keeps you relaxed, but still alert enough to get your job done.

>> Preparation time: 2 minutes

>> Yield: 2 ounces massage oil

>> Ingredients:

8 drops lavender

4 drops geranium

2 drops clary sage

2 drops spruce

2 ounces almond (or other vegetable) oil

1. Add the essential oils to the vegetable oil.

2. Mix everything together well and use as a massage or body oil.

Vary It! Use this same blend to scent the air.

Staying Calm and Carrying On: Fending Off Anxiety

Anxiety wears many different faces. It manifests in the nervousness you feel when giving a presentation, going for a job interview, or perhaps when flying.

A little anxiety is rarely a problem. Feeling a few butterflies in your stomach and getting energized from the burst of adrenaline that often comes with anxiousness may even improve your performance. However, if your anxiety level reaches the point where it turns your hands clammy from sweat and your mouth becomes so dry that you can barely speak, anxiety is not helping a bit.

If you feel anxious throughout the day, you probably have difficulty concentrating and then you can't sleep well at night. Anxiety can also make you fearful or preoccupied with problems at work and blow the smallest upsets way out of proportion. Some people become so anxious that they have panic attacks and become immobilized with fear and anxiousness.

Keeping your focus isn't just about staying mentally stimulated or remaining calm and relaxed. Get too hyper or chill out too much, and you can't keep your mind engaged. For optimum brain power, you need to be emotionally stable.

When you're feeling anxious, try sniffing one of these essential oils:

>> Chamomile

>> Clary sage

>> Fir

>> Geranium

>> Juniper

>> Marjoram

>> Melissa (lemon balm)

>> Orange

>> Petitgrain

>> Rose

WARNING

Severe anxiety points to an imbalance in brain chemistry. Besides trying aromatherapy techniques, ask your doctor and other health-care providers for suggestions on how to help your body and brain cope. If anxiety causes heart palpitations or chest pains or makes you feel dizzy, select a scent from the list in the "Lessening stress: Mind over matter" section earlier in the chapter. Good examples are ylang ylang, sandalwood, frankincense, and marjoram.

Keeping your cool

Aromatherapy offers gentle assistance to help you maintain and rebuild your emotional equilibrium. Just inhaling the scents of lavender and sandalwood increases the alpha waves in your brain. Alpha waves decrease the miscellaneous, idle chatter that runs through your mind and encourages your mind to relax. Lavender and sandalwood have a long history of creating meditative states.

Other alpha-wave inducing essential oils are eucalyptus, pine, and fir, which are stimulants, so they offer an extra element of increased attention when you sniff them.

Blood pressure rates jump when you're nervous, but just sniffing the scents of marjoram, orange, or geranium drops your pressure two to five points (both the systolic and diastolic rates).

WARNING

Sniffing marjoram, orange, or geranium can lower your blood pressure, but not to a medically significant degree. If you suffer from high blood pressure, don't rely on essential oils to manage your condition.

Reducing anxiety

If you have a tendency to get anxious or depressed, or when you just feel down once in a while, turn to the following essential oils:

>> Angelica

>> Bergamot

>> Cardamom

>> Chamomile

>> Cinnamon

>> Clary sage

>> Clove

>> Cypress

>> Lavender

>> Lemon verbena

>> Lemon

>> Melissa (lemon balm)

>> Orange

>> Orange blossom (neroli)

>> Petitgrain

>> Rose

>> Ylang ylang

Anxiety is considered a cousin to depression, so the antidepressants in this section work to ease you out of either condition with just a sniff.

Smelling Salts

You can make your own anxiety-relieving smelling salts.

>> Preparation time: 4 minutes

>> Yield: 1 tablespoon smelling salts

>> Ingredients:

    3 drops bergamot

    2 drops geranium

    1 drop neroli (or 3 drops petitgrain)

    1 tablespoon rock salt (or other coarse salt)

1. Combine all ingredients.

2. Carry in a closed container and sniff as needed.

Vary It! Add the same essential oils (in the same amounts) to 4 ounces vegetable oil to create a massage oil. If you can't get a massage, add a couple teaspoons of this massage oil to your bath water and enjoy!

Pepping Up Your Work Life

If you have a demanding job or home life, you need to keep your brain cranked up to your full capacity every day. I know, that's easier said than done. Sure, there's always another cup of coffee, but holistic health practitioners, including clinical aromatherapists and naturopaths, worry that a few cups of the java every day takes a toll on your adrenal glands. It's at least enough to give you jittery nerves, put you on edge, and make it easier to fall into depression, anxiety, and stress. That's not a good prescription if you're trying to stay on top of everything. Essential oils offer you an alternative: More energy and better focus with fewer unwanted side effects.

Improving focus

According to the research from the psychologists who study scent, aroma considerably improves your mental stamina, concentration, and efficiency. Besides, it makes for a pleasant work environment.

Your brain waves peak sharply in response to stimulants like coffee and energy drugs. You think more quickly and clearly as a result. The good news is that brain waves peak the same way when you sniff a stimulating aroma. Granted, scent isn't as powerful as the drugs, but it revs up your brain without the drug's negative health effects.

Scent can help with everyday productivity. It can

>> **Improve your mental performance:** Workers spent 40 stressful minutes identifying complicated patterns on a computer. Those in a scented room got 88 percent correct answers compared to 65 percent for those working in an unscented room.

The scents were peppermint (voted the favorite), benzoin, or cinnamon. Rooms scented with lemon have cut computer errors more than half. Aromatherapists also suggest lemon to keep focused and relaxed.

>> **Keep attention high:** Scent prevents the sharp drop of sustained attention that typically occurs after 30 minutes of concentration. It also sustains your mental energy by supporting your nervous system.

>> **Provide pep without side effects:** Essential oils don't over-amp your adrenal glands. Instead, they do quite the opposite. They can calm down your central nervous system and stop it from overreacting. This counters rushes of adrenaline that can make you too hyper and nervous. Calming essential oils such as lavender oil seem to reduce the nervous system agitation produced by caffeine.

Using common scents for increased brain power

The same essential oils that pep you up and reduce your drowsiness also decrease the likelihood of becoming irritable or getting headaches. These mind-stimulating scents work just by sniffing them:

>> Angelica

>> Basil

>> Benzoin

>> Black pepper

>> Cardamom

>> Cinnamon

>> Clove

>> Cypress

- » Ginger
- » Jasmine
- » Peppermint
- » Rosemary
- » Sage

If you're trying to stay alert and awake, or you need to stimulate your brain, sniff any one of these aromas every five minutes or so or use one or more to fill your room with scent.

Curiously, the scent of rose, neroli, and ylang ylang oils stimulate brain waves, even though aromatherapists use them to induce relaxation — the opposite of stimulation. Brains are complicated organs that operate on a variety of levels, and essential oils can stimulate and relax different parts of the brain at the same time.

REMEMBER

Some stimulating aromas are aphrodisiacs, but don't worry; they won't turn everyone's thoughts to love — except for jasmine. Jasmine on its own is such a potent aphrodisiac, you're better off leaving it at home and not sharing it in the workplace. (For more on the enticing subject of love potions, turn to Chapter 8.)

Gotta Go-Go-Go

This recipe helps keep you going. It's filled with stimulating fragrances, and I added bergamot to soften the aroma. It helps relax overworked muscles.

- » Preparation time: 4 minutes
- » Yield: 2 ounces massage oil
- » Ingredients:

    9 drops bergamot oil

    6 drops eucalyptus oil

    3 drops cinnamon oil

    2 drops peppermint oil

    2 drops ginger oil

    2 ounces vegetable oil

1. Combine the oils and stir or shake well.

2. Use for a massage or body oil.

SCENTING FOR PRODUCTIVITY AROUND THE WORLD

Someday, you may come to work and find the place filled with scent. That could happen in businesses all over the world if they follow the lead of several large corporations in Tokyo, Japan, that scent their office buildings. Throughout the workday, different fragrances circulate through the air-conditioning or heating system. The Shimizu Construction Company patented a computerized system to distribute scent. A refreshing peppermint is dispersed into offices and conference rooms to increase work efficiency, dispel drowsiness, and lessen mental fatigue. Lavender helps establish a positive mood.

At Kajima Construction Company, lemon is the morning wakeup call. This is followed by a midday rose to inspire contented work (or jasmine when the workers are women because women tend to prefer jasmine over rose). Then, after lunch, an invigorating cypress helps employees overcome the afternoon lull. Cypress also fills display areas and the public relation rooms to promote constructive work. Employees have even noticed that the scented rooms reduce their urge to smoke.

Keyboard workers made far less errors as they sniffed the aromas of lavender, jasmine, and especially lemon. These scents cut the rate of error in half.

In Tokyo aromatherapy doesn't stop at work. During the lunch hour, workers can partake in a peppermint refresher at a downtown aromatherapy bar. On the way home, they can stop off at atomizer-equipped booths that provide a mist of a stimulating scent. Even at home, their mattresses may have fragrance diffused into them. The next morning, scented alarm clocks begin another scented day.

Japan isn't the only country keen on scents on the job. A British firm offers a variety of fragrances to pump into the workplace and make employees feel better and less stressed. They even custom design individual corporate "odor identities" for the company to use much like a logo on their stationery and business cards. Not a bad idea when you want customers to remember you!

Taking scent to work

Sometimes, you need to be creative to employ essential oils. Sniffing an aroma sounds easy enough, but you can't introduce scent just anywhere. After all, you're not always the only one breathing the air. Others around you may or may not take kindly to the idea of having their moods changed even by a pleasant scent.

Try one or more of these ways to carry your healing fragrance with you:

» **Burn incense:** Consider burning incense if you work outdoors. Its powerful fragrance can scent large areas in cases where the smoke usually isn't bothersome, such as a construction or landscaping site.

» **Carry a scented hanky:** Bring back the era of high tea by carrying a handkerchief, which is the perfect vehicle to carry scent. Put a couple drops of essential oil on a hanky, or any piece of cloth. Every time you politely cover your nose with your hanky, you get an aromatic dose without anyone suspecting that you're really trying to keep your cool or need some energy.

TIP

This subtle technique works well when traveling on an airplane or train. It doesn't disrupt the person next to you, but you get the benefit of an aromatic lift and get to kill airborne germs.

» **Plug in an aromatherapy diffuser:** if you're fortunate enough to have your own office, an electric aromatherapy diffuser emits a steady aroma for hours.

» **Sniff an essential oils inhaler:** A subtle approach that improves just your own mood is the aromatherapy inhaler with blends that affect your emotions. Inhalers are convenient because they're small enough to slip into your pocket.

» **Spritz the air:** Air fresheners are okay in many workplaces, including most schools. I know several teachers who spritz a chamomile and lavender combo in their elementary school classrooms to keep the kids calm and focused. (Yes, it works!)

» **Wear as perfume:** At the risk of being downright sneaky, wear essential oils as cologne. Health-care workers, especially nurses, place a half drop of essential oil on their wrists or arms so that the fragrance surrounds their patients as they work on them. (If sage or rosemary isn't your idea of an appealing cologne, combine the essential oil with your favorite cologne or perfume. Yes, the oil will alter the cologne's fragrance, but hopefully in a pleasing way, and you get the therapeutic benefits.)

» **Use scented hand lotion:** Give yourself a mental or physical pick-me-up during a hard day with scented hand lotion. Lotion is perfect when you don't have much time to do anything else at work but rub your hands together. It's a great idea when you can't put fragrance into the air. Look for a lotion that contains the appropriate essential oils or add drops of your own essential oil to an unscented lotion.

OKAY, RUB IT IN

If you like massage, take advantage of it. Any stress-management consultant can tell you that taking even a short massage break increases your productivity. A massage also makes your body release pain-relieving chemicals called *endorphins*, that diminish pain similar to the pain-killing drug, morphine.

An office massage uses a portable, padded massage chair, so you can stay dressed and can be back at work in 15 minutes flat with your clothes and hair unruffled. This massage doesn't require oil. However, get extra mileage out of your massage by having massage oil or liniment massaged on your neck, your arms, or your hands. (How wonderful a hand massage feels after a few hours of typing!)

Look for massage oils that contain essential oils with brain-stimulating, muscle-relaxing, and circulation-increasing properties.

Lotion for Emotions

If you can find just a few minutes to spare in your busy schedule, create your own hand lotion to use in those minutes. To save fuss, muss, and time, buy an unscented hand lotion made with natural ingredients, or at least one with very little scent. You can even purchase an unscented lotion and mix in your own essential oils.

> » Preparation time: 1 minute

> » Yield: 1 bottle of lotion

> » Ingredients:

>   4 ounces unscented lotion

>   20 to 28 drops essential oil

1. Stir the essential oil into the lotion, and it's done! (I told you this was quick!)

   If you use a blend of several different essential oils, add 30 drops total (*not* 30 drops of each essential oil).

2. Use as a hand and body lotion whenever you like.

   Vary It! Use 12 drops ginger and 8 drops basil to perk performance. Use 12 drops lemon and 8 drops clove to improve your memory.

TIP

   Some essential oils are extra potent, so adjust the amount if you use rose, jasmine, or angelica oils. Use 1 drop for every 8 drops called for in the recipe. For clary sage, chamomile, or ylang ylang oils use 1 drop for every 5 drops in the recipe.

Going on a Scenti-Mental Journey: Boosting Memory

You depend on your memory. Think about it. Without your ability to recall data, you can't find your shoes in the morning, much less remember everything you're supposed to do that day. You can probably afford to forget where you laid your keys or to pick up bread once in a while, but it's a different story when you forget an important phone call or the boss turns to you with a question you should know the answer to.

You use your memory minute by minute. So, it's downright scary when important facts slip your mind. Not to worry, aromatherapy can help.

Taking a trip down memory lane: Putting scent to use

You know the experience: You encounter a whiff of a certain perfume or a fragrance you haven't smelled for years, and suddenly you're flying back in time to a long-forgotten experience you associate with that smell. The scent carries everything about that experience: the sights, sounds, and especially your emotional impressions at the time.

REMEMBER

Your sense of smell is closely connected to the areas of your brain that control both your short- and long-term memories. Aroma helps you remember important facts, places, and names.

Fortunately, memory is not a one-way street. Your brain not only associates stored information with scent but helps you retrieve it with fragrance. (For more on the brain and its relationship to scent, see Chapter 1.)

If you're like most people, you can recall an event twice as easily if aroma is involved compared to a strictly visual recollection. As time goes on, your scent memory stays sharp while your visual memory plummets. Years later, you sniff the same thing, and you're instantly journeying down memory lane. Take a hint from students who tried to memorize lists of words. They had better recall later if they sniffed a scent — even something that they didn't like — while doing the assignment and then smelled that scent again when asked to recall the words.

Aroma helps your memory in several ways:

>> **Remember better:** Work in a scented room. You notice and retain facts more quickly and easier and file them in your brain where they're easy to locate.

The connection of aroma to your brain's limbic system gives it a direct route to your thought processing and memory.

>> **Scent association:** Your recall of past events is much stronger when it's linked to scent rather than sight.

>> **Stimulate blood circulation:** Take a good sniff of an aromatherapy scent, and you automatically inhale plenty of oxygen. Not bad, considering that the number one reason for memory lapses is not enough oxygen reaching your brain. Too little oxygen makes you feel fuzzy-headed and easily confused. (See the sidebar "Stop and Inhale" for more on why taking a deep breath sends more oxygen to your brain.)

>> **Stop forgetful chemicals:** One of the ways sage oil alters your brain chemistry for the better is to stop the activity of an enzyme called *acerylcholinesterase* that contributes to memory loss and seems to play a part in Alzheimer's disease. A good thing about sage is that it doesn't disrupt other organs, unlike the drug tacrine, which slows degeneration from Alzheimer's but damages your liver in the process.

Having the scents to remember

Use your sense of smell to your advantage by inhaling fragrances that assist your recall and stimulate your blood circulation. These scents do other things as well, including promoting beta brain waves, which help make you alert and attentive. For an added perk, most of these essential oils double as spicy stimulants that help keep you alert — a dynamite combination for mental sharpness.

Some scents to spark your brain include

>> Basil

>> Bay laurel

>> Bay rum (pimento)

>> Clove

>> Lemon

>> Rosemary

>> Sage

If stress affects your memory, use these essential oils with the calming oils I recommend in the section "Lessening stress: Mind over matter."

Forget-Me-Not Liniment

You can whip up your own memory blend that also stimulates blood circulation and relaxes any muscle tension you have. Because it has an alcohol base, it's perfect to use for an office-chair massage. Liniment recipes usually call for rubbing alcohol — and use it if you want — but alcohol's strong smell interferes with the scent of the aromatherapy oils. I prefer using vodka, which is a combination of only alcohol and water. Don't forget: This liniment can get hot, and the heat increases the more you rub it on your skin.

» Preparation time: 4 minutes

» Yield: 2 ounces liniment

» Ingredients:

　8 drops lemon oil

　4 drops rosemary oil

　2 drops sage oil

　1 drop clove oil

　2 ounces vodka or rubbing alcohol

1. Combine all ingredients.

2. Use for massage as often as you can!

Vary It! If you prefer a lotion rather than a liniment, use any unscented or lightly scented body lotion instead of the alcohol. This lotion is also excellent for massage, and it's not as oily as a typical massage oil.

Traveling Tips

Travel can wreak havoc on your sleep schedule, especially if you're on the move a lot, and even more so if you're crossing time zones.

Flying through time zones can disrupt your body rhythms and lead to fatigue, dizziness, nausea, depression, and pressure in your head after the flight. You may spend a day or so adjusting when you'd rather be seeing the sights or actively participating in that meeting.

I don't think I could fly without my trusty essential oil inhaler in my carry-on. It counters the stuffy cabin's recycled air, not to mention being totally refreshing. Once traveling across the United States on a long plane trip from San Francisco to

Boston, I kept misting the businessman next to me. He was sound asleep, so I figured he wouldn't know the difference. When we landed, he kept commenting on how unusually refreshed he felt and then said, "It must be sitting next to you." (No, I didn't tell him my secret.)

Arrival Revival

Make your own aromatic spray for travel. Both essential oils in this recipe are excellent for making you relaxed yet focused — a perfect combination.

>> Preparation time: 5 minutes

>> Yield: 2 ounces of a delightful aromatherapy spritzer!

>> Ingredients:

12 drops lavender oil

5 drops geranium oil

3 drops rose

2 ounces distilled water

1. Add the essential oils to the water in a spray bottle.

2. Shake gently each time before spraying.

Vary It! If you're in need of a wake-up call, replace the geranium with peppermint oil.

Travel Companion: Eye Relax

Try this quick and easy way to relax your tired eyes and brain. As an added bonus, it helps get rid of early morning puffy eyes to keep you looking bright-eyed and alert.

>> Preparation time: 5 minutes

>> Yield: 2 eye bags

>> Ingredients:

½ cup water

2 tea bags (chamomile or regular black tea)

1. Bring the water to a boil.

2. Pour the boiling water over the tea bags, steep for a few minutes, and then let cool enough so that they don't burn your eyelids.

3. Squeeze the excess water from the tea bags and place 1 bag over each of your closed eyes. If handy, also place a small, folded cloth over the tea bags to hold them in place and block out light.

4. Relax with the tea bags over your eyes for at least three minutes.

Having the Scents to Unwind: Bathing Your Feet

It's all too easy to carry the problems of the day home with you. Just as they get you through the day, essential oils can help you unwind.

Use essential oils to be more focused with your friends or family, even when you're tired. Maybe after a long day you want to be alert to go over your child's school report or to take in that late night movie without falling asleep.

One aromatherapy treatment that feels really great at the end of the day is a foot soak. If you're on your feet a lot, soaking offers blessed relief to sore, tired, worn-out feet. And, in case you've had one of those overly cerebral days, there's nothing like focusing your attention on your feet instead of your head! It's a technique that sometimes even banishes a headache. A foot bath feels great and is perfectly safe, so you can indulge in it every day.

TIP

If your feet tend to get chilled, a foot bath warms them up, and that heat spreads to the rest of you. Because it improves the circulation in your legs, a foot bath may lessen the likelihood of you developing varicose veins from too much standing or even hemorrhoids from too much sitting. If you've already developed one of these conditions, use a foot bath as one of your therapies.

Soak Those Pups Foot Bath

A foot bath with essential oils is fast and easy. Choose oils to relax, wake up, or think better.

>> Preparation time: 2 minutes

>> Yield: 1 foot bath

>> Ingredients:

1 to 2 quarts water

5 drops tea tree oil

5 drops sage oil

2 drops peppermint oil

1. Heat the water or use hot water from the tap that is just cool enough to stick your feet in.

2. Fill a container big enough for both feet with the warm water.

3. Add the essential oils to the water and stir to distribute them.

4. Soak your feet for at least 15 minutes — and relax!

Vary It! Add ¼ cup Epsom salts — a common salt sold in grocery stores to relax sore muscles — when your feet are sore or just plain "dog tired."

Vary It Some More! Feel free to replace the essential oils in this recipe with your favorites to address whatever emotion you're experiencing. See the Essential Oil Guide for some ideas.

Sleeping Tight: Soothing Insomnia

Lack of sleep leaves you feeling tired the next day. If you don't get adequate sleep for weeks or months, you easily develop symptoms of sleep deprivation such as dizziness, confusion, agitation, and depression. If you travel for business as I do, then you really need a good night's sleep to do your best the next day.

Some aromas are so powerful they're comparable to sedative drugs. Some smell receptors in your brain are the same ones that activate sedative drugs like Valium and Librium.

Aroma has the advantage of having a direct route to relax you and put you to sleep. Napping in a scented room lulls patients in rest homes and hospitals to sleep as effectively as drugs for insomnia. And, after they do nod off, their sleep is less restless.

These aromas can send you, too, to dreamland:

» Bergamot

» Chamomile

» Citronella

- » Clary sage
- » Frankincense
- » Geranium
- » Lavender
- » Melissa (lemon balm)
- » Mandarin
- » Neroli
- » Rose
- » Sandalwood
- » Tangerine

TIP

Lavender makes a popular sleep pillow. If you don't care for the scent of lavender, then hops essential oil invokes good sleep just as well. Japanese researchers who conducted studies with pillows filled with hops found it to "facilitate falling asleep or to minimize stressful situations." Chamomile also makes you sleepy. As an added bonus, it is said to ensure good dreams.

Citronella isn't typically suggested to increase sleep. After all, it's a bug repellent. However, the essential oil has been shown to improve sleep, even for those who have a sleep disorder or nervous condition that keeps them up at night. In fact, it works better than taking repeated doses of hops extract, a well-known herbal sedative. (Check out the Sweet Dreams Sleep Pillow recipe, later in this chapter.) I've tried citronella, and it works. About 4 drops of the essential oil in a warm bath does the trick. That is, if the smell doesn't remind you of fending off bugs!

Nightly Night Blend

This blend enhances your sleep. Use it to scent your room or your sheets, or simply sniff it to send you off to dreamland. (Chapter 6 tells you how to scent a room and your sheets.)

- » Preparation time: 5 minutes
- » Yield: About 4 applications
- » Ingredients:

  3 drops bergamot oil

  3 drops geranium oil

2 drops chamomile oil

1 drop frankincense oil

1 drop rose oil

1. Combine the oils together and sniff the blend.

   Vary It! Add an ounce of distilled water and use it as a spritz to scent your room.

   Vary It! You can easily turn this blend into a massage or body lotion. Add the essential oil mix to 2 ounces vegetable oil or an unscented body lotion.

Sweet Dreams Sleep Pillow

Scented sleep pillows work amazingly well to knock you out at night. I travel a lot, so I always pack one. No matter where I'm sleeping, my pillow smells like home. By now, just the association of the scent with sleep is enough to send me to dreamland.

>> Preparation time: 20 minutes

>> Yield: One 7-square-inch sleep pillow

>> Ingredients:

   2 pieces of cloth about 8 inches square

   ¼ cup hops flowers (strobiles), dried

   ⅛ cup chamomile flowers, dried

   ⅛ cup lavender flowers, dried

   15 drops lavender essential oil

1. Make a small pillow by sewing the 2 pieces of cloth together on 3 sides, leaving 1 side open.

2. Blend the herbs together.

3. Sprinkle the lavender oil on the herbs and stir them to distribute the oil.

4. Spoon the herbs into the pillow through the open end and then sew up that side.

5. Put this little pillow under your regular sleeping pillow or tuck it inside your pillowcase.

Vary It! If you like, add dried basil leaves to your sleep pillow to prevent nightmares and agitated sleep. To dream more, add dried mugwort leaves to your mix, that is, if you're ready to have more dreams than sleep! Want to remember your dreams? Go for rosemary. (Remember, rosemary — that's for remembrance!)

TIP

The scent pillow lasts for many months. When it starts to get faint, crush it a little to release more of the scent. Eventually, when it no longer has much scent at all, add a couple drops of lavender to the pillow's corner and place the pillow in a plastic bag for several days. This allows the scent to permeate throughout the pillow. Re-scent as needed.

IN THIS CHAPTER

» **Understanding medicinal properties of essential oils**

» **Treating simple health problems**

» **Choosing a treatment method**

» **Playing doctor**

» **Using essential oils on infections**

» **Conquering indigestion**

» **Strengthening immunity**

Chapter **10**

Getting Well with Smell

Feeling a little queasy? Have a splitting headache? You've come to the right place. You already take care of these simple complaints without consulting your doctor. But, instead of using an over-the-counter drug to ease a cold, headache, indigestion, or bee sting, you can turn to essential oils as a natural alternative. After all, that's what aroma*therapy* is — a healing therapy.

The *aroma* part of aromatherapy refers to the scent of the essential oils derived from aromatic plants. The oils make the plants fragrant and give them medicinal properties. Read this chapter, and I bet you'll agree with me that essential oils are custom-made for healing.

This chapter covers how to use essential oils for medical aromatherapy. In it, I give you the information you need to treat all sorts of minor health problems.

Essential Facts for Healing with Essential Oils

TIP

Although essential oils are all slightly different, they're all variations on the same theme. Think of the array of muffins at your favorite coffee shop. The flavors vary, but they share basic ingredients, and they're all very much muffins. Likewise, an essential oil contains many ingredients but shares much in common with other essential oils. The basic structure identifies an essential oil, and this similarity gives many of them the same healing properties.

Aromatherapy is no stranger to researchers. Years of studying the properties of essential oils prove them to be strong medicine. It's no surprise to me that the healing properties of plants used by herbalists for centuries to treat infection and pain contain active essential oils.

Focusing on four areas of healing

When I consider how essential oils work to heal, four major categories stand out. Not every oil has all four aspects, but these four properties cover a lot of ailments. Look what essential oils can do:

>> **Kill microorganisms:** Oils target bacteria, viruses, fungi, and parasites.

>> **Improve digestion:** Essential oils can help relieve nausea, eliminate gas, increase digestive enzymes, and relax intestinal muscles. Some oils also stimulate digestive juices and increase appetite. In addition, the scent-relaxing essential oils help relieve nervous indigestion.

>> **Repair cells and stimulate immunity:** Enhance your immune system so that it better fends off and eliminates disease with essential oils. Oils can eliminate disease, infection, and waste from cells through your lymph system and help produce white blood cells. (See "E-lymph-inating metabolic waste" later in the chapter for information on the lymph system.)

Many essential oils encourage skin cells to heal and keep skin toned in several ways, including regulating its oil production. (See Chapter 7 for more on caring for your skin with aromatherapy.)

>> **Relieve pain:** Essential oils help with aches and pain by reducing inflammation, relaxing sore muscles, and dulling the pain response.

Some essential oils, being the versatile healers they are, cover even more than these four aspects. Many essential oils increase blood circulation, eliminate lung and sinus congestion, and alter hormones. For more on essential oils use for a certain condition and the essential oil formula, look up your specific problem in the Symptom Guide.

Making the cut

This chapter covers microorganisms, digestion, and cell repair and immunity ailments treatable with essential oils. I give you plenty of options for suitable essential oils to treat a specific condition so that you know which oils to look for during your next aromatherapy shopping spree. The lists also help you design your own products.

In deciding which essential oils to include on these lists, I looked at the results of many scientific studies and compared and compiled the findings. I also considered the results I've seen in my 50 years of practicing aromatherapy, along with observations from other aromatherapists. I left out essential oils that I consider too toxic to use and difficult-to-find oils.

TECHNICAL STUFF

The prestigious American Association for the Advancement of Science (AAAS) looked at the research from major U. S. universities and concluded that aromatherapy has genuine health benefits. AAAS concludes that the studies done so far show much promise and that more investigation is needed to discover how aromatherapy can be used in medicine.

Simple Cures for Simple Woes

Essential oils offer plenty of benefits over conventional drugs for many everyday woes. In some cases, they're even a better choice than medicinal herbs to heal minor health problems.

WARNING

Granted, essential oils aren't the answer to all health concerns — you need to look beyond aromatherapy to deal with heart conditions, kidney problems, diabetes, and any number of other serious disorders.

But what they can do is great! And you can still use essential oils as an adjunct remedy to help relieve some symptoms of serious disease and illness and feel more comfortable.

Reaping the health benefits of essential oils

Essential oils offer a variety of benefits in treating common ailments. That's one reason they've become so popular. Aromatherapy advantages include

>> **They're compact.** Traveling with your aromatherapy remedies, whether you're going to work or around the world, is easy. A few small, lightweight items are all you need, especially because many essential oils do double-duty by treating more than one condition.

>> **They're compatible with prescription medications.** In most cases, you can use essential oils along with pharmaceutical drugs. The oils carry a low risk of reducing the action of your medicines or of making them extra potent — which you can't say about combining most pharmaceuticals with each other. Because diluted essential oil is absorbed directly into tissues, only a small fraction goes into your bloodstream. Also, drug interaction is less likely with the conditions discussed here, such as indigestion, skin problems, and infections. When in doubt about using essential oils, check with an herbalist or aromatherapist.

>> **They act directly on the affliction.** Essential oils penetrate your skin to sink into underlying tissue. Many times, this is an advantage over ingesting an herb. Anything you swallow must travel through your digestive tract before it reaches your bloodstream and is distributed throughout your body. Instead of this indirect route, essential oils take the expressway to target the source of your problem. You simply rub a diluted essential oil on a painful or infected area, right where it's most needed.

>> **They're inexpensive.** A little essential oil goes a long way, making aromatherapy products reasonably priced. Compared to over-the-counter drugs, they're downright cheap.

>> **Your body eliminates them quickly.** Your body eliminates essential oils within several hours, so no residue remains. At first glance, it may seem an advantage for any medicine to linger in your body, but a substance that hangs around can accumulate and lead to an overdose.

>> **They have few side effects.** Stick to store-bought products that contain safe essential oils or use safe oils at proper dilutions when you make your own, and you'll rarely be bothered by unwanted side effects — unlike over-the-counter drugs.

>> **They work quickly.** Because essential oils don't pass through your digestive tract, they reach their destination in your body quickly and go to work almost immediately. So, you don't need to wait around for relief. Essential oils also encourage injured cells to heal, so you recover more quickly.

>> **They work with, not against, you.** The complex chemistry of essential oils means that they work with your body and its healing process. The emphasis is to assist your body to operate better and to eliminate the cause of your disease — not only get rid of your symptoms. This deep healing is holistic medicine's specialty.

Essential oils wipe out an infection but not the cells harboring it. They can stop injuries like burns from releasing toxins into the surrounding healthy tissue. They tend to not kill good bacteria, only the bad dudes, and do not create a resistance to bad bacteria as do many drugs. Simply put, essential oils promote health.

Healing it yourself (HIY)

You can purchase your essential oil remedies ready to use. But you can also make your own! I find the complexity of designing an essential oil formula an interesting and fun challenge. I enjoy choosing the best essential oils to treat both the medical condition and the individual. Sometimes it's just one oil; other times, a blend of oils works the best. Then I decide the best mode of application. The most fun comes at the end when I see the positive results.

If you feel creative and want to try your hand at making formulas but need a jump-start, find out more about an essential oil by looking up its properties in the Aroma Guide. I also give you simple formulas in the Symptom Guide.

This imaginary scenario shows how you might custom design your own aromatherapy blend:

> You have an uncomfortable lung infection. It began as a flu but has developed into a bacterial infection. You want a germ-fighting solution well suited for your lungs that also relieves your pain. Because your asthma's acting up, you need to avoid any essential oils that aggravate it and wouldn't mind using something to treat your asthma as well. In addition, you want to reduce the stress that made your asthma flare up in the first place.
>
> The answer to this one is easy. One essential oil, lavender, meets all these requirements.

Rather than run to the doctor or take unnecessary medications, you can HIY (heal it yourself) instead.

Treating chronic problems

You know all too many long-range, chronic health problems — the kind that can continue to plague you year after year. Conditions such as eczema, PMS, asthma, arthritis, and headaches can have your physician scratching their head trying to find the cause and figure out a cure. So many times, it's just when you think you finally have it licked that the problem comes back in full force.

Puzzling chronic conditions have at least one upside: When medical science can't offer you solutions, you're free to try alternative medicines such as aromatherapy. Plenty of people are happily helped with essential oils after unsuccessfully trying the medical route.

REMEMBER

You need patience when trying aromatherapy remedies, especially if you've had an affliction for several years. But, if you don't see any change after a month or so of aromatherapy treatments, you may be literally barking up the wrong tree (or some other plant). In that case, it's time to alter your remedy.

In your search for alternative ways to treat a chronic condition, start with essential oils, but don't stop there. As good as oils are for healing, they can't do everything. Use herbal medicine in conjunction with essential oils. As both an herbalist and aromatherapist, I go to whatever remedies are most appropriate. Many times, that means combining the dynamic duo of aromatherapy and herbalism. Together, they can be more effective than either one alone.

TIP

To work holistically on your health problems with herbs, diet, and lifestyle, turn to the Symptom Guide and look up your condition. (If you want more information, check out *Alternative Medicine For Dummies* by James Dillard and Terra Ziporyn, *Herbal Remedies For Dummies* by Christopher Hobbs (both Wiley), and my book *Herbs for Health and Healing* (Rodale Press).

Ways to Use Essential Oils

Now that essential oils are so popular, you can find medicinal products made with them almost anywhere. The best one for your condition depends on what you're treating.

REMEMBER

Essential oil treatments are all external applications, but the oils migrate through skin to the underlying tissue, so they treat internally, as well as externally.

Common ways to use essential oils medicinally include

» **As a body oil** with healing essential oils diluted into a vegetable oil you then rub on your skin. Fancy versions include salves, lotions, and creams. A large selection of body oils containing essential oils are available.

To make your own massage oil, add 6 to 8 drops of essential oil to an ounce of vegetable oil. To make your own body or lotion, add 8 to 10 drops of essential oil to an ounce of vegetable oil.

» **As a bath oil** that contains emotional and skin-healing essential oils to treat your conditions as you bathe. You can purchase a variety of bath oils containing essential oils. The number of drops you add to your bath water varies depending upon the strength of the oil you choose and the size of your bathtub.

For bathing, add 3 to 5 drops of essential oil to your bath water. For sensitive individuals or kids, dilute these drops in a teaspoon of a carrier oil like olive oil before adding to the tub water.

» **As a roll-on.** Handy dispensers let you apply your remedy to small areas of the body for "spot" therapy. The essential oils are typically diluted into a vegetable oil base, but sometimes other liquid bases are used.

To make your own roll-on, add 10 to 15 drops of essential oil to an ounce of vegetable oil and put it in a glass roll-on container. Try to get a container with an oil-resistant ball (that's the roll-on part.)

» **As a foot or hand soak.** For this soak, add 2 to 5 drops essential oil in a basin of either hot or cool water. These soaks are great for when you have issues with your hands or feet. Because the essential oils do penetrate skin and reach the blood system, they can also help other areas of the body.

» **As a liniment** you rub over sore muscles and joints to ease the discomfort. A liniment is made with a high concentration of essential oils that are diluted in an oil or alcohol base.

To make your own liniment, add 15 to 20 drops of essential oil to an ounce of witch hazel, rubbing alcohol, or vodka. Shake well before applying to skin. See Chapter 11 for more details on making your own liniment.

» **As a spray** you can spritz directly on skin problems like burns and poison oak. A spray can soothe and heal the skin and counter infection.

To make your own, dilute 10 to 15 drops of essential oils in an ounce of water, aloe vera, vinegar, or another water-soluble liquid.

>> **As a steam** you inhale. To do a "steam," add essential oils to simmering water and breathe in the steam, bringing the essential oils into your sinuses and lungs.

Add 3 to 5 drops of essential oil in a pint to a quart of steaming water and inhale. Be sure to keep your eyes closed.

>> **As a wash** for skin, as a mouthwash, air freshener, or body spray. How much water you use to dilute the essential oils depends on the application.

>> **As a compress** you place over a problem area. A *compress* is an absorbent cloth soaked in water with essential oil in it. You then fold the cloth and apply it directly to the area.

Add 1 to 2 drops essential oil to a cup or two of hot or cold water. Soak the cloth and fold it to make a compress. You then place this on the afflicted area with light pressure for a couple minutes. The process can be repeated several times.

>> **As a medicated powder.** Powders make a good base to carry essential oils. Use them on conditions that benefit from the drying action of the powder, such as an antifungal treatment. The essential oils kill odor-producing bacteria in a deodorant powder. You can buy aromatic powders made with essential oils.

To make your own powder, add 1–15 drops of essential oil to a base of arrowroot or another powder. (Put the drops in different areas of the powder.) Then leave the powder in a closed, plastic bag for a day to allow the essential oil's scent and properties to evenly distribute.

Whatever type of preparation you choose, repeat the application every few hours to keep a constant level of essential oils in your body to treat a temporary condition you want to knock out quickly. For long-range disorders, such as arthritis or eczema, you typically apply the treatment twice daily, although this varies with different afflictions.

WARNING

Always be careful when using this essential oil because they're so concentrated. Read Chapter 4 to learn which oils to use and not use.

You can find suggestions for specific uses for essential-oil treatments throughout this book:

>> For body, massage, and bath oils see Chapter 5.

>> To find out how to use essential oil sprays, go to Chapter 6.

Don't Bug Me: Natural Antibiotics

You co-exist with all sorts of microscopic creatures, some beneficial for your health and some not-so-much. Not to sound paranoid, but germs lurk everywhere, just waiting for someone to cough in your face, or for you to cut your finger or eat some less-than-fresh morsel of food. You've probably encountered your share of invasive attack organisms, so you're no stranger to the misery of a cold, an infected wound, or a bout of food poisoning.

Almost all essential oils counter infection to some degree. They attack bacteria, fungus, and viruses with amazing effectiveness because they easily enter tissues and cells that harbor infection. And they most often kindly leave the beneficial organisms alone. At the same time, essential oils make the environment (that's your body) healthier and, thus, a less hospitable home for them to hang out.

The three types of infection I address one by one in the next sections are

>> Bacterial

>> Viral

>> Fungal

Engaging in germ warfare: Treating bacterial infection

Bacteria grow in colonies. It wouldn't be so bad if they could be content with a small homestead, but no, give bacteria an inch and it wants to take over the world, or at least your body. If a bacterial infection that crops up in one place gets a strong enough hold, it sets its sights on more territory. Many bacterial infections aren't highly contagious, but with a little effort, they can move to someone else and give them the infection.

Essential oils are so important for treating infection. They destroy harmful bacteria, but they don't stop there. Some oils interrupt the growth cycle of bacteria and starve them by restricting their ability to use oxygen and other sources of energy.

REMEMBER

A big advantage of essential oils is that, due to their complex chemistry, so far bacteria haven't developed a resistance to oils as they can with antibiotics.

You may not realize it, but you're probably already using essential oils to destroy bacteria:

>> **Lemon oil:** If your dishwashing soap contains lemon oil, it's in there for more than just its pleasant scent — it's a strong germ-fighter.

>> **Pine oil:** As you can guess from its name, PineSol's ability to wipe out bacteria is due to pine oil.

>> **Eucalyptus, thyme, and mint oils:** This combination fights a variety of unwanted ailments:

  - I have aromatic memories from my childhood of my mother rubbing a balm on my chest when I had a cold. The antibacterial compounds in vapor rubs come from eucalyptus, thyme, and mint.

  - A popular mouthwash that won the American Dental Association award as the most effective over-the-counter plaque-fighter is a mix of compounds from these three oils that kill the germs responsible for bad breath, tooth decay, and gum disease.

  - An aromatic cream made with these essential oils kills the bacteria that accompanies acne.

TIP

Easily treat simple infections of the skin, gums, sinuses, throat, and bladder with essential oils. Look up your problem in the Symptom Guide for suggestions for a salve containing antiseptic essential oils for an infection or an antibacterial spray to treat a burn without touching it.

Killer good antibacterial essential oils

The most powerful antibacterial essential oils knock out common intestinal, skin, and lung infections, including staph, strep, and pneumonia. The test results on these killer oils are certainly impressive. Thyme oil proved as potent as standard antibiotic drugs!

>> Bay laurel

>> Cinnamon

>> Clove bud

>> Garlic

>> Oregano

>> Savory

>> Thyme

WARNING

These essential oils are strong antiseptics, but they can also be potent skin irritants. Use them carefully and always dilute them significantly. Rather than risk burning your skin with thyme oil, use a salve that contains it. Because using these oils safely is tricky, one alternative is to use the herbs themselves. (The whole herb contains the essential oil in a less abrasive state.)

Killer good oils, gentler versions

The oils in this next list of bacteria fighters tend not to be quite as strong as the killer oils in the preceding section, but they're still powerful. Their gentler nature makes these essential oils much more popular in skin medicines because they won't burn so easily. Instead, these oils reduce swelling and irritation. Lavender, helichrysum, marjoram, and geranium are especially potent.

The essential oils with asterisks are the most potent ones according to research. Even though these are gentler, they are still very concentrated essential oils that need to be diluted before you can apply them to your skin safely.

>> Bay rum

>> Cardamom

>> Eucalyptus*

>> Frankincense

>> Geranium

>> Helichrysum*

>> Lavender*

>> Lemon*

>> Lemongrass

>> Marjoram*

>> Myrrh*

>> Myrtle*

>> Pine*

>> Rose*

>> Sage*

>> Sandalwood

>> Tea tree

>> Vetivert

Spraying lemon essential oil into the air increases its antiseptic properties when compounds in the oil called *terpenes* combine with oxygen.

Inspecting infection: Treating viruses

Viruses are tricky and elusive little critters and not very polite. They take up residence and reproduce without invitation. They also love travel and gladly take up residence with someone with whom you're in close contact. Many viruses aren't inhibited at all about space travel, and propel through the air in search of new terrain to invade. The infections they cause include colds, flu, herpes, shingles, mumps, chicken pox, and even warts.

REMEMBER

Medical science can't touch most viral infections — even the common cold. If you've ever gone to your doctor for a bad cold, they may prescribe antibiotics, but that's only in case you develop a bacterial infection because the virus weakened your system. You get no cure for the cold virus itself.

Research results

Only recently are researchers investigating drugs to fight viral diseases such as herpes and severe acute respiratory syndrome (SARS) viruses like the one that causes Covid-19. Researchers know that quite a few essential oils destroy viral infections and are searching for oils that act against specific viruses in the hope of basing new drugs on these oils.

Some of the oils under investigation for SARS viral infections are many of those mentioned in this book: bay, eucalyptus, tea tree, cinnamon, ginger, bergamot, thyme, and lavender. People spray these oils on face masks worn for airline travel or for general use during an epidemic. Check the "Good antiviral essential oils" list in the next section.

WARNING

There's a limit to how much essential oil you can use safely. Essential oils on their own may not be adequate to treat serious viruses — or any disease.

For more tips on dealing with viruses, look up specific viral infections in the Symptom Guide to find the salve, lip balm, or oil that contains essential oils for viral infections. The Symptom Guide also advises adding a couple drops of an antiviral essential oil to steaming water and inhaling the steam to flush out a cold or flu virus.

GUT REACTION

Humans may have evolved a taste for spicy foods because the spices kill the microbes that make food spoil, according to Dr. Paul Sherman, an evolutionary biologist at Cornell University. He looked at more than 4,000 traditional recipes from 36 countries and found that the hotter the climate — and the faster food turns bad — the spicier the food. Cool climates, on the other hand, lean more toward less antiseptic flavorings, such as celery seed and caraway seed. When he tested 43 spices, he found that onion, garlic, oregano, and allspice did the best job in knocking out 30 different kinds of bacteria. Cumin, cinnamon, cloves, and cayenne hot peppers were pretty effective as well, taking out three-quarters of the bacteria.

In another study, of 21 oils tested, the essential oils of bay, cinnamon, thyme, and clove were strongest in destroying common sources of food poisoning: *E. coli, salmonella, staphylococcus,* and *listeria*. Marjoram is a runner-up in destroying *salmonella*. Bay and thyme oil destroyed the most common bacterial cause of diarrhea, Campylocbacter, which is also the most resistant bacteria. Adding garlic to meat almost completely eliminates *E. coli*, which is responsible for intestinal and bladder infections. The runners-ups against E. coli are cinnamon, oregano, and sage.

Note that many antibacterial essential oils are from kitchen spices. How appropriate considering that using these spices in your cooking puts them right where you need them to counter digestive tract infections. So, instead of trying to deal with using oregano essential oil safely, simply sprinkle oregano on your pizza for a therapeutic dose.

Good antiviral essential oils

Aromatherapy includes many essential oils that treat viral infections. Many antiviral oils do double time by also destroying bacteria. That's good news if you have both types of infections or aren't sure which bug you have. This full coverage also helps ward off a bacterial infection invading on the heels of a viral flu or cold. The essential oils with asterisks are the most potent antivirals according to the studies.

>> Bay*

>> Bergamot*

>> Black pepper

>> Cinnamon bark (be careful when using this potent oil)

>> Clove bud (be careful when using this potent oil)

>> Eucalyptus*

- » Garlic*
- » Geranium*
- » Holy basil
- » Juniper*
- » Lavender*
- » Melissa (lemon balm)*
- » Lemongrass
- » Lemon*
- » Marjoram
- » Myrrh
- » Oregano* (be careful when using this potent oil)
- » Rose
- » Rosemary*
- » Sage*
- » Tea tree*
- » Thyme* (be careful when using this potent oil)

Confronting the fungus among us: Treating fungal infections

After a fungal infection takes hold, it can spread like crazy. And that's only the beginning of the bad news. Fungal infections are quite social, spreading themselves from one person to another. Fungus also has the irritating habit of itching like crazy.

Common fungi

You may already know the itch and discomfort of a fungal infection if you've ever had ringworm, one of the most common fungal skin infections. It includes athlete's foot and the graphically named "jock itch." The athletic association comes from the fact that the fungi thrive in a warm, moist environment and athletes sweat a lot. Athletic sports gear with tight, look-at-these-muscles pants and triple-layered-for-high-performance shoes is a friend to fungus because it holds in all that sweat.

Another fungus that gets around is *candida*. This yeastlike fungus also likes warm, moist places. You very likely already have candida in your digestive tract playing a minor role in your digestive process. But when candida gets out of hand and multiplies like crazy, it causes you problems: indigestion, fatigue, and sometimes fuzzy thinking. Candida also thrives in the inside of your mouth (where it creates patchy spots called *thrush*), the vagina (where it is called a *yeast infection*), and your toenails and fingernails, which it discolors and cracks.

TIP

A product combining essential oils with vinegar or powder is an effective tool for treating skin and nail fungal infections. Both the powder and vinegar are very drying, so they discourage further fungal growth. You can also soak your nails in a foot or hand bath containing a few drops of an essential oil. Look up your condition in the Symptom Guide to find a simple formula.

Good antifungal oils

Happily, a long list of essential oils fights fungal infections. The essential oils with asterisks are the most potent ones according to the studies.

>> Basil (tulsi basil is especially potent)

>> Bergamot*

>> Black pepper

>> Caraway

>> Cinnamon* (be careful when using this potent oil)

>> Clove bud* (be careful when using this potent oil)

>> Garlic*

>> Geranium*

>> Lavender

>> Lemon

>> Lemon eucalyptus*

>> Lemongrass*

>> Marjoram

>> Myrrh

>> Oregano* (be careful when using this potent oil)

>> Peppermint*

- » Sandalwood
- » Tea tree*
- » Thyme* (be careful when using this potent oil)

WARNING

Go easy with essential oils, especially hot ones like black pepper, cinnamon, clove, and peppermint that can burn your skin. These oils can make skin already irritated by a fungal infection even more raw and tender.

Musta Been Something I Ate: Indigestion

Aromatherapy gets to work at the first stage of digestion, as the scent signals your brain that food is on its way. Simply sniffing pasta sauce, baking bread, or anything tasty sends your stomach grumbling in anticipation. Almost immediately, your digestive juices flow in your mouth, stomach, and small intestine. Just the smell of delicious food begins a chain reaction throughout your digestive tract. (Just think how bland a meal tastes when you have a stuffy nose and can't smell anything!)

Good digestive oils

Improving your digestion can be as effortless as adding herbs or spices to your food. Culinary spices are chock-full of essential oils that aid digestion.

Often described as stimulants, in reality most aromatic herbs are fairly laid back. They function to relax your intestinal muscles, which slows down the digestive pace giving your system time to help prevent gas from developing and stop cramping. Peppermint, the all-time star digestive heroine, relaxes your intestinal muscles within 30 minutes and prevents nausea. (Just don't overdo it; too much peppermint can *cause* nausea.)

The aroma from any of the essential oils in this section aids your appetite and digestion. They can also

- » **Decrease nausea:** Cardamom, lavender, rosemary, and juniper oils are examples of essential oils that help with nausea, often by blocking the signal in your brain telling you to vomit.
- » **Soothe stomach irritation:** Look to melissa (lemon balm), lemon, or fennel.
- » **Increase enzyme action:** Cinnamon spurs on the enzymes that break down food, and rosemary aids in its assimilation.

These essential oils not only help cure indigestion; they also address the source of the problems by destroying bacterial, viral, or fungal infections living in your digestive tract.

TIP

To treat digestive woes such as poor appetite, headaches related to poor digestion, heartburn, and plain ol' belly upsets, rub essential oils that are diluted into massage oil on your abdomen. The massage itself helps with digestive distress. Try an essential-oil belly rub on a child, or anyone, who has a belly ache but won't swallow a pill or drink an herbal digestive tea.

Sometimes, a less than direct approach can improve your digestion; you just need to reduce your stress. Tension restricts digestive juices, constricts muscles, and contributes to disorders such as colitis, stomach ulcers, and irritable bowel syndrome. Try the following essential oils to reduce stress and improve your digestion:

>> Anise

>> Basil

>> Cardamom

>> Chamomile

>> Cinnamon (be careful when using this potent oil)

>> Coriander

>> Dill

>> Fennel

>> Ginger

>> Juniper berry

>> Lavender

>> Lemongrass

>> Melissa (lemon balm)

>> Peppermint

>> Rosemary

>> Thyme

You'll find simple recipes for specific digestive problems in the Symptom Guide.

Tea time

Herbal teas such as peppermint, cardamom, thyme, melissa (lemon balm), and chamomile contain a dose of essential oils that get released into the hot water. In fact, herbal tea is my favorite way to take essential oils internally. Drinking tea is easier than trying to figure out how to get essential oils into your system without having much of the oil absorbed in your throat.

The herbs contain other compounds that help your digestion. You don't have to take straight essential oil; the tea becomes a complete healing package. Tea also goes right where it's needed, into the digestive tract.

Happy Belly Tea

One of my favorite herb blends makes a delightful tea, either hot or cold.

>> Preparation time: 12 minutes

>> Yield: 2 cups

>> Ingredients:

   2 cups boiling water

   1 teaspoon melissa (lemon balm) or lemongrass leaves

   ½ teaspoon chamomile flowers

   ½ teaspoon peppermint leaves

1. Pour the water over the chopped herbs in a pan or teapot.

2. Cover and let sit about 10 minutes.

3. Strain out the herbs and drink your tea. Keep any leftover tea in the refrigerator for a couple days.

   Vary It! Replace the herbs in this recipe with any combination of those in the section "Good digestive oils," earlier in this chapter. Just use a total of 2 teaspoons of herbs and follow the same instruction. Some of my favorite herbs for tea are cinnamon and ginger.

Chai Tea

If you're in a spicy mood and want to improve your digestion, try the East Indian drink chai. You can get chai in coffee shops throughout North America or use this recipe to make your own. Chai often contains black tea for the pick-me-up that the caffeine in it offers, but this version doesn't contain tea (which isn't easy to digest).

» Preparation time: 20 minutes

» Yield: 2 cups

» Ingredients:

3 cups water

2 teaspoons freshly grated ginger

2 two-inch-long cinnamon sticks, broken into small pieces

¼ teaspoon whole cloves

¼ teaspoon whole peppercorns

5 cardamom pods

½ cup milk (or substitute soy, rice, or almond milk)

1 pinch nutmeg powder

Honey to taste (optional)

1. In a medium saucepan, combine the water, ginger, cinnamon sticks, cloves, peppercorns, and cardamom pods.

2. Cover and simmer for 10 minutes on low heat.

3. Add the milk and heat on low for an additional 5 minutes.

4. Strain into mugs, sprinkle nutmeg on top, and sweeten with honey, if desired. Store any leftover tea in the refrigerator. It will keep a couple days.

Vary It! If you need that caffeine buzz, go for the green. Green tea offers more health benefits than black. Add ½ teaspoon green tea when you add the milk in Step 3. Then continue with the recipe. Try this blend as a substitute if you're trying to cut down on coffee.

Vary It Another Way! Rather than use a sweetener like honey or sugar, I prefer to use stevia, a sweet herb. Add ¼ teaspoon stevia leaves when you add the milk.

Seek Immunity: Immune System and Cell Repair

If your immune system goes out of whack, you can be in trouble. Having a healthy immune system is your insurance against coming down with any illness, short or long term, minor or serious. If your immune system is weak you can fall prey to a variety of ills including the common cold, viral disease, allergies, fungal and bacterial infections, cancer, and psoriasis — you name it. A strong immune system can protect you from contracting any or all these problems.

Your immune system is a complex group of several systems that communicate and coordinate with each other. If communication breaks down and the system gets confused, it can view normal substances in your body as invaders and wage an all-out attack. You may experience an allergic reaction such as hay fever, asthma, and food allergies. In some cases, your immune system responds by fighting against itself. Autoimmune disorders include lupus, infertility, rheumatoid arthritis, and Type I diabetes. Chronic hepatitis, atopic dermatitis, and degenerative disorders with no other known cause may well be autoimmune disorders.

A massage using appropriate essential oils is a great treatment option, especially a lymphatic massage that encourages the flow of lymph. (I talk more about the lymph system and its job of filtering out toxins in "E-lymph-inating metabolic waste" later in this chapter.

You lower your natural immunity through emotional or physical stress, poor diet (such as too many sweets), smoking, and alcohol overconsumption. Even "good" stress, like a vacation or getting married, can lower your immune response. This means that, as with so many other physical problems, you can make use of the antistress essential oils I cover in Chapter 9.

TIP

Be on an autoimmune alert if you tend to get sick often or are tired most of the time. These symptoms clue you into the fact that it's time to build up your immune system. But, hey, it doesn't hurt to try to be healthy all the time. View essential oils as preventive medicine that not only help to get you well but keep you from getting sick in the first place.

TECHNICAL STUFF

Problems related to immunity include allergic reactions such as asthma, dermatitis, psoriasis, fatigue, hives, insect bite reactions, poison oak and ivy rashes, lung congestion, and some bowel disorders.

Amping up the immune system

View essential oils as preventive medicine that not only helps to get you well but keeps you from getting sick in the first place. The following list includes essential oils known to increase your natural immunity to disease. With more research, other oils may join the list.

>> Bay laurel

>> Cinnamon (be careful when using this potent oil)

>> Eucalyptus

>> Frankincense

>> Oregano (be careful when using this potent oil)

>> Sage

Stimulating white blood cells

While they're busy revving up your immune system, many essential oils conveniently fight infection at the same time. A number of these oils enhance immunity by increasing your production of white blood cells, which are the cells that patrol your body, cleaning and literally gobbling up foreign invaders.

Some essential oils detoxify the substance in insect bites and stings so that you don't react so strongly. At least some of these oils undoubtedly perform other, still unknown, jobs associated with immunity. These essential oils work with the body to fight infection and heal itself.

>> Bergamot

>> Chamomile

>> Lavender

>> Lemon

>> Myrrh

>> Pine

>> Sandalwood

>> Tea tree

>> Thyme (be careful when using this potent oil)

>> Vetivert

Hastening healing

These essential oils work in conjunction with your immune system to heal individual cells. They repair skin damage and encourage new cell growth, which results in faster healing. Their ability to protect tissue lessens the further destruction of injured or infected skin and tissue. The regenerative properties of these oils also improve your skin's general condition and appearance, so you find them widely used in body products and cosmetics.

- » Carrot seed
- » Frankincense
- » Helichrysum
- » Lavender
- » Rose
- » Rose geranium
- » Sandalwood

E-lymph-inating metabolic waste

Your lymphatic system is your body's garbage collector. Somebody's got to do it, and the job falls to the lymphatic fluid. It floats through tissues to clean out the waste produced by natural metabolic functions. Your lymph nodes filter out toxins to keep your blood clean.

The garbage collection sites are the lymph nodes located throughout your body, with the main nodes in your throat, groin, breasts, and armpits. These hot spots swell up and get sore as they collect debris if you develop an infection near that area.

Essential oils that help your lymphatic system eliminate waste from your body include

- » Bay laurel
- » Grapefruit
- » Juniper
- » Lemon

Chapter **11**

Refrain from Pain

ain is no stranger to anyone. In fact, it's such a common complaint, I devote this entire chapter to it. The good news is that relieving pain is one of essential oils' special talents. You can choose from quite an assortment of pain-relieving essential oils. You can buy aromatherapy-based pain relievers to apply externally or others just to smell.

Just the scent of some essential oils can be a pain-relief treatment. Simply sniffing an oil isn't the strongest treatment, but it works quickly because it goes directly to your brain. Another advantage of using essential oils for pain is that you can sniff them over and over, as often as you need. Plus, inhaling the scent of essential oils has few side effects for most people!

In this chapter, I explain different types of pain and the treatment they require. I also show you just how essential oils can help you deal with all sorts of different pain arenas. You also can follow the simple recipes provided in this chapter for a DIY essential oil remedy. This chapter guides you through decisions about what to use on this or that type of pain.

Nip Pain in the Bud: Six Ways to End Pain

More than anything else, discomfort is what sends you searching for a cure to any disease. At least in that sense, pain is good because it alerts you to a physical problem in your body you otherwise may not be aware of. Even when you know that something's wrong, if it doesn't hurt, it's darn easy to put off dealing with it.

Okay, maybe you're not ready to embrace your physical pain, but you certainly must be ready to get rid of it. If you experience minor pain, essential oils usually help, sometimes as effectively as over-the-counter drugs. The oils can also be far safer to use and, used properly, don't carry the same risks of damaging your liver.

REMEMBER

Don't expect aromatic pain relievers to alleviate severe pain the way a prescription drug can. Dealing with serious pain is one of the times you can be grateful for medical doctors. You certainly wouldn't want to have surgery with a handkerchief scented with lavender and camphor over your nose as was done in the good ol' days.

The six typical ways to deal with pain are

>> **Numb it:** Dull nerve endings

>> **Reduce the swelling that causes it:** Reduce inflammation

>> **Heat and penetrate it:** Warm and relax your muscles

>> **Stop pain in your brain:** Dull your brain circuits

>> **Short circuit pain-causing substances:** Stop pain in its tracks

>> **Relax and sedate it:** Relax your muscles and mind

I talk about each of these methods in the following sections, along with the corresponding essential oil sidekicks. Some of the most versatile essential oils appear on more than one of the lists in these sections.

REMEMBER

You must always dilute essential oils before using them on your skin. Not sure how to dilute oils? Turn to Chapter 5. I mention a few essential oils in this chapter that you need to use with care, in most cases because they're very hot oils that can irritate or even burn your skin. Refer to Chapter 4 for guidelines on how to use essential oils safely.

While essential oils may not always completely eliminate your pain, they can do a darn good job of diminishing it. The good news is if you find you need to take pharmaceutical pain relievers, you can still safely sniff essential oils without causing an interaction. The oils may even allow you to reduce your meds — providing you have your doctor's approval to do so.

Having lots of choices is especially useful if you want to take pain-relieving essential oils for an extended time. Get better results by switching to a different blend of oils every week or so. Your body's pain sensors seem to become accustomed to essential oils and eventually don't respond as well to them. How long that takes depends upon the individual.

REMEMBER

Pain is a universal complaint. We all know it. Sometimes it's the source of the problem, but more likely it's a symptom of an underlying problem. Consider it a red flag that your body sends up to alert you that something is wrong. Be sure to always investigate the source of any pain and to visit your doctors when in doubt.

Numb it

One way to dull pain is to numb your nerve endings to temporarily shut down your pain response. The following essential oils are good at numbing pain when applied as a massage oil or pain-relieving liniment to the skin over the area that's hurting:

» Clove bud

» Frankincense

» Chamomile, German

» Helichrysum

» Lavender

» Lemongrass

Reduce swelling

You may not find inflammation a hot subject unless you have an infected cut or a bruise, but swelling causes pain, and decreasing swelling is one of essential oils' most important qualities.

If you get headaches, menstrual cramps, bruises, repetitive strain injury, sore throat, insect bite, or almost any type of infection, you have inflammation that pins down your nerves, and that pressure causes pain. Use the following essential oils in a massage oil, which are effective anti-inflammatory pain relievers:

» Chamomile, German

» Geranium

» Helichrysum

- » Juniper
- » Lavender
- » Marjoram
- » Myrrh
- » Rose
- » Tea tree

Heat and penetrate pain

Essential oils that produce heat relieve your pain by bringing blood to the painful area to warm it up and let your muscles, connective tissue, and nerves relax. The heat also provides deep, penetrating relief.

WARNING

Be sure to use these hot oils "gingerly" in small, well-diluted amounts, or they can burn your skin. Don't use them at all on a hot injury, such as a burn or a swelling. They'll only increase the inflammation. Instead use the essential oils in the preceding "Reduce swelling" section.

Essential oils that are both heating and penetrating include

- » Bay laurel
- » Bay rum (pimento)
- » Black pepper
- » Cinnamon
- » Clove bud
- » Ginger
- » Juniper
- » Peppermint
- » Thyme

The following essential oils are penetrating, but not heating:

- » Marjoram
- » Rosemary
- » Sage

Stop pain in your brain

Pain can happen anywhere in your body, but it takes your brain to register that it's happening. Essential oils can go right to the top of the command center to tell your brain to pretend that the pain isn't there.

TECHNICAL STUFF

Researchers don't yet know exactly how essential oils act on the brain. What I can tell you is that simply sniffing certain scents can decrease pain. Feel-good scents start a chain reaction. Neurotransmitters in your brain react to help you feel good. The reaction also acts to both raise your pain threshold so you can tolerate more discomfort and decrease your sensation to pain at the same time.

Some of the oils that effectively affect your brain are

>> **Chamomile:** Chamomile is a stronger pain reliever than most folks think. In several studies, it worked as well as pharmaceutical drugs to ease the discomfort of painful hospital procedures, including one study in which patients simply smelled the aroma of the essential oil.

>> **Lemongrass and ginger:** These oils act similarly to sedative opiate drugs without affecting your central nervous system.

Lemongrass oil depresses the higher, cerebral cortex, part of your brain (and its cough center) so that pain sensations don't register.

TECHNICAL STUFF

>> **Frankincense oil:** Frankincense has power of biblical proportions. It reduces pain sensations in your brain.

>> **Myrrh:** The wise men must have known something about essential oils. Myrrh seems to signal your brain that you're not in pain.

Short circuit pain-causing substances

Certain essential oils slow the action of pain-causing substances. The following are examples of essential oils that go through different routes:

>> **Birch** (which often masks as wintergreen when sold because the two smell so much alike) is an aspirin-like pain reliever. (Chapter 4 has the details on how to use birch safely.) In fact, birch oil contains the same compound as aspirin, making it useful to ease

- arthritic pain

- headaches

- menstrual cramps
- simple aches and pains

>> **Cayenne** oil lessens nerve pain by decreasing the amount of "substance P for pain" in your body. The substance carries pain messages from nerve endings in your skin to your central nervous system.

Cayenne oil's active compound *capsaicin* gives substantial pain relief to three-quarters of the people who try it. Yes, yes, this is hot stuff, but the burning sensation quickly goes away, and so does the pain of herpes, shingles, diabetic neuropathy, psoriasis, and surgery. Just don't hover over it or get it on your fingers, then ouch your mouth or eyes. You can buy over-the-counter skin creams with cayenne in any drugstore.

>> **Ginger** works to ease muscle contractions and arthritic pain. Both birch and ginger are good to relieve muscle cramps like menstrual pain. They also work to relieve painful joints, and some headaches when you make a liniment with them and rub it over the painful area.

Relax and sedate it

The essential oils in this section aren't exactly pain relievers, but they do relax sore and stiff muscles and, as a result, they lessen your pain. They also relax your mind through their scent alone. That's a convenient combination because you automatically smell their aromas as you use them. (Also look up the scents that reduce stress in Chapter 9.) Try it out for yourself.

The relaxing essential oils work when you sniff them individually. You can also combine several into a blend to ease mild pain and promote general relaxation.

Relaxing essential oils include

>> Chamomile

>> Clary sage

>> Helichrysum

>> Lavender

>> Lemon

>> Lemon eucalyptus

>> Lemon verbena

>> Marjoram

>> Melissa (lemon balm)

>> Myrtle

>> Petitgrain

Massage: Rub It Away

One of the most relaxing ways to relieve pain is with a massage using an aromatherapy oil or a *liniment* (a pain-relieving lotion made with essential oils). Massage is especially good for that slow, aching pain caused by long-term, chronic disorders. The massage itself not only relaxes you, but it subdues pain. It's thought to slow down the release of substance P that carries pain impulses to your nerves by stimulating substances (called *enkephalins*) that work like natural opiates.

If getting a massage is not an option at the moment, try these less enjoyable, but still effective alternatives:

>> Rub a pain-relieving massage or body oil or a liniment on yourself.

>> Place a compress soaked in a liniment over the area that hurts.

Fire or Ice? The Hot and Cold of It

Judging that fine line between full performance and injury can be difficult. Try to be realistic about how far you can push yourself. If you physically overextend your body, you have two treatment choices: hot or cold. That translates to one of two methods: an aromatherapy liniment or an aromatherapy anti-inflammatory. Although the actions of both preparations are due to the essential oils they contain, the difference between them is like night and day.

>> **Liniment for sore muscles:** Rub a liniment on your skin, and it brings blood to the underlying area and, as a result, makes the area very warm. This heats up sore muscles and relaxes them. It also warms up your muscles before you exercise.

WARNING

Don't use a liniment on a swollen area because the liniment will only make your swelling worse.

>> **Anti-inflammatory for swollen injuries:** An anti-inflammatory product has exactly the opposite effect of a liniment. You can apply it to sore muscles, but it's more often used on sprains, strains, or muscle cramps. These injuries are more severe, and more painful, than simple sore muscles. They almost always involve at least some swelling, making an anti-inflammatory suitable.

Warm up to aromatherapy: Liniments

A liniment contains hot oils, such as cinnamon and clove, that you dilute into either an oil or alcohol base. You then rub the liniment on your skin over the muscles that you plan to use the most.

Warming essential oils include

>> Bay laurel

>> Bay rum (pimento)

>> Cinnamon

>> Clove bud

>> Ginger

>> Juniper

>> Peppermint

>> Thyme

WARNING

These hot oils have the potential to be irritating. Be careful to wash your hands well after applying it and don't accidentally rub your eyes or mouth after applying a liniment. Remember, the idea is to warm the skin, not burn it. Not only are these essential oils extra strong, but a liniment needs a higher concentration of essential oils than a massage oil so that it heats up.

REMEMBER

Because it contains so much hot essential oil, a liniment is designed for what I call "spot" therapy. Unlike a general massage oil, use it only on the spots where you need it — not over your entire body.

Besides the hot-stuff essential oils, many liniments also contain muscle-relaxing essential oils. So, while a liniment warms a muscle to ease its tension, it also directly relaxes it. These muscle-relaxing essential oils are the most often used:

» Lavender

» Marjoram

» Rosemary

A liniment relieves pain by increasing heat. This requires creating a sensation of lots of heat, but you must do that without burning your skin. Liniments accomplish this by playing several tricks on the brain:

» **Liniment Trick #1:** Pain creates a reinforcing loop between the muscle and brain; your muscle is crying with pain, and your brain agrees. (It's like a mother telling her crying child how much a scrape must hurt, and the child crying all the louder.) All of this focus on pain makes it hard for a tightened muscle to relax.

However, as the heat from the essential oils increases, the brain starts getting nervous. It's forced to worry less about the muscle and concentrate on what appears to be the real emergency: Your skin is burning. Of course, you and I know that your skin is not really burning, but your brain doesn't. This gives your muscle a chance to relax. It increases blood flow to the underlying area by three to four times.

» **Liniment Trick #2:** A liniment has yet another trick up its sleeve to make it seem so much hotter than it really is. The trick is to include at least one of the following essential oils in the liniment formula:

- Camphor

- Peppermint

Both these oils increase the sensation of heat without actually increasing the heat. They do so by sending hot and cold nerve impulses to your brain. When the brain receives these confusing, alternating messages of hot and cold, the contrast between the two makes the heat appear to be more intense than it really is. As in trick #1, your brain is so worried about the possibility that your skin is burning, it hardly has time to care about a sore muscle.

I prefer using peppermint over camphor, which is potentially toxic. You don't need to avoid buying a liniment just because it contains camphor (many of them do) but go easy when you use those products.

Try an easy way to understand how peppermint can be hot and cold at the same time: Put a peppermint candy on your tongue and suck air in through your mouth. You feel the slight burning sensation produced by peppermint on your tongue and the refreshing coolness of it in the air you breathe in. The sensation is icy-hot.

>> **Liniment Trick #3:** You can increase the warming action of a liniment even more by rubbing your skin after applying the liniment. The more that you rub, the hotter it gets.

Heat Treat Liniment

Liniments come in many different types, and all are made with essential oils. You can buy them at drugstores or in natural-food stores (if you prefer one with better quality ingredients). You can also make a liniment at home.

Remember that rubbing alcohol is poisonous, so be sure to mark the container appropriately and don't use it on broken skin; use vodka instead.

>> Preparation time: 5 minutes

>> Yield: 2 ounces oil

>> Ingredients:

    8 drops eucalyptus oil

    8 drops peppermint oil

    8 drops rosemary oil

    4 drops cinnamon oil

    4 drops clove oil

    2 ounces rubbing alcohol or vodka

1. Combine ingredients in a bottle with a tight lid.

2. Shake or stir a few times a day to disperse the essential oils into the alcohol.

3. Shake the mixture before using and apply to the affected area.

Vary It! You can replace the alcohol with vegetable oil to produce an oily liniment that holds the heat-relieving properties better, although you have to put up with the greasiness.

A swell idea: Reduce inflammation

Inflammation, otherwise known as swelling, results when fluid from surrounding tissues seeps into a damaged area. It typically happens when you pull or tear a tendon, ligament, or muscle — all so common when participating in sports. You may also notice inflammation after surgery, but don't use these applications when there is open tissue until it heals. If the injury is discolored with the blue, red, or purple of a bruise, then you also have blood from broken blood vessels seeping in. (The blood makes the area extra warm to the touch.)

All this added fluid causes swelling. With the swelling comes congestion that restricts proper blood flow. You need that flow to bring nutrients and oxygen to your cells and to remove toxins to hasten repair. In addition, all the swelling pushes on your nerves and makes your injury hurt like crazy.

A sprain or a strain can happen when you exert your body past the strength of your muscles or joints.

>> A **sprain** occurs at your joints when the fibrous tissues called ligaments are stretched too much.

>> A **strain** happens when your muscles, or the tendons that hold them in place, are pulled or torn.

Confusing the two is easy because both cause rapid swelling, heat, and pain and restrict your ability to move. Often a sprain and sometimes a strain becomes bruised and discolored. Sound confusing? Don't worry, they both get the same treatment.

The benefits of reducing swelling are obvious, and two of the best ways to do so are ice and anti-inflammatory essential oils. The following essential oils reduce swelling and thus restore blood flow and diminish your pain:

>> Chamomile, German

>> Geranium

>> Helichrysum

>> Juniper

>> Lavender

>> Marjoram

>> Rose

I have to admit that pain has some helpful qualities. Pain alerts you to the fact that an injury has occurred and makes you want to deal with it — if for no other reason than to reduce your discomfort. The pain and swelling also work together to keep you from moving that area. This is one way your body can "talk" you into lying off exercise long enough to give your injury time to heal.

WARNING

A problem with using an aromatherapy anti-inflammatory is that it reduces swelling too well. Your injury often feels so much better that you have to remind yourself not to move the injured area or to keep it stationary with a sport brace.

Sprain and Strain Oil

St. John's wort and arnica are two well-known herbs that work as anti-inflammatories. For this formula, you can buy either one already extracted into a carrier oil. When you get hurt, you want to do everything that's possible to heal quickly. I like to combine the best of both worlds, herbalism and aromatherapy. The result is a double-strength formula that's so effective, that it seems to work like magic.

» Preparation time: 5 minutes

» Yield: about 2 ounces oil

» Ingredients:

2 ounces St. John's wort oil or arnica oil

12 drops lavender essential oil

8 drops marjoram essential oil

2 drops chamomile essential oil

1. Combine the ingredients.

2. Apply liberally to the skin over the injury, as often as needed.

   Vary It! If you can't come up with either St. John's wort oil or arnica oil, you can resort to using plain vegetable oil.

WARNING

Don't use arnica on broken skin.

Chapter **12**

Essential Oils to Up Your Energy and Enhance Your Workout

I f you're already a fitness buff, this chapter is for you. If you just want to stay in shape, this chapter is for you, too. It doesn't matter if you're pumping iron at the gym, pumping pedals on a bike, or even if you're lifting a toddler rather than free weights, essential oils fit into your workout regime. In this chapter, I show you how to go for the gold and avoid downtime due to a pulled muscle or fatigue.

Don't worry, I'm not talking "no pain, no gain" here. Most everyone wants to stop before it hurts. You want to avoid damage to muscles and connective tissues, so take it slow. Use the info in this chapter to incorporate essential oils into your basic training.

Inhaling essential oils has a recognized reputation for effectively promoting relaxation and a calming mood, but aromatherapy has another side. Instant aromatherapy pick-me-ups work for you both physically and emotionally. The best part is they don't over-amp your mind or body.

Boosting Your Basic Training

You need to move your body — your choice of dance, sports, yoga, or any other type of movement activity — to make it work properly. Movement encourages the blood flow from your hands and feet back to your heart for it to be repumped around.

Your muscles won't let you lift a finger without oxygen. Think of oxygen as the spark that ignites the energy to make movement happen. All that oxygen gets into your blood system via your lungs. That means you need healthy lungs to send oxygen to your bloodstream. What better way to encourage this deep breathing than the enticing aromas of essential oils? Breathing in certain oils before or even during a workout will improve your health and can even make your workout more effective.

Whether you're a dedicated decathlete or get your blood moving by walking around the block every day, your athletic capability relies on several factors. Each one is important for your performance, and they all need to work together for you to reach your highest physical potential, so it's a team effort.

>> **Blood flow** to provide oxygen to all your cells happens with deep breathing that's encouraged by pleasant scents.

>> **Concentration** is promoted by certain essential oils, such as rosemary and bay laurel.

>> **Muscle and connective tissue strength is aided by the increased blood flow and** feelings of more stamina that happens when you inhale essential oil. Massage oils and liniments encourage their repair.

>> **Stamina is increased** with aroma. It's that feel-good element that keeps you going. Add the aroma of some antidepressant essential oils to your exercise program, and you can change your entire outlook on life.

You typically feel on top of the world after a physical workout. Exercise affects your moods and your ability to think clearly in very positive ways. It can lift you out of the ho-hum doldrums and even help counter depression. This emotional uplift is partly due to your sense of accomplishment, and rightfully so! You also just got your blood circulating not just through your body, but also through your brain.

However, many people feel sore or stiff after a workout. You can help avoid this buildup by getting oxygen to your muscles. Use the essential oils in the "Improving Your Circulation" section later in this chapter.

There's not yet science to back the claim, but aromatherapists recommend a massage oil containing lemongrass essential oil to counter sore muscles due to the lactic acid buildup that happens in the body during prolonged exercise.

Summoning Energy with Essential Oils

To your body, tired is tired no matter where it originates. Work those muscles hard, and you feel fatigued all over afterwards. Put a lot of mental energy into whatever you're doing, and you probably have to push yourself to take your evening run since you really just want to veg out on the couch. Your muscles and brain rely on the same energy source, which involves a good diet and good blood circulation to get energy where it needs to go. (For more on mental fatigue and depression and countering stress, go to Chapter 9.)

Some essential oils that can help keep you going include the following. Notice that they all have very sharp scents.

>> Camphor

>> Cinnamon

>> Cypress

>> Eucalyptus

>> Peppermint

>> Pine

>> Rosemary

When you're feeling tired, either mentally or physically, these scents give you a lift.

You can carry your energizing fragrance with you. Try one of these ways:

>> **Plug in a diffuser:** An electric aromatherapy diffuser releases a steady aroma for several hours so you don't have to keep re-spritzing. You can even find diffusers to plug into your car.

>> **Sniff an essential oils inhaler:** Essential oils inhalers are something you can carry around since they're small enough to fit in your pocket. They provide a way to keep your scents to yourself. These inhalers are readily available for sale as aromatherapy products.

>> **Spritz the air:** Have your wake-up call floating in the air. Use a spray that contains energizing essential oils. Feel free to refresh the air as often as you need it. Driving on a long trip or late at night and not wanting to nod off? Spritz away! The only downside if you're not traveling solo is that you'll keep everyone else in the car awake.

>> **Use scented hand lotion:** If you don't have time to do more than rub your hands together, you can give yourself a mental and physical pick-me-up with a hand lotion that contains essential oils. It's a good alternative when you don't want to fragrance the air. Either get a lotion containing energy-boosting essential oils or add drops of your own essential oil to an unscented lotion. (Check Chapter 5 for recipes.)

Sniffing Perk-Me-Up Oil

This recipe combines peppermint to wake you up, lavender to keep you focused, and geranium to make you feel balanced while you're trying to stay awake or want to get some work done. It's true that lavender is used as a relaxing essential oil, but it also enhances focus.

>> Preparation time: 1 minute

>> Yield: 8 drops

>> Ingredients:

   5 drops peppermint

   2 drops lavender

   1 drop geranium

1. Combine all the oils.

2. Take a sniff.

Vary It! Add this 8-drop mix to one ounce of your choice of vegetable oil to make a body oil that you can rub on places like your temples and the back of your hands so you can wear your perky scent, if you like.

Improving Your Circulation

The secret to keeping physically fit is maintaining good blood circulation. You want to have blood cells flowing throughout your entire body. To achieve that goal, you need a strong heart to pump the blood and healthy blood vessels to carry it where it's needed.

In the long run, essential oils improve your performance by increasing blood circulation. And, guess what? Essential oils help improve your circulation somewhat even if your version of enjoying athletic competitions is from the bleachers or sitting in front of the TV. (I probably shouldn't admit this while I'm encouraging you to exercise.)

Your blood runs a constant course that carries the oxygen from your lungs to your individual cells. Your blood also runs nutrients for fuel from your digestive organs to your cells. It's vital for you as an athlete to have good blood circulation to bring your muscles the generous supply of the goodies they require to keep them pumping.

You also rely on blood to keep warm. If your fingertips or toes feel cold, you sometimes get dizzy when you stand up quickly, or you start panting just going up the stairs, the cause may be poor blood circulation. Although you may feel that cold fingers or a little dizziness is no big deal, these are little red flags going up to tell you that the time has come to give your body some attention before larger problems pop up.

If you're working to improve your circulation, getting a massage probably sounds like a good idea. And you're not wrong. A massage is an ideal way to get your blood flowing. While you're at it, use a massage oil designed to boost circulation.

TIP

To increase surface blood flow or warm up cold hands or feet, use friction. You instinctually do this when you rub your hands together to warm them up when it's cold outside.

These essential oils are sure to get your blood moving and give your performance a kick start:

>> Cypress

>> Eucalyptus

>> Fennel

>> Geranium

>> Ginger

>> Juniper

>> Lemongrass

>> Rosemary

Beefing up blood vessels

You have lots of good reasons to keep your blood vessels strong. Their flexibility and resilience allow them to withstand the force of the blood being pumped through them and keep it moving with the strength it needs to travel throughout your body. Develop a problem like hardening of the arteries, and the entire system won't work properly. Slow that blood down, and nutrients and especially oxygen don't reach their destination fast enough, leaving you feeling tired, both physically and mentally.

The oils listed here aren't quite as powerful in increasing circulation as those in "Improving Your Circulation" earlier in the chapter, but they have something else going for them: They tend to improve the integrity of your blood vessels to make them stronger and more fit. As your blood pumps more quickly and with more force, your blood vessels stay strong and flexible.

>> Bergamot

>> Cedarwood

>> Chamomile

>> Frankincense

>> Grapefruit

>> Lemon

TIP

If you have varicose veins or another specific problem, find formulas for your condition in the Symptoms Guide.

One of the most effective ways to improve circulation and ease stiff muscles is to take a hot bath — with essential oils, of course. For a bath, add three to four drops of circulation-stimulating essential oils to hot bath water. This bath isn't designed to put you to sleep, so probably not the best idea right before you're going to sleep. Instead, it gets your blood flowing, soothes your tired muscles, and it may energize you.

TIP

If you have sensitive skin, you can dilute the essential oils in a carrier oil before adding them to your bath. To do this, mix the three to four drops of essential oil in a tablespoon of olive oil or other vegetable oil.

Another way to improve circulation and to ease those stiff muscles is through massage by a massage therapist or self-massage. For a massage, buy massage oil that contains some of the essential oils I suggest in this chapter or make your own.

These same essential oils are great when used in a foot bath. You only need a couple drops in a pan of warm water. Consider taking a bath or a footbath and following it up by rubbing on an aromatherapy massage oil, perhaps using the following recipe.

Massage Oil for Circulation

If you don't get a massage, don't despair — you can still take advantage of this oil by rubbing it on your arms and legs.

>> Preparation time: 5 minutes

>> Yield: 2 ounces massage oil or lotion

>> Ingredients:

10 drops lemon

6 drops geranium

4 drops rosemary

2 ounces vegetable oil or lotion

1. Combine all the oils.

2. Use as a body massage oil.

Applying liniment

A liniment is an old-fashioned treatment that's ideal for today's fitness-crazed society. It's a product that's made by adding essential oils to either an oil or alcohol base to warm up your muscles and make them stretch more easily. This helps relieve pain and prevent injury in the first place. Drug stores usually have an entire shelf dedicated to different types of liniments, many of which contain essential oils.

If you're a weekend warrior, a do-it-yourself handyperson, or a gym rat, you're probably already very familiar with liniments such as Chinese Tiger Balm or the drugstore versions that alleviate muscle pain. Liniments not only relieve pain, but they also get your blood moving and increase your circulation.

The idea behind a liniment is that it heats a specific area just like a hot pack. Both a liniment and hot pack work by drawing blood to the area to warm it up. The heat then relaxes your tight and sore muscles with a "deep" heat as your blood circulates through your muscles.

It turns out that liniments are more than an afterthought. Fitness experts now suggest it's far better to apply a liniment before exercising than afterwards. You already know how important it is to warm your muscles up before participating in any strenuous physical activity. A warm muscle stretches and tightens much better than a cold one, which means far less pressure not only on the muscle itself, but also on your ligaments and tendons. When a cold or tight muscle can't stretch properly, it puts a tremendous pull on these connective fibers. They're not designed to do major stretching — that's the muscle's job — so if the muscle is cold, they're subject to being torn. So, warmups cut down tremendously on sports injuries. Find out more about choosing or making your own liniments and anti-inflammatories made with essential oils in Chapter 11.

WARNING

If you're engaging in a contact sport, say wrestling or martial arts, chances are using a liniment or anything that smells of essential oils won't be permitted. That's because your opponent may not appreciate a face full of smelly liniment when in an arm lock. You'll still benefit from using a liniment and other essential oil products afterwards.

To tend to your specific conditions caused by insufficient blood circulation, such as cold hands and feet, go to the "Symptom Guide" in the back of this book to look up individual conditions.

Going for the gold: Oils and athletes

You can take a hint from Ancient Greek athletes who were treated to special sports massages. You can follow their lead by buying or making a sports massage oil, as outlined in this chapter. They even designated a different massage oil for each part of their bodies. Mint was rubbed on their arms, thyme on their knees, almond oil on their hands and feet, and a heady blend of cinnamon and rose was for their chests and jaws. Even their hair and eyebrows were given special treatment with marjoram. I like this idea so much, I decided to also use a set of massage oils on different body areas when I give aromatherapy massages. Everyone who receives this specialized treatment feels like ancient royalty.

In India, athletes were also treated to aromatherapy baths and massage. A 12th-century text describes how this improves athletic performance. They used jasmine, clove, pine, cardamom, basil, and coriander with a sesame oil base. The modern day "Invincible Athletes" program adapted India's ancient aromatherapy, along with Ayurvedic medicine, into a sports program.

Rub a dub: Sports massage for everyone

If you work at a desk during the week and then lift weights all afternoon Sunday or go on that 40-mile, weekend bike ride, chances are you'll be plenty sore Sunday night. If you've been in full training, but need to push yourself to build up more, you'll probably feel it the next day.

Exercising past your conditioning ends up being painful, and it never hurts to plan ahead for a massage. The sooner you get your massage to work out the stiffness or inflammation, the better. If you're expecting to be sore, think ahead and schedule a massage. Having your body massaged Sunday evening is especially smart if you're planning to go to work Monday morning.

When I asked sports massage specialists about their techniques, most of them said they don't stick to one method. It depends on the shape you're in — or more likely how out of shape you are. If you're sore from overextending yourself or your muscles are cramping, you need a deep massage. This squeezes out the lactic acid that builds up in your muscles when you work them and lingers around creating soreness and stiffness. You don't always need to go to a specialist. A good Swedish-style massage typically goes deep enough.

The rubbing and muscle kneading of either Swedish or sports massage relies on using massage oil. If your massage practitioner isn't already using a muscle-relaxing massage oil, show them my suggestions in this chapter for essential oils or buy a suitable massage oil and ask them to use it on you.

TIP

If you pull a muscle or ligament or pinch a nerve, go to a sports massage specialist to straighten you out, literally. A sports massage practitioner then works around, not directly on the injury (although they may place an ice pack there) to release the areas that usually tighten up around an injury. If they know their aromatherapy, you can also expect an anti-inflammatory preparation. A sports massage practitioner can assist you if you're in regular training.

All wet: Hydrotherapy

The term *hydrotherapy* refers to the therapeutic use of water (*hydro* means water). It's an excellent way to get your circulation moving and helps to relax stiff muscles as well. To experience hydrotherapy, you expose your body to the extremes of hot and cold water by alternating back and forth between the two. You can do this by going into a sauna, a hot tub, or a bathtub of hot water. Then come out of the heat to hose or rinse yourself down with cold water every five or ten minutes. This may sound brutal, but ohhhh . . . it feels so good when it's over, and it certainly does get your blood circulating!

WARNING

If you have heart problems, take a pass on alternating hot and cold hydrotherapy. The shock of cold may be more invigorating than is good for you.

It's probably coming as no surprise that I suggest adding essential oils to your hydrotherapy regime to stimulate circulation. Add about ten drops to the hot rocks in your sauna or to a two- to four-person hot tub. To be on the safe side, go easy at first by adding a few initial drops to make sure that the essential oil you add isn't going to smell too intense or irritate your skin.

Unlike vegetable oils, the components in most essential oils are too small to gum up your hot tub — but make sure that you're using essential oil with no additives. Avoid resinous or gummy essential oils that might stick to the bottom and sides of the tub. Examples of these are myrrh gum and frankincense resin. These are probably not the essential oils you'd choose for a hot soak, anyway. You can recognize them because they have a thick, syrupy consistency.

Staying on Track: Boosting Stamina

Stamina is what keeps you going so that you can make that goal, play that last round, or ski one more slope before you quit or just make your daily loop around the block. It's one of the important aspects of your physical performance.

TIP

Maintaining your mental stamina is as important as building your physical stamina. If your mental focus and decision-making become blurry, you won't perform well at any physical sport or task. If you have problems with general fatigue, look it up in the "Essential Oil Guide" at the back of this book.

Several essential oils help you maintain your physical endurance and stamina. At the same time, they also keep you focused. Even more impressive is that they help you stay on track through their scent alone. That means you can carry an essential oil or even a sprig of the plant itself with you to sniff during training or a workout. (You can buy aromatherapy inhalers that contain scents designed to increase your stamina.)

Not surprisingly, most of the essential oils that increase stamina are the same ones that increase mental focus and your attention span. (Turn to Chapter 9 for more on these oils or if you'd like to make your own products.) Some essential oils that increase your stamina, just by smell alone, include

>> Angelica

>> Basil

>> Benzoin

>> Black pepper

- » Cardamom
- » Cinnamon
- » Cypress
- » Ginger
- » Peppermint
- » Pine
- » Sage

Just imagine; someday you may walk into the gym and smell cinnamon and peppermint to increase your stamina instead of everyone else's sweat. For now, whether you're working out at home or vacuuming the floor, you can fill the room with an invigorating scent or create your own blend of these stimulating, stay-on-track fragrances. See my suggestions for scenting rooms in Chapter 6.

TIP

Essential oils keep you alert, and some herbs can offer you stamina without dangerous steroids. Check out the benefits of herbs such as ginseng.

Stamina isn't just about keeping your focus, maintaining good blood flow, and having energized muscles. It has to do with how quickly your muscles recover from the stress of exercise. This is especially true when you push yourself beyond your muscle's limitations when trying to build up more muscle strength or to finish in first place.

Chapter **13**

De-Bugging Your Home, Garden, and Pets

When it comes to bugs, you probably don't think of aromatherapy. After all, essential oils are most often considered a therapy to enhance your emotional and physical health or complexion, not something that you'd use out in the garden. Nevertheless, essential oils offer plenty of ways to keep annoying insects out of your garden and your house and off of you and your pets. What could be a better form of therapy than making your home and garden a more pleasant and less stressful place for you to enjoy?

It's time to pull in the welcome mat and turn the insect's remarkable sense of smell to your advantage. A strong aroma can create a scent shield to disguise the smells that bugs rely on to locate a food source — your home or garden. Instead, they get hit with a strong waft of pine or citronella. It's not what they're searching for, so the annoying little critters go elsewhere. Covering up bug-enticing scents is a good start, but an even better ploy is to use scents that bugs actually hate so that you can send most any bug spinning in the opposite direction.

This chapter shows you how essential oils can help turn your living environment into a bug-free zone. My emphasis is on your first line of defense — aromatherapy repellents. I explain how you can use your scents on your family and pets and in your house and garden as an alternative to toxic pesticides and repellents. In this chapter, I also give you the aromas to use to keep away all sorts of pests, from moths to mosquitos.

WARNING

This chapter contains a few scents that I don't cover elsewhere because the plants are considered too concentrated and toxic to use in their essential oil form. Even drinking a tea made from herbs like pennyroyal, tansy, and wormwood comes with some cautions. However, toxicity is just what you want when you're dealing with bugs.

In Your House

Your home is a good place to start a bug patrol. After all, it is *your* house or apartment, not a parade ground for ants or an arena for flies to practice their dives. And your closets and cupboards are certainly not designed to host feeding frenzies of visiting grain and wool moths.

TIP

Find commercial bug repellants that contain essential oils. Look for those that don't have added chemicals that aren't good for your health.

This section lists the pests that are most likely to plague your happy home and tells you exactly what essential oils will send them packing.

Identifying and defeating common culprits

The following lists associate common pests with the essential oils they hate. Use one or a combination of these oils to keep pests away.

>> **Ants:** These critters are fairly easy to attack because they travel in regimented lines. I find that camphor and peppermint work well to repel ants. Make a spray to spritz along their trails, and ants will lose their way. You can also cut a sponge into small squares, add several drops of essential oil to the pieces, and stick them in the corners of your cupboards or wherever ants find an entrance to your home. (Replace the essential oils every week.) To rid your place of ants, try these essential oils:

- Camphor
- Orange
- Pine
- Peppermint
- Spruce

>> **Cockroaches:** It doesn't take a full invasion of cockroaches in your house before you want them out. Just one of these huge bugs is one too many to share your house with. Concentrate your repellent action in the dark, damp places where they like to hang out. Try these essential oils:

- Angelica
- Eucalyptus
- Peppermint
- Sage

>> **Flies:** These winged critters are a tough assignment because flies cover lots of territory. Because they fly, they can land anywhere, and you can't very well chase after them with a spray bottle. Keeping flies from coming into the house is difficult unless you scent it so heavily that you won't want to come in either. So, take a hint from yesteryear. In the days before window screens, people hung bunches of anise and bay by the open windows and doors so that flies wouldn't find the place inviting. Concentrate your efforts where flies enter your house and where they are most likely to land — around your windows and doors and on your kitchen counters. Scents that flies avoid include

- Anise
- Bay laurel
- Cedarwood
- Cloves
- Eucalyptus
- Orange

>> **Mice:** Okay, I know mice aren't bugs, but you have to admit that having mice move into your home can really bug you, so I'm including them among household pests. Spraying mint or even placing the fresh or dried leaves of the plant around keep mice away. Try these scents:

- Peppermint
- Spearmint
- Wormwood

>> **Moths (clothes-eating):** The commercial mothballs that ward off wool moths have an unpleasant odor and can discolor the very clothing they protect. Even worse, they contain some very potent chemicals — naphthalene and paradi-chlorobenzene. As a result, mothballs cause more than 5,000 poisonings a year, according to the American Association of Poison Control Centers. It's no wonder that insecticides are going natural.

These oils all work well when you're battling clothes-eating moths:

- Bay laurel
- Camphor
- Cedarwood (use the essential oil or a cedarwood chest for clothes storage)
- Lavender
- Patchouli
- Sage

» **Moths (grain/pantry):** *Grain* or *pantry moths* are tiny greyish moths that look like little sticks when they're not flying and otherwise flutter around the pantry searching for cereal and other grains to dine on. An old tradition that still works as good as it did 200 years ago is to stick a few bay laurel leaves in your grain jars to keep these moths at "bay."

REMEMBER

You may notice that peppermint appears on every list of pest deterrents. Experts on natural bug repellents — yes, they're out there — recommend peppermint as the over-all best essential oil to detract bugs, both indoors and out. Peppermint also has the advantage of having the opposite effect on us people. To most of us, it smells great!

Sashay Away Moth "Balls"

Make your own herbal sachets to fend off clothes moths. Toss them in your storage chest or chest of drawers and hang them on ribbons from your clothes hangers. I find that lavender is a very effective moth repellent and smells wonderful, but cedarwood is even better, so I combine the two. Fabric stores sell small squares of material for quiltmakers. You can buy these ready-to-go squares at craft stores or online if you'd rather not cut your own.

» Preparation time: 20 minutes

» Yield: 8 moth repellent sachets

» Ingredients:

¼ cup lavender flowers

8 fabric squares, each about 6 inches square cut with pinking shears

10 drops lavender oil

8 pieces of string (or ribbon) about 6 inches long

10 drops cedarwood oil

1. Add the essential oils to the lavender flowers.

2. Place the scented lavender in a glass jar for a day or so to give the scents from the essential oils time to permeate them.

3. Lay out the 6 fabric squares with the design (or outside) facing down.

4. Place a heaping teaspoon of the scented lavender on each piece.

5. Bring the edges of the fabric together and tie with the string.

6. Place your "moth balls" in with your woolens.

Household Spray

I use a homemade bug repellent spray to deal with household. Use this spray to discourage pests inside your home. It contains some of the most versatile essential oils. I use vinegar because bugs don't care for it at all. It's also cheap, easy to spray, and evaporates without leaving a trace. This recipe is for an all-purpose spray. If you want, alter the ingredients if you have your sights set on a particular bug you want to attack.

» Preparation time: 10 minutes

» Yield: 4 ounces

» ½ teaspoon eucalyptus oil

» ¼ teaspoon peppermint oil

» ¼ teaspoon lemon oil

» 4 ounces vinegar

1. Put all ingredients in a blender and mix.

2. Store in a spray bottle.

3. Shake well before use and spray away!

Disinfecting your home fragrantly

Most essential oils are antibacterial, antifungal, and antiviral, so they disinfect your house to eliminate a much smaller bug: germs. The household tips in this chapter may not make your chores more enjoyable, but they certainly will be more fragrant.

TIP

If you're too tired to get the housework done, then make sure you've added a drop of an essential oil with an energizing scent. If you're feeling depressed because you'd rather be doing anything but these chores, then go for an antidepressant essential oil. See ways to counter depression in Chapter 9.

Ways to keep the germ population in your household down and have your home smell good at the same time include:

>> **All-purpose spray:** An all-purpose disinfectant spray goes a long way to declaring your home a germ-free zone. Use it on floors, countertops, and sinks (and walls if they're painted with glossy paint) in your kitchen and bathrooms. Add ¼ teaspoon eucalyptus and ¼ teaspoon lemon oil to ¼ teaspoon vinegar and ½ cup water.

>> **Clothes dryer:** Next time you do laundry, take a small scrap of fabric and put 20 to 30 drops of an essential oil of your choice on it. It will lend its scent to all the clothes, towels, or sheets, and it certainly makes folding the laundry an aromatic experience!

>> **Dishes:** It's likely that your dishwashing detergent already has a citrus scent. If not or if the scent is very mild, increase its disinfecting ability by adding 15 drops of lemon, lime, or orange oil to a 10-ounce bottle of detergent. (To keep your hands looking like they never did all those dishes, use the pricier bergamot oil instead.)

>> **Dishwasher:** Add 2 drops lemon or orange oil to the detergent in your dishwasher's soap compartment. This won't do much to scent the dishes themselves, but it works wonders on a smelly dishwasher.

>> **Hand-washed fabrics:** When washing your delicate woolens or lingerie by hand, add 1 to 2 drops lemongrass, petitgrain, or bergamot oil to the wash water.

>> **Refuse pails and garbage cans:** Dab a few drops of tea tree or eucalyptus oil on a scrap of paper and throw it in the pail or can to cover any stale smells.

>> **Sponges:** Place 3 drops lavender oil on a couple of your kitchen sponges and clip them securely in your dishwasher with clothes pins the next time you wash your dishes to freshen them.

>> **Vacuum cleaner:** Take a small scrap of fabric and place about 10 drops of an essential oil on it. Throw this into the bag of your vacuum cleaner. Even if you have an airtight model so that you can't enjoy the fragrance, it will help to disinfect your vacuum bag.

A WARNING ABOUT INSECTICIDES

The case against using household and garden chemical insecticides and cleaners has strong evidence. The products are still on the market because the findings are still unproven, but be especially careful in using household and garden chemicals if you're pregnant.

Studies show that some of the chemicals used in these products may promote cancer and damage organs including the kidney, spleen, and liver. Being exposed to even small amounts over the long term may have health consequences, resulting in nausea, diarrhea, nervous system problems, and skin eruptions. You absorb most chemicals through your skin, but you can also inhale them.

When you read the labels on household cleaners, don't confuse the names of chemicals with some of the compounds found in essential oils or in the oils themselves. For example, benzene, which is classified by the United States Federal Drug Administration as the fifth most hazardous air pollutant, is different from the essential oil benzoin (profiled in the Essential Oil Guide). The powerful germ fighter phenol, which rapidly corrodes skin, is produced from coal tar and is not the same phenol compounds found in essential oils. (Chapter 15 explains all this chemistry talk.)

In the Great Outdoors

My first experience with aromatic bug repellents wasn't to keep the bugs off me but out of my garden. I lived in a community where almost every yard had a vegetable garden, left over from the World War II days of victory gardens. My garden was unusual because I grew so many medicinal and fragrant herbs among the vegetables. I gave my first herb walks through my garden for curious neighbors.

My garden soon gained a reputation for more than herbs. Unlike everyone else's garden, it attracted almost no bugs. I could peer over the fence into my next-door neighbor's garden to see it crawling with wildlife — the unwanted kind! Tomato hornworms, cabbage worms, aphids, and Japanese beetles all happily munching my neighbor's vegetables. These same pests weren't bothering my vegetables. It didn't take rocket science to figure out that the scent emanating from all my herbs was either too annoying or simply covering up the signals that these pests rely on to seek out food.

This success with keeping bugs out of my garden got me thinking how well some of these same herbs might work to keep bugs off me. That's when I started making my own liquid insect repellents. Nowadays, you have it easy. You can choose from dozens of natural bug repellents, not only for you, but for your dogs and cats, too. But if you'd rather play mad scientist in your kitchen, I give you a few ideas so you can create your own concoctions.

On you: Bug out

There's something disconcerting about being outdoors enjoying the fresh air and the beautiful plants and then hearing the high-pitched whine of a mosquito zeroing in on some patch of exposed skin. It's enough to make you not want to venture past the protection of your screen door. That's where nature's insect repellents come in handy to distance yourself from flying pests such as mosquitoes.

I'll be the first to admit that, when it comes to mosquitoes, essential oil bug repellents don't always work better than the standard drugstore variety, but they're good alternatives to putting the chemicals found in those repellents on your skin. Considering the potent chemical insecticides that are used in bug repellents, aromatherapy is far safer.

TIP

A citronella candle is one way to reduce the number of insects hovering around you without wearing a repellent. Impregnated with citronella, these candles release the scent as they burn. They're available from most camping and household stores and online. (Also, see how to scent your own candles in Chapter 6.)

You can try these essential oils as insect repellents:

>> Cedarwood

>> Citronella

>> Eucalyptus

>> Geranium

>> Pennyroyal

>> Sandalwood

All-natural Insect Repellent

The good news is that mosquitoes hate the smell of eucalyptus, pennyroyal, and citronella. Unfortunately, so will many of your friends. I like to add a touch of geranium to give the brew a little better aroma. Geranium is a minor bug repellent itself. Use this flea, mosquito, fly, and tick repellent sparingly because it's potent stuff. This repellent lasts more than a year after it's made. (If you're pregnant, eliminate the citronella and pennyroyal and, even then, use this concoction very sparingly.)

WARNING

Keep your insect repellent away from your eyes and mouth because it can sting. (Be careful that you don't rub your eyes right after applying the repellent with your fingers.) Also, remember that rubbing alcohol is poisonous to drink.

>> Preparation time: 10 minutes

>> Yield: 2 ounces

>> Ingredients:

¼ teaspoon citronella oil

¼ teaspoon eucalyptus oil

⅛ teaspoon pennyroyal oil

⅛ teaspoon cedarwood oil

⅛ teaspoon geranium oil

2 ounces vodka or rubbing alcohol

1. Combine all ingredients. Be sure to store it in a glass container because such a strong concentration of essential oils can eat through plastic.

2. Use by dabbing on here and there. Dab wherever mosquitoes tend to hover, such as around your head and ankles.

Bites and stings

Of course, even with careful prevention, bugs can sneak through your defense systems at times. If you're their target, and you get bit or stung, aromatherapy again comes to your rescue with remedies to ease your discomfort. Nature provides as many remedies as she does insects. Use essential oils that reduce inflammation to stop the itching and swelling of bites and stings.

WARNING

If you tend to have an allergic reaction to that type of sting or bite or show any signs of impaired breathing, faintness, or shock, then get professional help right away instead of depending solely on aromatherapy first aid.

Insect Bite Solution

A simple dab of essential oil of lavender or tea tree provides relief for a few mosquito bites or other insect bites that don't demand much attention. Chamomile, lavender, helichrysum, and tea tree oils reduce swelling, itching, and inflammation.

This oil lasts at least a couple years if you store it in a cool, dark place.

>> Preparation time: 4 minutes

>> Yield: ½ ounce

>> Ingredients:

   ½ teaspoon lavender oil

   ½ teaspoon tea tree oil

   1 tablespoon vodka or rubbing alcohol

1. Combine ingredients.

2. Store in a bottle with a tight lid. A glass container is best to store this oil, but if you prefer a lightweight, plastic container, choose one made of stiff plastic, which is more resistant to essential oils.

3. Dab directly on bite as needed.

TIP

Keep a bite oil handy. That way, even when you've just been stung and you're in a hurry to slap on a remedy, you can avoid dabbing undiluted essential oil directly on your skin.

In Your Garden

Whether you have acres of crops, a little garden patch out back, or just a few tomatoes in pots on your balcony, if you grow vegetables or flowers, you certainly encounter bugs. They may be small, but, as you've surely discovered, bugs have colossal appetites.

If you put the time and effort into planting and growing a garden or crops, you'll want to do everything you can to keep your plants healthy so you can reap all that you sow. That includes protecting your flowers, veggies, and herbs from pests. In this section, I tell you how to use essential oils in your battle for the harvest.

Table 13-1 lists the essential oils that fend off garden pests. Of course, the oils are in both the fresh or dried plant, so use either the herb or essential oil. To make a spray, you can throw the plants or the essential oils into a blender with vinegar and water. (You can find a recipe following this table.)

TABLE 13-1   ## Essential Oils to Make Your Garden Pest-Free

Pest	Herbs
Aphids	Cayenne, garlic (Coriander, eucalyptus, fennel, garlic, hyssop, and peppermint are slightly less effective.)
Asparagus beetle	Basil
Beetles	Eucalyptus, rosemary, geranium
Cabbage looper	Clary sage, dill, eucalyptus, garlic, hyssop, nasturtium, onion, pennyroyal, peppermint, sage, southernwood, thyme, wormwood
Cabbage maggot	Garlic, sage, wormwood
Carrot fly	Onion, rosemary, sage, wormwood
Codling moth	Garlic, wormwood
Colorado potato beetle	Catnip, coriander, eucalyptus, French marigold, nasturtium, tansy
Cucumber beetle	Catnip, nasturtium, rue
Japanese beetle	Garlic, tansy
Mexican bean beetle	Catnip, French marigold, rosemary, savory
Nematodes	French marigold
Peach borer	Garlic
Slugs and snails	Fennel, garlic, rosemary
Spider mite	Anise, coriander, cumin, oregano
Squash bug	Catnip, nasturtium, peppermint, tansy
Tomato hornworm	Basil, dill, nasturtium, peppermint, thyme, wormwood
Whitefly	Nasturtium, peppermint, thyme, wormwood

You can plant these herbs amongst your other plants to repel pests in your garden. Then, harvest them to make a garden spray! Catnip, nasturtium, and French marigold aren't readily available as essential oils. However, these aromatic herbs are strong enough insecticides and deterrents in their plant form.

The essential oils from a few plants have been developed into natural-ingredient pesticides. One new herbal pesticide contains cinnamon oil, which counters infections in people. (See Chapter 10.) Cinnamon wipes out many insect pests and fungal diseases on your garden plants as well.

INDIAN NEEM TREE KNOCKS 'EM DEAD

The neem tree *(Azadirachta indica)* is a tropical tree from India, where the strong-smelling, highly antiseptic leaves are used on skin diseases and placed in strategic areas to discourage insects. Look for garden insecticides that contain it.

Neem oil kills young aphids, thrips, whiteflies, and the Colorado potato beetle by stopping their development and making it impossible for them to feed and/or digest their food. Although it doesn't instantly wipe out these pests, it's very effective after a few weekly applications. It also repels the Japanese beetle.

Even though it's an effective toxin for some pests, neem oil doesn't harm most beneficial insects, it's toxic to some fish. It's not toxic to people but read the instructions for its safe use.

Enough Already! All-Purpose Garden Spray

This all-purpose spray is made with both essential oils and herbs that contain essential oils. Spray it on your vegetables and flowers. (It works on your garden plants to keep off bugs.)

Any extra solution keeps for several days if stored in a cool place.

>> Preparation time: 15 minutes

>> Yield: 4 ounces

>> Ingredients:

   5 cloves garlic

   1 cup water

   ½ teaspoon cayenne powder

   ¼ teaspoon peppermint oil

   ¼ teaspoon rosemary oil

   ½ teaspoon biodegradable liquid dishwashing detergent

1. Put the garlic, cayenne, and water in a blender and mix.

2. Strain through a fine strainer.

   If you don't have a fine strainer, re-strain the mixture through a coffee filter.

3. Stir in the essential oils and soap.

4. Put the solution in a spray bottle and head out into the garden.

In the Doghouse: Aromatherapy for Your Pet

Essential oils don't just benefit you. They can also be used to protect your pet from pests like fleas and ticks. However, talking about what essential oils to use on your pets becomes as much of a discussion on what to not use on your pets. Keep in mind that their bodies are different from yours, not to mention smaller, and that essential oils are concentrated and powerful. This section explains how to safely use oils and herbs to help your pets, where to apply your remedies, and what oils are superstars at kicking fleas and ticks to the curb.

Using oils on your pets safely

Essential oils are potentially toxic if you use too much. They're even more toxic for dogs and cats because their organs aren't designed to clear the oils quickly from their bodies. Your pet may not show signs of essential-oil overdose immediately. It can take years before your pet shows noticeable symptoms.

The American Society for the Prevention of Cruelty to Animals, Animal Poison Control Center database says to watch out when using essential oils around your pets, especially cats. Pets can experience weakness, vomiting, depression, muscle tremors when exposed to essential oils. Cats that ingest or are exposed to essential oils can even die.

TECHNICAL STUFF

When exposed to natural flea preventatives, 92 percent of cats had adverse effects within 24 hours. These lasted up to 6 days. Three-quarters of the owners had applied the products according to the label. Half of the animals recovered after a bath while others received intravenous fluids, muscle relaxants, and anticonvulsive medications. Of the cats that had products containing essential oils like tea tree, peppermint, cinnamon, lemongrass, and clove applied to their fur, an average 7 percent had poisoning symptoms.

Whatever you do, don't dab essential oil right on your pet because it will go through to their skin. Dogs, and especially cats, are smaller than us and have thin skin far more porous than yours. They may have thick coats, but essential oils and other chemicals seep right into their skin. Essential oils on fur can also be a problem since chances are your pet will lick their fur and paws.

I've heard too many sad stories from pet owners who accidentally caused their beloved pets to overdose with essential oil. They all end the same way with the owner saying, "If only someone had told me." So, I'm telling you that it's wise to use essential oils on your pet with discretion. Avoid them altogether on animals who already have liver or kidney conditions, are pregnant or nursing, and on kittens and young puppies.

Despite potential dangers, you see essential oils recommended for all sorts of pet conditions. I've worked in the natural pet product industry to design products that use a safe amount of essential oil. That's made me keenly aware of all the products you can buy that contain way too much essential oil. For more on using essential oils safely for both you and your pets, be sure to read Chapter 4.

REMEMBER

Make safe products for your pet by using aromatic herbs instead of their essential oils. Some effective oils are too toxic to use on your pet in their essential oils form, wormwood being one example. Use herbs like this in their powdered form. You can powder herbs yourself by grinding them in a coffee grinder.

Getting the dosage right

The standard way to figure how much essential oil you need for a pet takes a little easy math. First, take the average adult person, who is considered to weigh 150 pounds. You simply divide the pet's weight into that of the person. For example, if your pet weighs 10 pounds, their dose is $\frac{1}{13}$ of yours. One dose for a person is typically one drop. That makes your 10-pound pet's dose only $\frac{1}{13}$ of a drop diluted in a carrier.

WARNING

Cats are even more sensitive than dogs, so cut a dog dose in half for a cat. If the safe dose is that small, you may wonder whether you should use essential oils at all on your cat. The safest answer is simply "no."

Have you ever used an essential oil diffuser to scent your house and watched your cat flee to an unscented room? Even if your cat tolerates a scented room, that's not saying they're enjoying it. A cat's natural instinct is "no!" Diffusers are great for scenting your house (see Chapter 6 for more about them), just not for kitty, even though they put just a little scent into the air.

WARNING

Be sure to keep kitty's sleeping rooms scent-free.

Sending fleas and ticks fleeing

No one likes the idea of having fleas in their house or on their pets, and especially on them! However, dosing Fido and Puss with conventional flea powders, soaps, dips, and collars is rough. These flea deterrents contain some of the most potent chemical insecticides.

REMEMBER

When they groom themselves, your pets are likely to ingest residue from anything you put on their fur. Flea killers can make them sick, causing nervous system problems, depression, hyperactivity, diarrhea, and vomiting.

Fleas may be tiny, but they can smell. The good news is they hate the scent of powerful oils like eucalyptus and bay laurel. Fortunately for your pet, researchers have put the most popular essential oil flea repellents to the test.

Although essential oils won't kill fleas and ticks unless the oil is on them, they hate certain scents. Ticks drop off clothing and blankets that carry those scents. Oregano and spearmint on clothing prove as effective for ticks as the commercial DEET repellent. An impressive tick repellent is sweet basil — you know, pesto basil. What gets the blue ribbon for killing all the stages of a flea's life is African basil (*Ocimum gratissimum*). The following scents help make ticks and fleas flee off your pets (and off you). Don't put the essential oils directly on your skin or doggie's fur. You can place a drop on clothing or the outside of a collar. You can also purchase sprays that contain them.

» Basil (African basil for ticks)

» Citronella

» Eucalyptus

» Geranium

» Lemongrass

» Orange

Your pet's neck is the perfect place for a flea repellent because fleas like to congregate around a pet's warm and cozy neck. Fleas like this location not only because it's warm but because it's a place where your pet can't nip at them.

You can purchase an essential oil collar in a pet store or online. Read the ingredients to make sure that it contains essential oils without any of the toxic chemicals usually found in flea collars.

Another place to use flea repellent is in your pet's bed. You can make them a pillow that contains the appropriate herbs and/or essential oils. Or, mist your pet's existing bed and the surrounding area with an aromatherapy spray. (These are good ideas even if you don't have a flea problem to improve the smell of your pet's quarters.) Try a little at first to see your pet's response.

Pets may not care for the same aromas you do. They prefer more organic smells that you probably consider downright foul. (You know exactly what dogs sniff when they're out on a walk.) One scent that usually goes over okay with a pet is cedar. In fact, you can buy dog beds filled with cedar chips. (If you happen to have a wood shop at home you can make your own supply of cedarwood chips. Go ahead and stuff them into a homemade dog pillow and save yourself 60 bucks.)

TIP

If you love both dogs and gardens, plant thyme — the same common thyme you use in cooking. Protect the plants when they're young, but when they're established, let your dog roll on them. A dog's natural instinct is to de-flea themselves with aromatic plants. My dog Pepper made a daily visit to the thyme patch. My current dog, Ginger, has flattened out a yarrow patch growing near my front door. Both are good choices considering the scent of thyme and yarrow repels fleas.

Orange-icide: Killing fleas on your pet

Repelling fleas to keep them off your animals is a good idea, but if your pet already has fleas, a repellent may not be strong enough to make them retreat. In that case, you need to outright kill them. You can do this by using one of the citrus oils, which contain a compound deadly to fleas.

You can't douse your pooch with essential oils, but you can use shampoo and wash those fleas away. Several pet shampoos available now contain citrus oil or the active compound in it to do the deadly deed. You can also make your own antiflea shampoo by adding a 1-2 drops (per shampoo) of orange oil to unscented pet shampoo.

Your cat may be a different story. I've had cats that tolerated a cat shampoo, although barely and with constant reminders that this is not an appropriate way to treat a cat. Kitty may have a point here since it's not just the water and soap that offends them, but the essential oils themselves. It's debatable if it's even safe to shampoo a cat with any product containing essential oils. If you do, go lightly and don't do it very often.

REMEMBER

Give your dog an essential oil flea bath only occasionally. Opinions on how often it's safe vary, from every other week to only once a month. When in doubt, ask the vet.

De-fleaing your home

So, you convinced the fleas to flee from your pet with a flea bath, but your work isn't done yet. Flea eggs are likely lying anywhere your pet hangs out, and they can stay there a couple of years before hatching.

Only about 20 percent of a household's flea population resides on your dog or cat at any one time.

Fleas are especially fond of warm humid places, so they can rapidly multiply in the summer months. The same day that you give your pet the bath, vacuum your floors and furniture, especially around your pet's favorite hangouts. Then sprinkle the Flea Away House Salt (see the next recipe) behind the furniture and in areas where dust tends to collect. You might need to do this several times.

A repellent salt is one way to keep fleas from taking up residence in your house. It prevents them from laying their eggs in dark, dusty, unseen, and untrampled areas. You simply sprinkle it on the carpet. Don't worry, the ingredients are harmless and won't trash your carpets.

One caution about using Flea Away House Salt: If your pet's diet is lacking and they're attracted to salt, they may make up for it by licking up your flea powder and overdose on both salt and essential oils. Keep an eye on your pet to ensure they don't eat your flea powder. If you suspect your pet gobbled it up, contact your vet.

Flea Away House Salt

Even though it contains only two ingredients, this is a well-tested recipe with a great track record. The salt absorbs the essential oil so it retains the flea-discouraging scents longer and lasts in the jar for months.

>> Preparation time: 2 minutes

>> Yield: 1 cup salt

>> Ingredients:

1 cup table salt

1 teaspoon lavender oil

1. Add the essential oil to the salt drop by drop to evenly distribute it.

2. Lightly sprinkle under your couch or in hidden corners — just the kind of out-of-sight places that fleas like to hide.

3. Store the extra in a glass jar.

4. Reapply if needed every day.

If you're wondering if a lavender bath salt you already happen to have on hand will work instead, the answer is yes! Just be sure it doesn't contain additives that could stain carpeting or be toxic to animals.

3

How Essential Oils Work

IN THIS CHAPTER

» **Understanding how essential oils are produced**

» **Steaming the oil out with diffusion**

» **Squeezing out oil**

» **Soaking out the oil with enfleurage**

» **Going elemental with carbon dioxide**

» **Defining and using hydrosols and aromatic waters**

» **Making your own kitchen distiller**

Chapter **14**

Distilling Essential Oil: Extraction Methods

I f the fragrance of plants has captured your imagination, you're not alone. Interest in essential oils and how they are made is a popular topic these days. If you're asking, "what exactly is an essential oil?" this chapter answers your question. I discuss where essential oils come from and how they're created. I explain how essential oils are extracted from aromatic plants through the process of distillation and discuss other methods of extracting essential oils.

Besides extracting essential oils, the process of steam distillation often yields water-based hydrosols. You may not be familiar with them yet, but hydrosols are becoming more and more available. In this chapter, I explain what they are, how they're made, how you can make them, and, of course, how you can use them.

If you're interested in creating your own essential oils and hydrosols, but don't want to spend the bucks to buy a distiller, follow my instructions for putting together your own distiller for a fraction of the cost.

Extracting the Essence

The goal of early alchemists was to capture the "quintessence" or the "essential" part of a plant that makes it aromatic. Along the way, they designed several ways to distill essential oils. Fast forward to modern times.

To obtain essential oils in their pure form requires elaborate laboratory equipment to separate the oil from the fresh plant. The method used depends upon the plant, but steam distillation is most common. The most common ways to extract essential oils are

>> **Carbon dioxide:** Using gas to extract

>> **Distillation:** Using water and/or steam

>> **Pressed or expressed:** Extracting oil with high pressure

>> **Solvent:** Soaking plant matter in chemicals

I explain each method in the upcoming sections.

Noting who uses oils

Most essential oils go to either the perfume industry or to the food industry to flavor prepackaged foods. In fact, essential oils would cost you much more if it weren't for the demand from the industries that use them to scent various products.

All sorts of products get their scent from essential oils, either to make them appealing to consumers or to cover up an objectionable industrial smell — plastic, a preservative, or a smelly adhesive.

TECHNICAL STUFF

Until the 1990s the only essential oils you could find on store shelves were the peppermint and wintergreen oils sold at drugstores. Nowadays, you can visit a natural-food or specialty shop or look online and find a large selection of essential oils readily available to use for aromatherapy purposes. Yet, that wide array represents only about five percent of the essential oils produced today.

Looking at ratios

When you sniff a plant, it usually smells very aromatic. It may surprise you that even the most fragrant plants contain only minute quantities of essential oils. So, it takes lots and lots of plant material to produce even one vial of essential oil.

Essential oils are extremely concentrated. This potency is why you need to use them carefully. To make sure you use essential oils safely, read Chapter 4. Due to their small size, essential oils easily escape from a leaf to float into the air or come off a steaming cup of aromatic tea. It's their tiny size that makes them move easily out of an aromatic plant or your cup of tea.

Several factors determine how much essential oil you can derive from a plant:

>> **The plant itself:** Not all aromatic plants contain the same quantity of essential oil.

See the nearby sidebar, "An Oily Situation," for information on the inherent amount of oil in typical aromatherapy plants.

>> **Where and how a plant grows:** Unsurprisingly, plants cultivated for their oil tend to produce more of it. The same type of plant grown in different regions or different soils produce different amounts of oil.

>> **The harvest and storage process:** Essential oils are easily released into the air, so precious oil can be lost during improper harvesting and storage.

>> **How it's distilled:** The type of distiller, how well it works, and if it's tightly sealed and properly adjusted can all make a difference in how much essential oil it produces.

>> **Temperature during distillation:** Some plants have optimum temperatures to use during distillation.

Bringing the Heat: Distillation

Distillation uses steam to pull essential oils from the plant. Chances are that the essential oil you purchase is steam distilled because more than 80 percent of essential oils are produced this way.

Steaming things up

With *steam distillation*, plant matter is suspended over boiling water in a closed container so that the steam rises through it. (Envision a covered vegetable steamer.) The essential oils are quick to hitchhike a ride with the hot steam, which is carried up a long tube surrounded by a cold-water bath. The cold forces the steam to rapidly cool and condense back into water. Water and most essential oils do not mix, so the two go their separate ways — the essential oil into a small collection vial and the water into a large vat. Figure 14-1 is a diagram of a steam distiller.

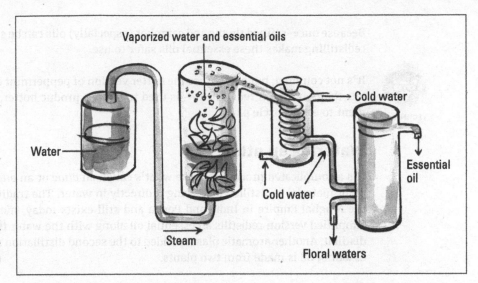

FIGURE 14-1:
An oil distiller
apparatus for
steam distillation
in operation.

The figure is labeled with: Vaporized water and essential oils; Cold water; Water; Cold water; Steam; Essential oil; Floral waters.

Steam distillation can happen in a number of ways:

» **Steam distillation:** The plant material is suspended above boiling water as shown in Figure 14-1.

» **Water distillation:** Plant material is placed directly in the water.

» **Pumped steam distillation:** Steam is pumped directly into a chamber holding the plant material, so there's no contact with water at all. This modern technique is fast but can't be done at home.

Distilling then redistilling

Some oils require a second distillation. Peppermint oil, for example, is commonly *redistilled* or *rectified* — run twice through a steam distiller to extract the oil.

When distilled the first time, peppermint oil smells like peppermint, but the scent is harsh, and so is the taste. Distill the oil a second time, and one sniff reveals that the harshness is gone in favor of the lighter, fresher smell and taste that most people associate with peppermint. The lighter version is considered superior and worth the extra work and expense of distilling the oil twice. Almost all peppermint oil offered for sale is redistilled.

Thyme and camphor oils also are almost always redistilled. This process converts the much hotter, brownish essential oils into a clear version. It alters the aroma of these oils, making them smell less harsh and more refined.

Because once-refined thyme and camphor (especially) oils can be somewhat toxic, redistilling makes these essential oils safer to use.

TECHNICAL STUFF

It's not common, but sometimes the hotter version of peppermint or thyme — the one that's not been redistilled — is used to make a produc hotter, such as a liniment to ease muscle pain.

Watering an attar

It's a complicated process to make what's called an *attae* or an *otto*. The aromatic plant material is distilled by placing it directly in water. The tradition dates from the Mughal Empire in India and Persia and still exists today, mostly in India. A simplified version redistills an essential oil along with the water that was used to distill it. Another aromatic plant is added to the second distillation so the resulting essential oil is made from two plants.

The term attar is also used today as a general term to describe any rose essential oil, as in "attar of rose."

Touching on turbo and other methods

Some essential oils you buy may be made with newer methods that take less time than regular steam distillation and use industrial-size units. They are often used for hard plant materials such as roots, seeds, and barks that are difficult to steam distill.

>> **Turbo distillation** uses *cohobation* — a process in which the water is recycled back into more steam to collect additional essential oil.

>> **Hydrodiffusion** forces steam in from the top of the still rather than from the bottom.

>> **Fractionation distillation** uses different levels of heat to capture and separate the different compounds in an essential oil.

>> **Vacuum distillation** extracts individual compounds in a vacuum.

Pressing and Expressing Oil

You get essential oils from citruses, such as orange, lemon, lime, and grapefruit, by pressing it out from the peels and seeds of the fruit. That's right. You may eat the inner, juicy sections of the fruit, but it's the peel that gets distilled because that's where the essential oil is.

Making citrus essential oil requires a lot of citrus peels, but they're left over from manufacturing citrus juice, so they're readily available.

The technique for extracting citrus oil is similar to the technique used to press olives to make olive oil. The process is simple enough, although you can't do it at home, because it demands a fancy press that operates under pressure.

Citrus oils usually pressed include

>> Grapefruit

>> Lemon

>> Mandarin orange or tangerine

>> Orange

Pressed oils are quite likely to retain the pesticides and herbicides used on the fruit crop. So, if you want to avoid them, go for citrus essential oils produced from organic peels or ones that are steam distilled instead of pressed. During the distillation process, only the tiny essential oils are picked up by the steam. This leaves behind the heavier materials in the peel, as well as most of the pesticides.

Soaking It In: Enfleurage

An ancient method of extracting oils that's still done by a few cottage industries, *enfleurage* is a long process. Flowers are layered by hand on solid sheets of warm animal or vegetable fat, which absorbs the essential oil. The "exhausted" flowers are removed and replaced several times to produce a very fragrant fat. The essential oil is then separated out or left in the fat as a solid perfume.

Enfleurage is mostly used to extract jasmine and tuberose. Their delicate scents can't withstand the heat used during steam distillation and they both continue to exude fragrance after they're picked. Jasmine and tuberose oils you find for sale today are almost always extracted using a solvent (see below for that process) instead of enfleurage.

Pumping the Gas: Using Carbon Dioxide

Carbon dioxide (CO_2) extraction uses non-toxic carbon dioxide gas under high pressure at a constant temperature to extract essential oil. (It's also called supercritical fluid extraction.) Because carbon dioxide is a gas, it can be completely removed from the final product. And, because the process doesn't use high heat, the essential oil retains a scent very close to the plant's natural aroma.

The equipment for this process is expensive, and so are the resulting essential oils so it's done with high-end oils and oils like cannabis that are too resinous to easily steam distill. Several culinary essential oils are produced with CO_2 extraction, because they're in high demand for the flavor industry.

Extracting with Solvents

In *solvent extraction* a liquid solvent solution is used to dissolve the dried plant matter and pull the essential oil from it. A solvent-extracted essential oil is called an *absolute.*

After removing the plant matter, the solvent is boiled off under a vacuum or in a centrifuge to separate it from the essential oil. Because the solvent has a lower boiling point than the essential oil, the solvent evaporates, leaving the oil. When it cools down, the solvent becomes a liquid again and is reused.

At this stage, the semi-solid absolute is appropriately called a *concrete* because it's thick. It sometimes goes into perfume, but usually, the concrete is dissolved into warm alcohol, which is removed. What's left is the absolute.

Because this process is expensive, it's most often reserved for costly oils, many of which cannot be distilled, such as jasmine and vanilla.

A *resinoid* is a thick tree sap, gum, or resin. The resinous frankincense and gummy balsam of Peru are so thick, they are usually produced using either solvent or alcohol extraction.

WARNING

The essential oils produced are said to be relatively free of the toxic solvents. However, some absolutes may retain a residue. Because solvents are odorless, this is difficult to detect. Methods that recover all the solvent or that use non-toxic solvents are being developed. Absolutes are not used to flavor foods or recommended for internal use.

It's your choice. Some aromatherapists avoid using absolutes (solvent-extracted) altogether while others restrict their use to small amounts or use them exclusively to smell. Most perfumers find they can't live without absolutes and the popular highly floral scents that can't be distilled.

Retaining Water: Hydrosols and Aromatic Waters

A lot of water runs through the still during steam distillation. Usually, the water and the essential oil separate, but many essential oils contain water soluble compounds that refuse to separate during this process. Instead, these aromatic compounds stay in the water and make it very fragrant and therapeutic. This oil-water combo is called a *hydrosol*, literally, "water solution." It's also known as a hydrolat, especially in Europe.

Finding and using hydrosols

Hydrosols have many uses and have the advantage of being ready to use. Unlike essential oils, you can put undiluted hydrosols directly on your skin and use them in cooking.

Finding hydrosols is easier than it was 20 years ago, but you still may need to track them down. Look for them in spray bottles. The following hydrosols are the ones most readily available commercially:

>> Chamomile

>> Geranium

>> Lavender

>> Lime

>> Orange blossom

>> Rose

>> Rosemary

>> Sandalwood

>> Lemon verbena

>> Yarrow

Hydrosols are especially good skin moisturizers because they contain essential oil compounds along with water.

Common ways to use hydrosols include:

>> Aftershave

>> Animal flea spray

>> Breath freshener

>> Face moisturizer

>> Freshener for sheets and towels

>> Fruit rinse

>> House plant spray

>> Ironing spray

>> Room freshener

>> Sore throat spray

>> Spray disinfectant

>> Therapeutic mist for massage

A spray bottle makes a great hydrosol dispenser and makes it easy to spritz them on your skin or around the room. I carry hydrosols on my many seminar trips to refresh myself, as well as freshen the places I stay.

The most common hydrosol is rose water. You can find it, along with orange water, in East Indian groceries and liquor stores to flavor alcoholic drinks. The quality of these products is only fair, but they work fine for cooking. Rose water also flavors the Indian yogurt drink lassi.

Storing and keeping hydrosols

Because hydrosols are water based, they lose their scent more quickly than essential oils.

Oxidation changes the scent so the hydrosol smells slightly sour or a little off, or what I can best describe as "flat." The water causes them to oxidize and mold more rapidly, making them unsuitable for skin care when they get old.

Depending on which plant you talk about, most hydrosols last from six months to a year when carefully stored. A few types of hydrosols contain such strong antioxidant essential oils that they last even longer. Examples of these long-lasting hydrosols are rosemary, juniper, bay laurel, and sage.

Some hydrosols don't last very long at all. When I distill lemon-scented hydrosols, such as melissa (lemon balm), they don't last very long even when I store them carefully.

TIP

To retain the quality of hydrosols for as long as possible, store them in super clean bottles in a cool place like a lower shelf in your kitchen. You can even refrigerate them if you want them to last longer. Even if they're brand new, I put my bottles, lids, and sprayer tops through the dishwasher before I pour hydrosols into them. If that's not possible, hand wash everything with soap and hot water. Sterilize lids and sprayer tops in any alcohol, even rubbing alcohol. Just be sure the alcohol is completely evaporated before using the containers.

Shaking up some aromatic waters

Add essential oil to distilled water to produce a fragrant water, and you have an *aromatic water*. Aromatic waters are often confused with hydrosols because both are water-based and are used for the same purposes. (See the preceding section for a list of hydrosol uses.)

Unlike hydrosols, aromatic waters tend to separate, so you must shake the bottle well before each use. The oil and water don't readily mix, but after a few days and lots of shaking, some water becomes scented while the remainder of the oil floats on top. Commercial aromatic waters often contain an emulsifier to keep the oil and water blended.

Aromatic waters are less moisturizing to the skin because the essential oil molecules float around in the water instead of being fully broken down and incorporated with it.

On the plus side, aromatic waters are less expensive than hydrosols. They're a really good deal if you make your own. You can also make a much larger selection.

Doing It Yourself: Distilling Aromatic Waters and Making a Diffuser

If you want to produce your own essential oils, you need to either buy or make a steam distiller. You can purchase ready-made stills — see the Appendix for sources. You can also rig up a makeshift distiller in your kitchen.

REMEMBER

Don't expect your tabletop distiller to produce much, if any, essential oil. With most of the plants you can distill in your kitchen, you end up with scented water and can siphon off a few drops of essential oil floating on top if you're lucky. These few drops may not seem like much reward for all your efforts, but it's still an exciting process to distill your own aromatic plants.

Dishing on distillers

When I bought my first distiller, the only way to get one was to custom order it from a scientific glass blower. Nowadays, you may have a hard time deciding which distiller to get from the wide selection available.

I now appear to be collecting stills because I own two copper distillers, a tabletop brass still, and an assortment of glass distillers in various styles. I've used large stainless-steel distillers and seen a ceramic one in action. Copper distillers are quick to assemble and very attractive, but they don't always have the tight seals of a glass distiller. Sorry, I don't have a favorite. As you can imagine, there's a lot of discussion among distillers about which style is the best, with no consensus.

After you choose the type of distiller you want, keep a couple other considerations in mind. Your distiller must be

>> **The appropriate size:** Before you purchase your distiller, determine what you want to distill and how much. See the upcoming "Choosing what to distill" section.

Distillers range in size from small tabletop units to large, free-standing models. They can hold anywhere from a single cup to many pounds of chopped plant matter.

It's not very efficient to put a quart of plant material into a distiller designed to hold several gallons.

>> **Quick cooling:** The process of the steam reverting to water is what pulls out the essential oils and that depends on rapid cooling. Ask the manufacturer about this.

>> **Well sealed:** You don't want the steam carrying your precious essential oils away.

Choosing what to distill

You need a supply of fresh or dried plant material to distill. You can collect plants from your garden or order dried plants in bulk. Even plants that contain an abundant quantity of essential oils, such as eucalyptus and rosemary, require several buckets of plant matter to produce just a quarter ounce of essential oil. Most fragrant plants contain even smaller amounts of essential oils so distilling less than a few gallons of chopped plant material can result in no essential oil.

REMEMBER

Fresh aromatic plants contain more essential oil than dried ones. Oil evaporates into the air when a plant is dried — up to 40 percent of the essential oil can be lost. On the other hand, you can fit two to three times more dried plant than fresh in a distiller, and the more plant material you distill, the better your chance of obtaining essential oil.

Many essential oils are too fragile to endure the heat of steam distillation. This includes many floral scents, such as jasmine, carnation, lilac, and wisteria. I tried a few of these just to make sure this is true; it is. That's why I don't discuss these oils in this book. However, you can use the plants themselves to make your aromatherapy concoction. The perfect book on using the plants themselves when the essential oil isn't available is my *The Aromatherapy Garden* (Timber Press/Hachette), which is filled with photos of my fragrance garden.

Steam distillation may be a simple technique, but all that hot steam alters the compounds that make up many essential oils. You may notice that some essential oils don't smell exactly like their plant counterparts. That's also why you can't distill sweet floral scents like carnation and violet.

It's a magic act, but plants some times change their chemical composition during distillation. An example is the German chamomile's daisy-like, white and yellow flowers that produce a deep blue essential oil. That blue essential oil is more anti-inflammatory than the flowers before they were distilled. Roman chamomile contains a different set of compounds so it comes out of the distiller as a pale-yellow color.

Assembling your DIY stovetop distiller

You can easily set up a stovetop essential oil distiller in your kitchen. In fact, you might find almost everything you need already in your kitchen. All you need is an old-fashioned pressure cooker. You know, the contraption you slid to the back of a cupboard when you got your instant pot. A pressure cooker makes for a perfect distiller, because the seal on the lid prevents steam from escaping.

TIP

You want a stainless steel pressure cooker rather than aluminum, which might interact with the essential oil.

Other supplies you need for your pressure-cooker distiller include the following:

» **A five-gallon bucket** about half filled with water

» **An open glass quart jar** to catch the essential oil and water you distill

» **A steamer basket** that fits inside the pressure cooker. Ideally, you want one with 3-inch legs. If you can't find a basket with legs that long, fit some metal or silicone tubing around shorter legs to make the steamer basket taller. The goal is to lift the steamer above the water level.

» **Four to five feet of silicone tubing** that fits over the end of the pressure cooker's top spout. The tubing needs to be long enough to drop into the 5-gallon bucket and hang off the end down to the jar on the floor. For this process to work the tubing has to descend.

   You can get the tubing at a hardware store. Buy silicone because it's heat resistant and won't melt or put particles into the hydrosol. Make sure it has an inside diameter of about ¼ inch so that it fits over your pressure cooker's outlet gasket, which is the next item you need.

» **A thin, flexible gasket** made from heat-resistant material. This is also from the hardware store. You put this gasket over the outlet in the pressure cooker cover. Then, slip the silicone tubing over that. This assures a tight seal, although you may be able to slip the silicone tubing right over the outlet without it.

When you have all the equipment assembled, you need a 5-pound bag of ice and the plant material you want to distill. Then, follow these steps:

1. Put the pressure cooker on your stove burner.

2. Add three inches of water.

3. Set the steamer basket inside the cooker and place the aromatic plant material on top of it.

4. Tighten on the pressure cooker lid on the pan.

5. Pop the gasket over the pressure cooker's outlet on its lid.

6. Fasten one end of the tubing to the pressure cooker's air release on the lid.

7. Set the 5-gallon bucket on a stool or chair next to the stove.

8. Place the glass jar on the floor.

9. Curl the rest of the tubing into the bucket, leaving a length hanging over the edge and drop it into the jar.

10. Add ice to the water in the bucket.

11. Turn the burner on high to start boiling the water, and then turn it down but keep the water constantly boiling so it keeps making steam.

Steam signals that the distillation process is starting. Scented water starts to drop from the tube into the jar. Keep an eye on the amount of water in your jar. Turn off the heat when the jar contains about three-quarters of the amount of water you poured into the pressure cooker. Your water is done. Store it in a very clean glass jar.

IN THIS CHAPTER

» **Discovering essential oil chemistry**

» **Meeting the compounds**

» **Looking into variations on the theme**

» **Using chemistry for buying, blending, and storing**

Chapter **15**

Exploring Essential Oil Compounds

I've always been fascinated by knowing how something works, and that extends to my interest in essential oils. So, if you're like me, you want to do more on your essential oil journey than just memorize a list of useful oils for various disorders. You want to know why particular oils are important so that you can decide which scent is really the best choice for each situation. If you, too, are curious about essential oils, then there's no better place to start than discovering what makes scent in the first place.

In this chapter, I give you a peek into the chemistry of essential oils. Before you panic and flip to the next chapter, remember that there isn't a test at the end. And I'm not your mad-scientist chemistry teacher. This chapter helps you make sense of the scientific jargon. I give you a just-the-facts overview so you can get a deeper understanding of how aromatherapy works. True, you don't have to study chemistry to enjoy and reap the benefits of essential oils, but your journey into aromatherapy is much easier if you understand a thing or two about the makeup of fragrant plants. Essential oil chemistry is often a neglected topic, but it's the nuts and bolts that can make more sense out of scents you use.

Journeying into Essential Oil Science

Knowing some simple — with emphasis on the word simple — chemistry helps you select the best aromatic plants for the job. An oil's chemical constituents dictate its fragrance, therapeutic properties, and safety. It guides you in which oils you purchase and in creating blends that are effective *and* smell great—an important consideration because aromatherapy is so much about fragrance! You can rely on a simple understanding of chemistry to help you select and purchase essential oils or substitute one oil for another. You can make wise choices when using them therapeutically and discussing their virtues with other essential oil enthusiasts. Plus, knowing all this technical stuff makes it easier to spot misinformation, which is sadly prevalent in the essential oil field. With a basic understanding of the chemistry behind the smells, you can say, "Ah, that's how they work!"

The mystifying molecules of aroma

An essential oil isn't just one element — each oil is composed of many very tiny aromatic molecules. That's important to know because chemistry mixes and matches these compounds in various combinations. Every time Mother Nature rearranges the pieces, she comes up with a new design fragrance.

REMEMBER

Essential oils are like a giant jigsaw puzzle in which many of the pieces are interchangeable. The compounds described in this chapter are only the pieces of a puzzle. What's most important is how these pieces come together as a whole to make an essential oil. Each component contributes to an essential oil's properties and aroma, but how they come together to act synergistically is what's most important.

Come step with me into a miniature but vast world of chemistry that holds an amazing number of different aromatic compounds.

TECHNICAL STUFF

So far, researchers have identified more than 30,000 aromatic compounds. Some essential oils contain hundreds of different compounds — each contributing its own scent and therapeutic properties! Do the math if you like but take it from me — a mind-boggling number of possible combinations exist. Plants that have a similar aroma are likely to also share some of the same aromatic compounds and healing properties.

Ask a chemist what makes chamomile relaxing or why thyme essential oil is such a potent antiseptic or why so many essential oils have relaxing effects, and they will point to research showing how the individual aromatic compounds in an essential oil work on the body. After all, an essential oil's therapeutic uses depend on which compounds it contains and how much of each one.

Fortunately, it turns out that you carry around a highly accurate sensor: your nose. You can sniff out a lot about which individual molecules are in a plant just by smelling it. Compare the smell of a lemon peel to lemon verbena, lemon balm, lemongrass, lemon thyme, or lemon eucalyptus — either the essential oil or the plant itself. You've probably guessed from their names, before even inhaling their scent, that all these plants smell like lemon. They do. That's because their essential oils contain at least one type of lemon-scented component giving each one its own unique slant on the lemon theme.

But that's only the beginning. You can sniff a whole array of lemony plants that smell distinctly different from each other because their essential oils contain other aromatic components in addition to the lemon-scented ones. For example, lemon thyme essential oil has a component called *thymol* that makes it smell like thyme mixed with lemon. The leaves of the lemon eucalyptus tree contain *eucalyptol* and combine the smell of lemon and eucalyptus.

Keep in mind that essential oils have complex chemistry and that they can contain more than one type of component and fall into more than one category. As you work more and more with essential oils, you'll find yourself recognizing the similarity in the essential oils that are within a category.

REMEMBER

If you understand how essential oils work, you can make better educated decisions on how to use them properly.

The world within the plants

Trust me, you don't have to memorize a bunch of chemical compounds to practice aromatherapy, but being familiar with them helps you realize why essential oils work.

Thank goodness science helps out by grouping essential oil compounds into categories, which makes it easier to see what's what and to compare and contrast the essential oils. Each group shares similar structures. The more a compound resembles another, the more likely it is that it also has similar scent and medicinal properties.

TIP

Each essential oil has a chemical profile. Envision a pie with different sized slices, each representing a different compound. You can determine the percentage of each compound and then make an educated guess how that complete pie, or compound, acts on the body.

I describe the following chemical compounds in this chapter. They aren't the only compounds found in essential oils, but they're the most important ones because they're used to compare the quality, fragrance, and safety of oils. When you go to purchase essential oils, these are the terms you see most often:

>> Alcohols

>> Aldehyde

>> Esters

>> Ketone

>> Phenols

>> Terpenes

Like most compounds, those in essential oils lead a very active life. They charge reactions in the body and mind; they interact with each other; they morph; and they age. Lab analysis can figure out the percentages for each compound in an essential oil, but that only gives the average. These oils all have a history with all sorts of things changing their composition. Growing conditions, how well they've been stored, how old they are, and things they've touched all factor into their composition. (For more on the factors that determine essential oil quality, go to Chapter 3.)

Getting Acquainted with Essential Oil Compounds

Your life is filled with aroma. If you've ever sniffed your way through your kitchen spice rack or held a flower to your nose, you're already acquainted with the many compounds in essential oils used to produce the scents. Smell the fragrant leaves and flowers in a garden and a potpourri of fragrance hits your nose. One rose smells different from another; peppermint is distinctly more peppery that spearmint; and thymes and scented geraniums come in entire fruit bowl selections of scents that range from lemon to rose.

If you'd like to meet the aromatic compounds that make up the world of scent, let me introduce you to them by name. In this section, I also tell you a little about them, how they work, and what they can do for you.

Some of these chemical compounds have names that you already know but in another context. Let go of what you know when I start naming compounds. They may be structurally related but are not the same.

Alcohols: Fighting germs and soothing the body

Alcohol essential oils? Yes indeed, but I'm not talking gin and tonic here. Alcohol comes in many different forms, including the type found in essential oils. In fact, alcohols are abundant in therapeutic essential oils. They occur in the oils most often used in aromatherapy. These gentle compounds have several good qualities:

>> They're safe to use.

>> They rarely cause allergies.

>> They're relatively easy on the liver in the essential oil lineup.

>> They destroy bacterial and viral infections.

>> They're anti-inflammatory.

All these qualities make essential oil alcohols popular ingredients in skin-care products. In fact, many of them are excellent skin toners suitable to heal skin injuries, damage, infections, mature skin, and skin conditions like eczema. I add these essential oils to skin creams and lotions I make.

Even the scent of alcohol is considered a tonic to the nervous system. It relieves anxiety, nervousness, and insomnia and reduces both emotional and physical pain.

Examples of the many essential oils that contain alcohol compounds with the approximate percentage are

>> Basil 50%

>> Coriander: 70%

>> Geranium: 50%

>> Jasmine: 45%

>> Lavender: 35%

>> Marjoram: 55%

>> Neroli (orange blossom): 40%

» Palmarosa: 85%

» Rose: 60%

» Sandalwood: 80%

These are my go-to essential oils to put in massage oils. I choose these oils when I want to see someone feeling so relaxed that they seem to melt into the massage table. It works every time! They're also helpful in massage oil to move lymph so it can better travel around your body picking up toxins and eliminating infection.

TIP

You don't need to have a full-on massage to enjoy the benefits of these essential oils. Rub a massage or body oil containing them on sore muscles, and you'll begin feeling much better in only ten minutes!

Check the labels on your aromatherapy body products, and you'll spot essential oils from this list. For more on using these essentials for skin care, see Chapter 7.

Meet cineol. It's one example of an alcohol compound found in tea tree, bay, and cardamom. This may seem like a diverse group of essential oils with different smells but use your smell imagination to think of what each one smells like. Can you imagine the sharp smell they all share? It's cineol that gives eucalyptus such a sharp smell (although it goes by the name eucalyptol to indicate that it comes from eucalyptus). Cineol destroys bacterial infections and clears lung congestion. You can see why eucalyptus and other oils that contain it are so popular to treat lung problems.

Another alcohol compound is linalool. You see it as a component of popular essential oils, including lavender, bergamot, marjoram, basil, coriander, and neroli (orange blossom), to name a few. Linalool contributes relaxing and sedative properties to these oils, which help ease insomnia and nervousness. Linalool is antifungal and antiseptic. It's considered about five times more effective than the hospital antiseptic phenol.

Aldehydes: Using a bit of citrus

If *aldehyde* sounds like the chemical *formaldehyde*, you're not too far off. But there's no need to be concerned about these essential oils. It's like talking about apples and oranges.

Aldehydes tend to have a citrus-like scent.

» They reduce inflammation and destroy bacterial and viral infections.

» Most produce a light sedative effect when inhaled, so they increase relaxation.

IDENTIFICATION CLUES

Notice how the endings of individual essential oil compounds match the endings of the name of the type of compound itself. The ending designates who's who in the essential oil world.

- Alcohol compounds end with the suffix -ol. An example is cineol.

- Terpenes end their compounds with -ene to match the end of their name, like terpene.

- Ketones end in -one. An example is thujone.

- Phenols tag ol at the end so their names have the same ending as alcohol, as in eugenol

- Aldehydes use the "al" at the beginning of their name to end their compound, resulting in citral.

- Esters get a little more creative. They typically have two names with the first ending in -yl and a second name ending in -ate. An example is methyl salicylate.

At the same time, some aldehydes also have an energetic effect. You can find both actions in lemon, eucalyptus, and cinnamon essential oils.

REMEMBER

A little goes a long way with aldehydes, both smell-wise and for safe use. Sucking on a cinnamon stick can make your tongue feel like it's burning, so you can imagine how much the essential oil can burn. It's suggested to use ¼ to ½ the number of drops of aldehydes compared to gentler oils. They are so strong, some aldehydes can be harsh on the skin. Apply these essential oils to your skin with caution, because they can produce skin irritations and allergic reactions. Citruses, such as lemon, fall under this category. Orange oil is especially notorious for reddening skin.

Relatively unstable, some aldehydes easily oxidize as the oil ages, giving essential oils that contain them a short shelf life. Oxidation (See Chapter 4) increases the skin-irritating effects of the oil. If you have aged oils, sniff them only and don't use those oils on the skin.

TIP

Store aldehyde oils carefully in airtight glass containers away from heat. I purchase expensive aldehyde oils like melissa (lemon balm) in small quantities. Even when well stored, melissa may last a year at best. Still, all's not lost with old oils. They retain much of their antiseptic properties, so you can use them to make a DIY antiseptic cleaning solution: Simply add a half teaspoon of essential oil to a cup of vinegar. I use it on the kitchen counter and floor and put it down the drain to cleanse it.

Essential oils that contain aldehyde compounds include

>> Cinnamon: 76%

>> Citronella: 80%

>> Lemon eucalyptus: 80%

>> Lemongrass: 75%

>> Melissa (lemon balm): 50%

One aldehyde compound with a powerful lemon scent is *citral*. Citral not only makes lemon smell . . . well, lemony, but is also responsible for the lemon scent in lemongrass, lemon verbena, lemon myrtle, and lemon-scented tea tree. Melissa, aptly called lemon balm, contains citral. If you have a preceptive nose, you detect just a hint of lemon from lemony citral hidden in basil oil; lemon basil contains so much citral it's almost all you can smell. It contributes potent antibacterial properties to these oils. The downside is that some people's skin is sensitive to citral.

When it comes to natural insect repellent, citronella essential oil gets top billing. Check out the label on any bug repellent you have on your shelf, and chances are you see citronella listed. It owes both its lemon-like scent and ability to fend off bugs to a compound that's named after it: *citronellal.*

Eucalyptus and tea tree obviously like variety. There are several types of both trees, each producing a different scent. The ones with a powerful lemon scent owe their aroma to the citronellal they contain. It also makes both excellent insect repellents. For more on getting rid of bugs, see Chapter 13. While citronellal is a relatively minor constituent in melissa essential oil, only composing about a third of the essential oil, it's responsible for its lemony fragrance.

Esters: Healing the skin and mind softly

The thought of something fruity may conjure images of fruit salad, but I'm here to tell you about another fruity aroma. *Esters* are strongly aromatic compounds that often have a very fruity aroma. They can also smell floral and herby. that's also described as herby or "green" and often slightly sharp. They're common in therapeutic essential oils. I like how these gentle compounds have a friendly name, like a great Aunt Ester.

REMEMBER

Esters tend to be super safe to use, although you still need to dilute them before use.

Esters are some of the most emotionally and physically relaxing — as well as most loved — essential oils. Traits include

>> Relaxing when inhaled

>> Considered balancing to the mind

>> Fast-acting nervous system and muscle relaxants that help release spasms when you're in pain

>> Antibacterial and often antiviral, making them good choices when your skin is infected

>> Great at countering fungal infections

Feeling uptight or depressed? Take a sniff of an ester essential oil. These are the oils I turn to for an emotional feel-good response. The small compounds of esters easily float through the air, so just one strategically placed drop is enough to help. Simply crushing a lavender flower from the garden or inhaling a cup of chamomile tea will do the trick.

In addition, esters soothe your skin, helping to repair it when it's injured or irritated. Use essential oils that contain esters on acne and other skin blemishes, as well as skin conditions like eczema. Lavender and chamomile are two popular skin-care essential oils. Helichrysum is expensive, but it rivals lavender in the skin repair department.

Esters are exceptionally small and fleeting. Crush an aromatic leaf or put a vase of aromatic flowers on the table, and these are the first essential oil compounds to greet your nose. They're also the first compounds to leave essential oils that you're storing. When you can no longer smell the full bouquet of an essential oil and it smells "flat," you know the esters have begun to evaporate out of the oil. It's not spoiled so you can still use it, although it may have lost some of its properties.

Examples of essential oils that contain esters with their approximate percentages are

>> Benzoin: 70%

>> Bergamot: 40%

>> Chamomile, Roman: 75%

>> Clary sage: 65%

>> Helichrysum: 40%

>> Jasmine: 50%

>> Lavender: 50%

>> Petitgrain: 55%

>> Neroli (orange blossom): 22%

A good example of an ester is *linalyl acetate.* Despite its tongue twisting name, this ester smells great and makes you feel good. It's the perky highlight aroma in lavender, bergamot, clary sage, petitgrain, and helichrysum essential oils. It also lightens up deeply scented jasmine essential oil. Plus, it helps relieve pain caused by inflammation.

When your muscles, joints, or connective tissue are hurting, chances are you reach for a pain-relieving liniment, which certainly contains pain-relieving essential oils like wintergreen. It is almost solely composed of an *ester* called *methyl salicylate.* (If that name rings a bell, that's because it's related to aspirin.) This ester produces a slight warming sensation in massage oils and liniments. To discover more about how liniments work, go to Chapter 11. For guidance on using oils and liniments safely, see Chapter 4.

Ketones: Stimulating your senses

Have you ever sniffed a sprig of rosemary or a bay leaf to improve your memory? Try it, and you'll find the scent mentally stimulating and physically energizing. You can thank the ketones in the plant's essential oils.

TECHNICAL STUFF

Like many of the compounds found in essential oils, ketones share a name with something you want to avoid. You don't want your lab tests to detect high ketone levels, because they signal complications of diabetes. Ketones in the blood are related to the compound found in essential oils, but are manufactured in the body.

Ketones carry a distinctive, camphor-like and sometimes minty aroma. These essential oils are often stimulating to inhale.

Sniffing a ketones-containing oil usually can

>> Perk up your mental and physical energy

>> Enhance your memory. Rosemary and sage have an age-old reputation as scents to improve memory, and they still work just as well today. I use them individually or in tandem. Simply stick a sprig of these fragrant herbs in your pocket or behind your ear, and I bet you feel a little sharper. I put them on my desk next to my computer.

>> Help you think faster

>> Improve lung and bronchial conditions because they thin out congestion to improve breathing. They are often inhaled in a steam to reach deep into the respiratory tract.

>> Promote good digestion, as you might already know about peppermint and fennel seeds

Ketones are also wound healers that promote skin regeneration, so they find their way into first aid products and cosmetics.

WARNING

For all the good they do, just the mention of ketones sends up a red flag to aromatherapists. That's because you need to use some of them cautiously. It's good to review the toxicity of any ketone essential oil before using it. Wormwood and hyssop have such toxic ketones, they aren't used in aromatherapy. If you're a gardener, you can use ketone's toxicity to your advantage as natural insecticides. See Chapter 13 to de-bug your yard.

TECHNICAL STUFF

The problem with the toxic ketones is that they can overstimulate the nervous system. They may become toxic to the nerves or adversely impact the liver. Some ketones build up toxicity in the body. Others are not easily metabolized in the body, which is rough on the kidneys.

While some ketones can be toxic, not all of them are so worrisome. Rosemary and peppermint oils have only small amounts of less toxic ketones. The ketones in dill, caraway, and fennel oils are also less toxic. Juniper and cedarwood's ketones are stronger, so use small amounts of these essential oils on your skin to avoid reactions.

Examples of essential oils that contain ketones with their approximate percentages are

>> Caraway: 54%

>> Dill seed: 50%

>> Rosemary: 25%

>> Sage: 40%

>> Thuja (sometimes sold as cedar): 60%

Some ketones are powerful. The ketone compound called *thujone* can be toxic to the nervous system and liver, so essential oils containing high amounts of it — thuja, tansy, and wormwood — are rarely used. Even culinary sage contains thujone. It's fine to use sage off the spice rack but think twice before using the essential oil. While acting as a consultant to aromatherapy companies, I've had to suggest they limit the amount of sage they use in their commercial products.

Camphor essential oil contains a lot of the camphor ketone. Drugstore liniments designed to ease sore muscles and joints contain camphor for its hot-cold, pain-relieving action. However, don't overdo it. Your skin absorbs camphor, can over-excite the nervous system, and an overdose can even cause convulsions. Find more about liniments in Chapter 11.

Phenols: Heating things up

Phenols are not found in therapeutic essential oils as much as the other groups. They do offer a powerful antibacterial action. They also warm the skin and stimulate blood flow. This heating action lands them in liniments that warm the skin to relieve underlying pain. However, too much, and they irritate or burn the skin. Use them in small amounts both for safety and so that their sharp smell doesn't overpower a blend.

Speaking of burning sensations. Think twice before you put clove oil on the gums of a teething baby. It will dull the pain but not until it causes a lot of pain and irritation. The result? A fretful baby turns into a screaming baby.

Examples of essential oils that contain phenols are

>> Clove: 80%

>> Oregano: 90%

>> Thyme: 50%

The phenol compound called eugenol produces the familiar scent of cloves. So, it's no surprise that it makes up about 90 percent of clove oil. Eugenol gives a clove aroma to allspice and bay rum. If you have a keen sense of smell, you'll detect a clove scent in bay laurel, basil, nutmeg, and marjoram. Even myrrh and ylang ylang have a slight spiciness due to eugenol.

Thymol is a phenol that is used in vapor balms. All of the variations of thyme contain thymol, giving them their characteristic scent mixed with whatever other compounds they contain. Marjoram essential oil contains about half of the thymol as its relative oregano, so its aroma is softer and the action of its essential oil is less toxic.

Terpenes: Feeling good scents

Terpenes are divided into small monoterpenes and the larger sesquiterpenes. Both of them reduce bacterial infection, inflammation, and relieve pain. Quite a few in both categories are feel-good scents that work to influence mood in several ways. Monoterpenes are usually mood uplifters, but they boost your mood in a relaxing way rather than in an energizing way. Sesquiterpenes usually produce feelings of deeper relaxation and contemplation.

Monoterpenes: Keeping you smiling

Monoterpenes are essential oils' largest chemical family. That means you find these compounds in most essential oils. Many of them reduce bacterial and viral infections, inflammation, and pain. Some of them reduce sinus and lung congestion. A few of them even show anti-cancer activity, at least in the lab.

My aromatherapy students often mention that they feel happy just peeling an orange, grating ginger, or scraping lemon zest. It's no wonder when you consider how monoterpenes tend to be mentally stimulating just through their scent. Quite a few of them appear to act directly on the brain's neurotransmitters to increase serotonin, dopamine, or GABA — substances that have a big impact on your mood and sleep.

Monoterpenes can perk you up or relax you. When I first began working with essential oils, a lot of people said the actions of these oils was "all in your head." It turns out the effects are in your head but are due to real physical changes in your brain rather than imagined.

While you may think hot spices like black pepper, ginger, and nutmeg should be stimulating, these essential oils also have a relaxing component.

REMEMBER

Monoterpenes tend to have a sharp scent so a dash of any one of them brightens the fragrance of an essential oil formula. They also make wonderful room scents in an essential oil diffuser. More ideas for scenting your house are in Chapter 6.

Monoterpenes' small and light structure evaporates quickly and produces top notes. They have a relatively short shelf life because they readily oxidize, so they break down when exposed to air. That's especially true of the citrus essential oils.

Examples of essential oils that contain monoterpene compounds with their approximate percentages are

- >> Black pepper: 60%
- >> Cypress: 75%

- » Fir, silver: 90%
- » Ginger: 55%
- » Grapefruit: 96%
- » Helichrysum: 46%
- » Juniper: 87%
- » Lemon: 87%
- » Nutmeg: 75%
- » Orange: 85%
- » Patchouli: 65%
- » Pine: 70%

If you've ever walked through a pine forest, you already know the familiar smell of the terpene compound pinene. A less fun association with it is the smell of pine-scented cleaning solutions like Pine-Sol. Take a sniff of rosemary, frankincense, cypress, or juniper, and you'll detect that same piney scent in the background.

CANNABIS "TERPS"

Terpenes are potent medicines in cannabis essential oil. Yes, cannabis has an essential oil, which is responsible for its strong, characteristic smell. In fact, cannabis contains a few different terpenes.

Several strains of cannabis have been developed, each one with a different terpene make-up and each one working slightly different on the mind and body. Typically, that also gives it a different smell to the discerning nose.

The anti-epileptic and anti-cancer properties in cannabis are at least partially due to its terpenes.

One of the primary terpenes, or "terps" as they've been nicknamed, in cannabis is myrcene. Some strains contain up to 60 percent myrcene in their terpene profile, which gives them a musky, earthy scent. Myrcene has a pine-like but almost floral scent. Studies show it sparks the activity of a cannabinoid receptor. It acts as a sedative and relaxant that also is a strong anti-inflammatory. It appears to block peptic ulcers and even carcinogens from getting a hold in the body. Small amounts of myrcene also occur in the essential oils of bay, thyme, eucalyptus, and lemongrass, and in citrus. Some other cannabis terpenes are helladrene, pinene, and limonene.

The terpene limonene is found in lemon, grapefruit, and orange oils. As you may have guessed, it has a citrus scent, but one that unmistakably hints of turpentine. You'll have to smell carefully to find it, but this light lemon-turpentine scent is also buried in the diverse-smelling essential oils of marjoram, fir, and caraway.

Sesquiterpenes: Keeping you mellow

Sesquiterpenes are larger than monoterpenes. In Latin, *sesqui* means "double." The large, heavy molecules make these essential oils thicker. They go through the skin into underlying tissue more slowly than other essential oil compounds and take a while to evaporate. Sesquiterpenes are often excellent wound healers that encourage cell regeneration. Like monoterpenes, most of them reduce bacterial infection, inflammation, and relieve pain. German chamomile, a favorite to reduce inflammation, is a constant in my skin-care products. I use helichrysum to heal damaged skin.

Sesquiterpenes have a long shelf life; they tend to be stable and do something we dream about: They get better with age. Use them in perfumes, potpourris, and body oils to make the aromas last longer.

Even the scent of sesquiterpenes is heavy. Their scent is typically described as low notes, and aromatically, they are considered emotionally grounding and balancing.

Although used in perfumes, the fragrance of ylang ylang is described as cloying. Descriptions of vetivert smelling like wet soil are even less complimentary. You may be among those who downright hate the heavy scent of patchouli. Yet, the heavy sesquiterpene scent in these oils is invaluable to high-end perfume. Almost every perfume I make contains at least one of them, but only a tiny amount. Perfumers know that a little bit goes a long way. Examples of essential oils high in sesquiterpenes with the approximate amount they contain are

>> Cedarwood, Atlas: 50%

>> Cedarwood, Virginian: 60%

>> Chamomile, German: 35%

>> Cypress: 75%

>> Helichrysum: 40%

>> Ginger: 55%

>> Patchouli: 55%

>> Sandalwood: 90%

>> Ylang ylang: 45%

>> Vetivert: 65%

While most essential oils are more complex, sandalwood contains a whopping 90 percent of *santol*. This sesquiterpene plus alcohol combines the best of both worlds. It's gently healing on the skin and has a calming, meditative scent. Because it is a sesquiterpene, it gets better and thicker with age.

Patchouli oil is rather unique among essential oils because it consists of more than 24 different sesquiterpenes. A 40-year-old patchouli sample I have has turned thick and dark as molasses with an amazing fragrance thanks to all its sesquiter-penes. Even those who dislike patchouli don't recognize it and love the richly aged scent.

Typecasting: Chemotypes

Sometimes plants look like identical twins that only a mother — or in the case of essential oils, a chemist— can tell apart. Botanists identify plants according to how they look visually. Chemists divide plants by their chemistry. That's a big difference. Sometimes a botanist says that two plants look identical, but the chemist steps in to say, "Wait! According to my lab analysis, they have slight variations in their chemical structure." The chemists decided to create their own category and called it a *chemotype*. That's simply shorthand to say, chemical type.

Chemotypes are quirks of nature that develop to help a plant survive. Perhaps a plant needs to adapt to changing weather patterns, a new insect in the area, or a change in soil; maybe a plant migrates to a new environment and finds itself in a different climate. Plants encounter new environments when birds or the wind distribute their seeds, or they get transplanted. When that happens, the plant needs to adapt to its new surroundings.

REMEMBER

Plants are focused on survival, so it doesn't take them long to. These changes can happen from one generation to the very next one. Sometimes a plant doesn't wait and changes itself and then passes those traits on to its offspring. Plants unable to change may die off. This means that the region a plant — and the resulting essential oil — comes from can make a difference.

So, if the new version of the plant looks just like the previous one, what *is* the difference? What changed is the combination of compounds. That change often occurs in the plant's essential oil, altering its aroma. That's valuable to know when you depend upon an oil to have a certain fragrance or effect.

This chemotype talk may all sound overwhelming, but there's no need to panic. You can use aromatherapy in your daily life just fine without knowing the chemotypes. But they do come in handy when you're making your own products and looking for a specific use. For example, maybe you prefer to use a chemotype that's gentler on the skin or one that decreases inflammation better or is more antiseptic. Or you want to use a particular oil in a blend you're making, but you need it to be more lemony or minty. There may be a chemotype waiting for you.

The label should have the essential oil plant's genus and species followed by the abbreviation "ct" (for chemotype) with the chemotype name following that. The thuyanol chemotype of thyme reads *Thymus vulgaris* ct. thuyanol.

Not all species make chemotypes, but some, including basil, thyme, eucalyptus, and rosemary, are quite good at it. You won't run into all of the essential oil chemotypes that nature produces when you're shopping, but here's a list of the ones you're most likely to see.

>> **Thyme:** Grown at sea level in alkaline soil, thymol chemotypes contain strongly antiseptic compounds. Other climates produce the gentler *linalool* chemotypes.

>> **Eucalyptus:** A chemotype of eucalyptus, *cineol,* specifically treats sinus and bronchial congestion.

>> **Rosemary:** The *verbenone* and *cineol* chemotypes of rosemary are sweeter and gentler compared to the harsher camphor chemotype.

>> **Basil:** Tulsi or holy basil can be the herby-smelling *thymol* or clove-like *eugenol* chemotype. Both are strongly antiseptic.

The availability of chemotypes has increased along with the number of online essential oil companies. With a little chemotype knowledge, you'll be better equipped to maneuver your way through the vast selections of essential oils. Otherwise, beginning aromatherapists, and even those who are more practiced, can be baffled.

REMEMBER

To avoid surprises, be aware that chemotypes are not always labeled properly. I've encountered an obvious chemotype with no indication that it's a chemotype. So, one time you might buy rosemary essential oil and find it smells a little harsh and another time it's sweeter. Maybe a eucalyptus essential oil seems a bit too minty or lemony compared to what you've been using. Let your nose lead the way!

4

The Part of Tens

Explore ten underused essential oils to create unique, personal blends.

Add fragrance to your life in ten easy ways

Grow ten great aromatic plants in your own garden.

Chapter **16**

Ten Unique Oils for One-of-a-kind Blends

When you go shopping for aromatherapy products, you'll quickly notice that most of them use the same oils. If you want your aromatherapy experience to be unique, you'll need to experiment with some off-the-beaten path oils.

In this chapter, I introduce you to ten essential oils that probably won't be in your starter kit, but they're all good oils to know. Though they may not be as popular for use in aromatherapy products as the ones you read about in the Essential Oil Guide, you'll find them in some store-bought aromatherapy products, and they're all available for sale as essential oils.

REMEMBER

These essential oils have several unique features that make them valuable, yet they have limited use for several good reasons. Some of these oils have an unusual scent that needs to be carefully worked into an aromatherapy product. You may want to use some of them because they possess a property that's not found in many essential oils.

Here's your chance to make creative choices and create something different and more interesting to stand out above the rest. Just a little bit of these underrated oils can really spice up whatever you're making.

Some of these oils can be somewhat toxic so you'll need to be extra careful. But don't assume you need to avoid these oils. Their toxicity also gives them some unique medicinal properties.

Angelica

Angelica (*Angelica archangelica*) is a tall, stately herb that grows wild throughout much of Europe. Thought to have originated in Syria, angelica was one of the first aromatics to be exported to Asia. It still flavors *Cointreau* liqueur and Benedictine, which is derived from an old monastery brew. There are two similar angelica essential oils. You'll find their scent is pungent and spicy, almost peppery with the root oil smelling a bit more "rooty." The fragrance is aromatic but so potent, you'll probably want to blend it with a softer smelling essential oil.

Angelica works well to aid breathing and relieve coughing. Besides being antiseptic, you can add angelica to massage oil to help regulate menstruation. The scent alone counters depression and helps snap anyone out of shock. Victorian ladies relied on this scent to stop them from fainting. This is an ideal essential oil for those who experience nervousness associated with menopause or hormonally related problems.

Before you start using it liberally, be forewarned that angelica's strong scent easily overpowers any formula that includes it. Chances are that you'll not use much anyway because this is a pricy essential oil. A little does go a long way. That's a good thing because both the seed and root essential oils need to be used carefully and in small amounts. While a small amount of this oil helps conquer nerves, use too much and it might overstimulate the nervous system.

Be especially careful with the essential oil distilled from the root because it contains a compound called *bergaptene*. This compound can cause photosensitivity, or sun sensitivity, and can give some people a rash. So, you don't want to apply a product that contains angelica root essential oil directly on your skin and then venture out into the sun.

Camphor

Camphor (*Cinnamomum camphora*) is a tree from Asia with aromatic inner bark and leaves. The scent is often compared to the sharp, synthetic smell of mothballs. However, camphor is more aromatic with a pleasant woody scent and a spicey hint of cardamom.

If you've enjoyed pain relief from any drugstore liniment, chances are it contained camphor essential oil. That's because camphor's unique hot-cold action on nerve endings increases the sensation of heat in a liniment. For more on how camphor tricks pain, refer to Chapter 11.

Camphor's scent is potent enough to counteract shock and depression. In China, the wood is burned as ceremonial incense. More about hydrosols is explained in Chapter 14.

WARNING

Camphor needs to be used with some caution because it is a heart stimulant and skin irritant. You should even be wary of rubbing on a lot of liniment containing camphor if you have a heart or nervous system condition. Stay away from the toxic brown camphor from heavier parts of the oil and yellow Borneo "camphor" (*Dryobalanops aromatica*). You can also turn to Chapter 4 to learn more about how to use essential oils safely.

Ravintsara (*Cinnamomum camphora ct. cineol*) is the camphor that I prefer. It's what's called a *chemotype* because it's a camphor tree, except this particular tree from the island of Madagascar contains little camphor compound. It does have a highly antiseptic compound called *cineole*, which is abundant in eucalyptus essential oil, giving it a eucalyptus-like scent. Ravintsara is safe for treating skin, respiratory, viral infections like shingles, and for acne and oily skin problems. A massage oil containing ravintsara helps with muscle fatigue and lymphatic problems. It costs a little more than the super cheap camphor essential oil. Don't confuse it with the related ravensara (*Ravensara aromatica*) oil, which has different chemistry and properties.

Coriander

You may think this humble herb belongs more on your kitchen spice rack than in your essential oil collection. To tell you the truth, it's happily at home in both spots. Coriander (*Coriandrum sativum*) seed and leaves may not be the topmost choice for aromatherapy, or even for cooking, but a little dash adds the perfect hint of spice in either scenario. The seed scents aromatherapy soap. You'll find it gives a subtle, spicy punch to other essential oils in your aromatherapy product blends. The aroma is uplifting and motivating and helps relieve stress.

TIP

It makes a surprisingly good substitute for the rose-woody aroma of rosewood (*Aniba roseodora*) oil because the two share a similar chemistry. You can bring it even closer to rosewood by adding a little rose geranium, or palmarosa essential oils. I use this substitution because the rosewood tree is verging on being endangered in the wild. See Chapter 3 to learn more.

You're most likely to find coriander's spicy, sharp aroma in a natural deodorant because it's particularly good at neutralizing body odor. It's a good antiseptic and antifungal. Coriander also soothes inflammation, rheumatic pain, and headaches. The main commercial use for coriander essential oil is packaged foods and flavoring liqueurs like Cordial Medoc and Danziger Goldwasser.

Lemon Verbena

Lemon verbena (*Aloysia triphylla*) is a popular garden herb that I bet you'll love as much as I do. The leaves often find their way into a tasty herbal tea for my herb classes. You'll find it adds its unique scent to commercial hair rinse products and hand lotions. The scent is lemony and pleasantly herbal so not as sharp as lemon. It isn't cheap, so lemon essential oil often sneaks into lemon verbena "products" to cut the cost. While this is a sneaky practice, it's a technique you can use yourself when putting together your own lemony blends. For more on making your own essential oil blends, see Chapter 5.

Lemon verbena is a relaxing and downright happy scent that works in two seemingly opposite directions. It perks you up and improves your concentration while also treating nervous conditions and encouraging sleep.

Other attributes of lemon verbena are its ability to counter infections, such as *staph* and *E. coli*. It's used for colds, offering sinus congestion relief. In parts of South America, lemon verbena tea is one of the most popular remedies for asthmatics. Even inhaling the scent coming off a hot cup of lemon verbena tea is helpful to do in between asthma attacks.

The essential oil is used in products that are designed to help oily complexions and to scent bodywash and hair rinse. The diluted essential oil works well on hard-to-heal wounds.

WARNING

For all its good smells and properties, lemon verbena can irritate skin, so always be sure that's it's well diluted before you use it.

Litsea

The litsea (*Litsea cubeba*) tree is in the same laurel family as bay laurel that produces the well-known bay leaves. You can spot the similarity between the two plants as you sniff the peppery scent that they share. The obvious difference is how a delightful citrusy lemon predominates in litsea. The tree grows in India, Southeast Asia, and China, where it is known as May Chang. Often sold under this name, the essential oil is distilled in China from the aromatic leaves. The tea made from the scented flowers is both calming and somewhat mentally stimulating.

Traditional Chinese medicine says the scent of both leaves and flowers encourages the flow of *chi*, or vital energy, through the kidney and bladder area. Litsea essential oil eases physical pain. Just taking a sniff of it helps to relieve emotional turmoil, anxiety, and even shock. I carry litsea in my herbal first-aid kit to have it on hand for this purpose. I also put a little bit in a remedy when the injury or condition has been caused by trauma.

Litsea is an antiseptic on bacterial and fungal skin infections and acne. It also treats asthma and bronchitis, and it helps counter allergic reactions. One way to use it is in a throat spray. It does need to be used in small amounts and always greatly diluted because the essential oil can be a skin irritant. Always use it diluted.

WARNING

Don't use litsea at all on sensitive skin or anyone who has glaucoma because it is known to increase eye pressure, at least in animals.

Oregano

If you enjoy eating pizza and pasta, you're already familiar with this ultimate Italian seasoning. In fact, oregano (*Origanum vulgare*) smells so much like dinner, it found little use in aromatherapy until it was popularized as a cure-all. The claims were exaggerated, but since then it has become a go-to oil for some people.

Oregano essential oil is a powerful antiseptic agent that destroys many viral infections, as well as almost all bacteria that it has been tested against, including *Salmonella* food poisoning and *staph* skin infections. It is also effective against respiratory infections.

WARNING

The problem is that this potent oil isn't the safest choice because it is a skin irritant. Plus, continual use can be rough on the liver and kidneys. Eating oregano as a spice is perfectly safe, so do enjoy your pasta! It's only the highly concentrated essential oil that can lead to trouble.

Capsules are designed to destroy digestive infections like candida in the digestive tract because they contain only minute amounts of the essential oil. Make sure they are in *enteric* capsules because these capsules don't open until they reach the intestines. Otherwise, the essential oil is absorbed long before it reaches its destination. See more on safety in Chapter 4.

TIP

I often prefer using the closely related marjoram essential oil over oregano oil. Much gentler, marjoram still packs a punch and reduces inflammation. When strong antibiotic action is needed, I think of eucalyptus, lavender, or tea tree because they reduce inflammation yet don't contain the worrisome compounds found in oregano essential oil.

Rosewood

This South American rainforest tree often goes by its French name *bois de rose*, or "wood of rose." The fragrance is a beautiful combination of sweet rose with woodsy aroma that's complimented by just a hint of spice. The aroma of rosewood (*Aniba roseodora*) eases headaches, nausea, depression and helps balance emotions. It fights many types of infections including colds. Because rosewood helps rejuvenate cells, it's suitable for use on all complexion types.

TECHNICAL STUFF

Rosewood is distilled from the woodchips of the fallen tree. It was first distilled in 1875 in French Guiana, but the essential oil became so popular that almost all the trees were cut down. As much as I love this essential oil, I don't use it due to ecological concerns. I'm including it here in the hopes that a more sustainable solution to its production is on the horizon so we can all enjoy it. See Chapter 3.

Rose geranium, palmarosa, and even coriander serve as a substitute for rosewood's aroma and some of its properties.

Sage

Sage (*Salvia officinalis*) essential oils come from the same sage you grab off your kitchen spice shelf to flavor your food. You likely know its distinctive sharp, but very herby scent as a flavoring in turkey dressing, but small amounts of this seasoning creep into other foods. Sage essential oil is an ingredient in some deodorants. It not only destroys bacteria responsible for body odor, but it also reduces perspiration.

Sage's antioxidant properties are on a par with another seasoning, rosemary. Both of these help preserve food.

Inhale sage essential oil as steam because it's a decongestant with strong antiseptic properties. It treats throat and mouth infections in sore throat gargles.

It's also used on oily skin and acne, and it is said to encourage hair growth. It has a reputation for alleviating hot flashes.

Put the aromatic sage water or the hydrosol (the aromatic water portion that remains after the oil is distilled) in a spray bottle.

New research shows that loss of short-term memory, Alzheimer's disease, and possibly other degenerative brain diseases may be helped by just sniffing the scent of sage.

WARNING

It isn't recommended to use the essential oil if you're prone to seizures because it brings them on in some people. Sage essential oil contains high quantities of a compound called *thujone* that can be toxic to the nervous system, injure the kidneys, and irritate the skin and mucous membranes.

The closely related clary sage essential oil, with many of the same properties, is profiled in the Essential Oil Guide.

Spikenard

Spikenard (*Nardostachys jatamansi*) has an earthy and heady scent that's reminiscent of its herbal relative, valerian patchouli. Add this intense oil to your aromatherapy blends with a light hand.

The sedative scent treats nervous conditions, headaches, insomnia, emotional tension, and anxiety. In a body or massage oil, it relieves muscle pain. Studies indicate that spikenard essential oil may even promote the growth of damaged nerve endings — something that wasn't known to be possible a decade or so ago.

Other uses are to counter skin inflammation, rashes, psoriasis, and a dry or mature complexion. It's been used for hair loss and scalp irritation.

However, there are ecological concerns about this oil's sustainability in the environment. See Chapter 3 for more on this.

Tuberose

The intensely aromatic tuberose (*Polianthes tuberosa*) flower hails from Mexico where it was prized by the Aztecs for its use as both fragrance and medicine. In Hawaii, the flower leis worn around the neck are often made with it.

The name comes from its tuberous root. The scent is a very sweet and heady floral that's rich and honey-like with a slight hint of camphorto that resembles jasmine.

Its main use is in perfumes like White Shoulders and Chloe and other perfumes that are so popular, you might already be wearing tuberose. It's considered an aphrodisiac. In fact, its name in India is *rat ki rani*, meaning "mistress of the night."

As one of the most expensive floral oils, when you see it in a product, it's almost always a synthetic oil. The solvent-extracted oil has a slightly "green" scent. This process is described in Chapter 14.

Chapter **17**

Ten (or so) Ways to Add Fragrance to Your Life

Throughout this book, I offer dozens of ways to incorporate aromatherapy into your life without ever stepping out your front door. In this chapter, I give you ten or so ways to have aromatic experiences by venturing a little farther.

Each of these ideas is a particularly nice experience to either share with a friend or explore on your own. My advice is to be adventuresome, and you can really go places with aromatherapy!

Plant Your Own Fragrant Herb Garden

Growing your own herbs for use in aromatherapy not only gives you a good supply of aromatic material, but it also makes your home and its surroundings more beautiful and fragrant. I love having my own fragrance garden, but if that's sounding a little too ambitious for now, you can plant some aromatics in your existing landscaping.

TIP

The next time you lose a plant, need to tear out a section of your garden, or spot an empty space amongst your plants, consider filling in that spot with fragrance in the form of an aromatic plant.

You can buy plants at plant nurseries, herb farms, and farmer's markets. If you're looking for unusual herbs not offered at these places, track down mail-order companies that carry a large selection of plants or seeds. You can also search the web for an individual plant you're after, preferably by its botanical name.

Get an Aromatherapy Facial

Take the time to give yourself a real treat. You and your skin will enjoy and benefit from a facial that incorporates essential oils. Some esthetician-aromatherapists offer facials, as do salons and spas.

You can buy aromatherapy products containing essential oils. You can also really get into it and use the directions in this book to make your own aromatic facial products using the aromatherapy products and techniques I describe in Chapter 7.

TIP

If you can't splurge right now on a professional facial, trade with a friend and give each other facials.

A facial can make a very thoughtful gift. It may seem like an unusual present, but give a friend their own, customized aromatherapy facial, and I guarantee they'll love it. You can give a facial through a gift certificate to a salon or offer to give one yourself.

Get a Massage with an Aromatherapy Massage Oil

Most massage practitioners use an oil or lotion when they give a massage, usually a scented one. For the ultimate experience, seek out a practitioner trained not only in using different essential oils for their aromatherapy effects, but also in different aromatherapy techniques.

Try a custom-designed massage Ayurvedic-style. This uses oils and techniques based on ancient healing practices from India. It is an aromatic experience that you won't forget.

You can find many massage oils made with essential oils available for sale. If you're feeling that creative bug, make your own massage by adding essential oils to a vegetable oil base, using the recipes in Chapter 5.

TIP

If you make your own massage oil, find a bodyworker willing to use your blend instead of their standard one. Some masseuses liked my version of massage oil or body oils to relieve pain and cramping so much, I supplied them with it to use on their other clients. I've heard similar stories from others, so it could happen that you end up selling your own exclusive line.

Take an Aromatherapy Class

As the popularity of aromatherapy grows, so does the number of educational possibilities. Aromatherapy classes and seminars are certainly an aromatic experience in themselves!

Some courses offer certificates to show that you completed the course, although at this time, the United States doesn't require or provide a license to practice aromatherapy. Many aromatherapists like myself offer certificates based on guidelines from national organizations like the National Association of Holistic Aromatherapists and the Alliance of International Aromatherapists. I provide a list in the Appendix to help you find these courses.

Web and mail-order courses offer ample opportunity to study from home. Still, learning about aromatherapy in a classroom setting really brings it to life because you can sniff the oils and aromatic plants as they're discussed. There's nothing like having a hands-on course in which an instructor guides you through creating your own blends. If you're interested in distilling oils yourself, seeing a live demonstration of distilling essential oils offers invaluable tips. I tell you about distillation methods that extract the essential oils from aromatic plants in Chapter 14.

Visit a Fragrance Garden

Whenever I travel to conduct a seminar, my first question is whether I can visit a botanical garden, an herb farm or shop, or some other aromatic place while I'm there. By now, I've seen the United States by following my nose. Most major cities have a botanical garden, and these gardens usually include a fragrance garden. I've had the good fortune to live close enough to visit the Los Angeles County Arboretum in Arcadia and the San Francisco Botanical Garden Arboretum in Golden Gate Park many times. Both have fragrance gardens as a part of their herb gardens. These aromatic gardens are purposely set in a raised bed on a hillside, placing the fragrant plants at your fingertips and at nose level. I love how the fragrance gardens are designed with the low-vision visitor in mind. The Los Angeles Arboretum's aromatic herb garden is even dotted with easy-to-reach signs that identify each plant in Braille, which made it a favorite haunt for me and my blind mother.

TIP

To find a botanical garden near you

>> Do a web search for "public garden" plus the name of the city or other area.

>> Ask at the local university or college. You can often find a small public botanical garden associated with a university. Even if you don't, the botany department can usually point you in the right direction.

>> Call a local plant nursery. The staff often knows the whereabouts of public gardens.

>> Tap into the local chapter of the Herb Society of America.

You almost always find at least one public garden in a major city in the United States. This is also true in many other countries throughout the world.

Some private herb farms and gardens are open to visitors, although often only when they hold classes or events or by appointment. Private gardens likely have many fragrant plants, even if they don't devote an area specifically to them. Some large gardens — like my own — do have a fragrance garden.

Take an Aromatherapy Tour

You can join a special tour to visit aromatherapy hot spots, such as the aromatic lavender fields, herb fairs, and essential oil distilleries of Provence, France, or Tuscany, Italy. I've led tours to both spots, and what an amazing experience to travel with a group of like-minded plant lovers. Provence and Tuscany are the aromatic hotspots to visit, but you can find other smell-worthy destinations. Perhaps you fancy the rose distillation and fragrance bazaars of Turkey or incense making and the fragrance gardens and forests in Japan.

REMEMBER

International aromatherapy conferences often tour local spots related to essential oils either before or after the conference so that you can see the aromatic sights of the area. If you enjoy immersing yourself in everything botanical, you can join tours organized by botanical gardens, botanical organizations, garden magazines, and garden clubs. The Appendix can help you follow your nose to track down these opportunities.

Since fragrance is my thing, I always search out aromatic hotspots so I can organize my trip to visit them. You can follow my lead by adding some interesting side trips to your vacation or business trip. On the web, search for terms such as "botanical tour" and "aroma tour."

Take an Aromatic Bath, Ahh!

One fragrant experience to try at home or when you finally get away and have the time to luxuriate is a warm, aromatic bath. An aromatic bath is a great way to relax and takes just 30 minutes— but please, take as long as you like! If you're like many folks these days, finding even that much time to relax may not happen very often. But, go ahead and splurge. It's good for your health and peace of mind.

Follow these steps for a great, relaxing bath experience.

1. **Arrange your bathing supplies: thick scented towel, warm robe, slippers.**
2. **Put on soothing music. Your choice, of course!**
3. **Make a soothing cup of chamomile tea and drink it while the tub fills.**
4. **Add half a cup of scented bath salts to your hot bath water.**
5. **Light a candle and turn off the lights.**
6. **Step into your bath and relax for 30 minutes with no thoughts of the outside world.**
7. **Emerge and dry off, then dust with a fragrant powder or apply a moisturizing cream to your entire body.**
8. **Wrap up in your warm robe and carry the candle to the bedroom.**
9. **Place a fragrant dream pillow under your bed pillow, slip into scented sheets, and enjoy fragrant dreams and a restful sleep.**

   (See Chapter 6 for directions on making your own dream pillow.)

Bring in a Fragrant Bouquet

This room-scenting solution may seem too simple to work, but adding a bouquet of fragrant flowers can scent an entire room. Mostly flowers emit scent out into the air (in case a bee flies by), although some leaves like eucalyptus and rosemary are strong enough to use for room scenting. And, you get to enjoy their beauty, as well.

People have been scenting their homes this way for a long time. The healing nature of floral scents has been appreciated for centuries. An "ailing" person's friend or loved one would choose or create a bouquet with a scent that was appropriate for the situation. They might choose lavender to cheer someone up, stick in a few sprigs of rosemary to help them get through grief, or declare their love with roses.

Giving fragrant flowers is a custom that still works today. (We still take flowers to ailing friends and family in hospitals or use floral arrangements to pay our respect at funerals.) Follow your nose to decide what scents you like best and then add some of the flowers and plants that are recommended in this book to treat different moods. See the descriptions in the Essential Oil Guide for help.

Scent a Message

The greeting card industry still thrives even in the digital age. You can make giving someone a card even more personal by adding scent.

It takes just one drop of the essential oil of your choice. Place a drop on a piece of paper and tuck it into a box of cards or stationery overnight to subtly scent the whole batch. Want something more potent? Take a glass rod or toothpick, dip it in an essential oil, and dab each card. Once scented, keep your cards and stationery in an airtight container.

Scent is a way to connect with more than friends and family. One of my students said they'd been sending letters to their congressional representatives for years and receiving form letter responses. Then, they sent a scented letter and received a personal reply — and have for each subsequent letter since.

Chapter **18**

Ten Herbs to Grow for Fragrance

For many years, herbs have perfumed the air around my house. They adorn the landscaping with color and textures. An assortment of butterflies and hummingbirds come to visit them. Herbs are a cinch to cultivate. Even if you don't think you have a green thumb, you'll probably be surprised how easy it is to grow herbs. They're much less demanding than vegetables or flowers. If you already have a flower or vegetable garden or plot, simply tuck in a few fragrant herbs. If not, you can grow a good selection of herbs in a few square feet of ground or in a planter. Many of the essential oils I discuss in this book come from fragrant herbs that you can grow yourself. You can use the herbs you grow to cook and to make the many different aromatherapy products I describe throughout this book.

In this chapter, I describe ten fragrant herbs that are especially easy to grow, even in a small area or in a container. In the following sections, I give you the basics to cultivate each one. I tell you whether the herb plant is an *annual* (lives for only one season), a *perennial* (lives for many years), or a *biennial* (lives for two years and doesn't flower until the second one). I also let you know how much sun it needs, the best soil conditions, how big it will get, and some special tips in case you want to grow your herbs in containers. For how to use these herbs and their essential oils, look them up in the Essential Oil Guide.

TIP

You may discover your green thumb when you plant some of these herbs, or at least understand why so many people love to grow plants. If you find yourself interested in cultivating an aromatic herb garden, check out my book, *The Aromatherapy Garden* (Timber Press). It covers 100 fragrant herbs and even more varieties — all the favorites I've grown. The colored photographs in the book are of my garden, so you can see what they'll look like when you plant them in your garden.

Basil, culinary

Bushy basil grows so rapidly it fills in empty spots in your garden and forms an attractive, low border along a pathway. Or follow the example of the Italians, Moroccans, and Greeks and set pots of basil on a sunny porch or windowsill to repel flies and mosquitoes. (Basil is also rumored to attract lovers!)

You can choose from 150 to 350 basil species (no one can agree) in a variety of fragrances, including lemon-scented and anise-scented types.

You may as well plant basil from seed because it sprouts in about a week. If you cut back the flower stalks, your plants stay compact and continue to produce more leaves throughout the summer for culinary delights like pesto, as well as for your aromatherapy projects.

Facts about basil:

>> **Type:** Annual

>> **Sun needs:** Full sun

>> **Soil needs:** Dry, medium rich, and well-drained soil

>> **Size:** Grows to 2 feet tall by 1 foot wide.

>> **Notes:** Basil grows especially well in a container, even a small half-gallon-sized pot. It even thrives indoors if placed in a sunny window. When it's growing in a pot, keep the herb trimmed down and be sure to use all the leaves you trim off to flavor your meals.

Bay Laurel

This attractive plant's main feature are its shiny, leathery leaves; its clustered yellow flowers, which bloom in June and July, are very small. The tradition of potting bay began in Europe, to make it easier to bring the plant indoors to winter and avoid the possibility of a hard winter (below 28 degrees F) killing it. Potting bay also stunts its growth, so the scented leaves are easier to pick. Otherwise, bay grows into a huge tree. Add the leaves to your beans and soups, use them to keep the bugs out of your grains, and use them in your aromatherapy projects. The seeds seem to take forever to sprout, so start bay from a plant.

Facts about bay:

>> **Type:** Perennial.

>> **Sun needs:** Sun or partial shade

>> **Soil needs:** Well-drained and sandy

>> **Size:** If not planted in a pot, it can grow into a 25- to 60-foot-tall tree. The milder the climate, the taller it grows. In a pot, it can grow several feet tall.

>> **Notes:** If you plant bay in a pot, make sure that the pot is large enough. It can start off in a gallon-sized pot and grow very slowly but eventually graduates to at least a 5-to-10-gallon pot. Be sure to keep it trimmed back so it doesn't outgrow that pot. All the bay leaves you trim off come in handy to flavor your soups and stews.

Chamomile, German and Roman

Both Roman and German chamomiles are spindly, feathery plants. They bloom in early summer with a profusion of small, daisy-like flowers. Roman chamomile makes a fragrant ground cover.

TIP

If you're planning on using chamomile for tea, grow the sweeter German chamomile. It prefers seeding directly where it will grow and comes up within a couple of weeks. Sow it early in the spring, or the plants become leggy in hot weather. Water the young seedlings gently so that they don't fall over into the mud.

Facts about chamomile:

>> **Type:** German chamomile is an annual; Roman chamomile is a perennial

>> **Sun needs:** Full sun

>> **Soil needs:** A rich soil produces lush growth, but fewer flowers. For more flowers, use a light, sandy, and well-drained soil.

>> **Size:** Grows to 1 to 2 feet tall by 1 foot wide (German chamomile) or 6 inches tall by 6 inches wide, and then it spreads out (Roman chamomile).

> **» Notes:** If you're growing in a pot, Roman chamomile is a better choice than German, but either works provided it has a fairly sunny location and adequate moisture. Be prepared for the annual German chamomile to become thin and wispy in a pot. It probably won't last long and may not flower.

Clary Sage

Clary sage's large, heart-shaped leaves grow from a central stalk that eventually bends with the weight of its showy, lilac or pale blue flowers in June and July. The resinous flowers are where you find this herb's fragrance. Clary sage is effective when planted in isolated groups, with other herbs in a mixed border, or by itself in a container. Start it from seeds — they sprout in less than two weeks — or from plants purchased at a nursery. Read about the different types of sage in the Essential Oil Guide.

Facts about clary sage:

» **Type:** Biennial

» **Sun needs:** Full sun

» **Soil needs:** Likes well-drained, fertile soil. It prefers slightly moist soil but can tolerate dry spells in between waterings.

» **Size:** Grows to 3 to 5 feet tall by 1 to 3 feet wide

» **Notes:** A two-gallon pot is best for clary if you're doing container gardening. That gives it enough room to look good and produce some flowers. It needs at least a 5-gallon pot to reach full size and flower abundantly.

Lavender

Try to plant lavender where your garden visitors can sniff its fragrant buds and admire its soft, gray foliage. The very fragrant, vivid purple flowers cluster on tall spikes in the summer. They contrast well in your garden with pink-flowering herbs such as pink yarrow or roses. Collect the flower stalks when the buds are still tight, and they'll hold their scent for years.

Lavender is difficult to grow from seed or cuttings, so buy plants. Once established, the plants live at least 12 years. Of the many subspecies and cultivars, English lavender is the most fragrant and the hardiest. French lavender is the best choice if the soil isn't well drained. If you live where the winter temperatures drop below freezing, surround the base of the plants with straw or leaves and be sure that your plants are in a well-drained area.

Facts about lavender:

>> **Type:** Perennial

>> **Sun needs:** Full sun

>> **Soil needs:** Sandy, very well-drained soil

>> **Size:** Grows to 2 to 3 feet tall by 2 to 3 feet wide

>> **Notes:** The dwarf Munstead lavender is better suited for a container, rather than the much larger, standard-size lavender. Munstead is only about 2 feet tall and doesn't tend to flop over like standard lavender. Most nurseries sell this or another type of miniature lavender for this very reason. You can start off putting it in a half-gallon container the first year. It needs a 5-gallon pot in a couple of years to keep it from becoming stunted.

Marjoram

Marjoram is a small, bushy herb that looks nice when placed near the edge of a bed or terrace. Plant it where it's easy to reach so that you can pinch its leaves and release its scent — unlike many culinary herbs, marjoram doesn't automatically perfume the air.

The slightly hardier "pot" marjoram that hails from southeast Europe and Turkey is often considered a substitute because it can make it through a winter if the ground doesn't freeze (although this type is less aromatic with a coarser flavor).

Sowing marjoram from seed is tricky because, although the seeds sprout easily, the young plants are fragile and subject to damping-off disease or being knocked over by a forceful watering. Go the easier route and buy plants and then divide the roots when they're established. Tiny white flowers appear throughout the summer, but keep marjoram cut back to encourage leaf growth and to keep it from getting "leggy."

Facts about marjoram:

>> **Type:** Perennial (although in cold climates, it's usually cultivated as an annual).

>> **Sun needs:** Full sun

>> **Soil needs:** Well-drained, dry soil

>> **Size:** Grows to 2 feet tall by 1 foot wide, and then it spreads out.

>> **Notes:** Marjoram prefers at least a half-gallon container. In a hanging basket on your porch or patio, it gracefully hangs over the edge. It's a spreader, so it eventually covers a wide container or becomes ground cover.

Melissa (Lemon Balm)

Lemon balm flowers are inconspicuous, but their yellow-green, lemon-scented foliage looks good in your garden growing next to deep greens. The cultivar golden lemon balm has especially attractive, variegated leaves.

TIP

If you live in a climate where the ground can freeze, plant lemon balm in a protected location and put straw or leaf mulch around its roots during the winter.

You can start it from plants or seeds or divide the thick root clumps into individual plants. Melissa is a prolific self-sower when it gets established. (In fact, if any of your neighbors have lemon balm, chances are that they have extra plants that they'd love you to take.)

Facts about lemon balm:

>> **Type:** Perennial

>> **Sun needs:** The plants grow lusher in full sun but tolerate partial shade.

>> **Soil needs:** Fertile and moist, but very well drained because soggy ground kills it.

>> **Size:** Grows to 3 feet tall by 2 feet wide.

>> **Notes:** Melissa seeds like crazy and seems to grow almost anywhere, including in a pot. Use at least a 3-gallon pot for a full-sized bush.

Peppermint

Peppermint is common and grows so easily that you may want to curb its growth to keep it from taking over your garden by planting it in a container. The easiest way to grow peppermint is to separate the roots and replant them.

The couple dozen species of mint have been hybridized so much that you can now choose from quite a selection. Very small, lilac-pink flowers bloom on short flower stalks throughout the summer.

Facts about peppermint:

>> **Type:** Perennial

>> **Sun needs:** Partial shade is best because full shade or full sun reduce peppermint's oil content.

>> **Soil needs:** Moist-plus soil is best. It can even handle excessive wetness.

>> **Size:** Grows to 3 feet tall by 1 or so foot wide, and then it spreads out.

>> **Notes:** Peppermint grows in just about anything, even a small, 4-inch container, but use something larger if you want lush growth. If you go bigger, peppermint is beautiful cascading over the edge. I have most of my mint collection in 4-to-10-gallon pots to keep all the different species contained and separated. Otherwise, they'll try to take over my entire fragrance garden!

Rosemary

Rosemary is a tall, graceful bush and an early bloomer, with its pale blue flowers appearing in late winter in mild climates. It lends itself to pruning and being formed into interesting topiary shapes or trimmed into a hedge. To imitate the Tudor style, train it into patterns against a wall or fence. If you try this, be sure to get an upright or standard rosemary. The other, low-growing ground cover rosemary is nice to cascade over a hanging pot or terrace.

The easiest way to start either one is to purchase the plants. Once it is established, you can propagate it by *layering*. For this technique, lay a few branches on the ground and cover them with a little mound of dirt. Keep this mound watered, and eventually roots will sprout. After a few months, cut the new plant off of the "mother" plant and replant. Mulch the roots in the winter with straw or leaves if your ground freezes and temperatures dip below 20 degrees F.

Facts about rosemary:

>> **Type:** Perennial

>> **Sun needs:** Full sun

>> **Soil needs:** Well-drained, fairly dry soil

- » **Size:** Standard-size rosemary grows up to 5 feet tall by 4 feet wide in a mild climate. Creeping rosemary is 8 to 12 inches tall, depending upon the variety. It's about 10 inches wide, and then it spreads out.

- » **Notes:** Rosemary makes an attractive picture in a container due to its swooping branches. Grow it in a 1-gallon pot or choose a 5-gallon container if you want a larger plant. You can use either the standard, upright plant or creeping rosemary, depending on which height you like. Creeping rosemary is easier to grow in a small pot.

Thyme

Thyme looks great when planted along a pathway, in a rock garden, or as a fragrant ground cover. It's particularly attractive cascading over a raised terrace or the side of a hanging pot.

Choose from a couple hundred different species and numerous cultivars, including lemon, caraway, and creeping thyme. Planted together, different thyme plants play off each other's colors. Tiny, white to lilac flowers bloom profusely throughout the summer.

Thyme's delicate root system makes it difficult to transplant except from a nursery pot. If you must transplant it, give the plant several months to re-establish its fine root system before a freeze. Even established plants can be damaged if the ground freezes solid, but a layer of sand on the soil helps prevent frost damage.

Facts about thyme:

- » **Type:** Perennial
- » **Sun needs:** Full sun
- » **Soil needs:** Well-drained, light, rather dry, soil
- » **Size:** Grows to 8 inches tall by about 8 inches wide, and then spreads out. (The height varies with the different types.)
- » **Notes:** Because thyme spreads, grow it in a wide container, although it can be shallow — say only 7 inches deep.

5

The Guides

Heal your body and mind with therapeutic and medicinal essential oils.

Turn to popular and useful oils to improve your daily life.

Symptom Guide

This Symptom Guide is a practical reference to using essential oils to treat many common conditions. In this guide, I share my favorite essential oil remedies. I've seen them work reliably over my five decades of working as an aromatherapist and herbalist with holistic medicine. The problems that I describe typically are ones that you already self-diagnose and then treat yourself without seeing a doctor. Instead of using over-the-counter drugs, I suggest the essential oil products and treatments for you to use. In case you're feeling creative, I also give you recipes for making your own simple aromatherapy preparations.

Aromatherapy, like other forms of holistic healing, treats the individual. Most clinical aromatherapists prefer to custom-design a formula for an individual. Because that's not always practical, I am providing you with generic formulas. However, don't hesitate to be creative and change a suggested formula to better fit your personal needs. Refer to the Essential Oil Guide to find out more about oils that are appropriate substitutes.

Many disorders that I don't describe can be helped with essential oils even though it doesn't offer a cure. For example, if you have diabetes, multiple sclerosis, a kidney or liver disorder, or some other serious problem, essential oils can still help relieve your symptoms. One of the many advantages of essential oils is that, unlike many herbs, there have been no problems reported when the appropriate amounts of essential oils are used in conjunction with pharmaceutical drugs you take.

It's an empowering thing to take your own health in your hands. It's your body, and the more you learn about it and the various healing modalities, the better position you are in to make good choices. When you do so, be responsible. Make sure that you seek out more advice whenever you feel unsure of a treatment that you're pursuing.

WARNING These suggestions are intended to complement your health but not replace the advice and care of a qualified health-care practitioner. If you don't know what's ailing you or suffer from serious disorders that would normally send you to a doctor, get professional help before you embark on your self-healing methods. A medical diagnosis can often determine whether or not you are treating the right thing. If you're treating a condition that would normally find you making a doctor's appointment and using prescription drugs, you're beyond the scope of this book for using essential oils and herbs to heal it.

Essential oils are powerful healers, but their use needs to be respected. The safe way for you to use them is in tiny amounts. That's all you need. Before trying any of the following remedies, be sure you read about using essential oils safely in Chapter 4.

I've organized the information on each condition into four categories to help you find an essential oil remedy easier:

>> **Medical description:** This defines the condition or symptom.

>> **Essential oil remedies:** In this category, I give you the specific aromatherapy solutions to treat your conditions and symptoms with essential oils, and I suggest the type of essential oils products for you to buy or make.

>> **Essential oil formula:** In this section, I provide simple recipes that use essential oils in case you'd like to create your own formulas instead of buying them. In some cases, the remedy is so simple (say, an essential oil is added to water) you won't be able to buy it in a store, so you do need to prepare it yourself.

>> **Healthy habits:** Essential oils are remarkable healers, yet they are not always the only path to health and healing and don't do the job alone. They work far better in conjunction with herbal medicine, and dietary and lifestyle changes. Combing therapies will almost always be more effective. In most cases, you can also use essential oils along with your regular medications. In addition, follow general healthy guidelines like eating a good diet, exercising, and getting plenty of sleep to boost your immune system and avoid stress.

The herbs suggested in this chapter for internal use are typically ingested in whatever form you find most convenient, as tea, pills, herbal extracts like alcohol-based tinctures. To make herb tea, pour boiling water over the herbs, steep them for about five minutes, and then strain and drink. For the rest, follow the directions on the package. Investigate holistic ideas for healing your condition and for staying healthy.

REMEMBER

Be patient using aromatherapy and herbal remedies. They make quick and effective first-aid remedies, but chronic conditions can take weeks or even months to resolve.

Because so many physical and emotional disorders exist, you may not find the condition that you're looking for in this guide. If you don't, look up any of the symptoms that you experience. For example, if you have diabetes, no aromatherapy cure exists for the disease, but my suggestions on improving circulation can help you. If you suffer from cancer, look up what you can do to treat your immune system. Other conditions that I list here, such as insomnia and headaches, are symptoms of many different problems. Use my ideas to ease your symptoms.

TECHNICAL STUFF

To translate the formulas in the guide (and throughout this book) into European measurements

1 teaspoon (1/10 ounce) equals about 5 milliliters

1 tablespoon (1/2 ounce) is about 15 milliliters

1 cup (8 ounces) is 250 milliliters

Acne

Medical description: Acne is a skin inflammation that develops in the pores of your skin. It produces blemishes that can become infected, creating small sores. A hormonal imbalance is most often blamed as the cause, although holistic practitioners suspect that toxicity circulating in the blood can play a role.

Essential oil remedies: When shopping for aromatherapy products designed for acne, you'll encounter a large assortment that are sold in natural-food stores and some drugstores, as well. Get a product that you can apply directly to your acne. A general skin toner that will reduce future breakouts is also a good idea if you have an oily complexion. (Refer to my suggestions under Oily Skin or Dry Skin for other essential oils that aid your type of skin.) If you have a severe case of acne, use an herbal paste so you can dab it directly on the offending spot. Look for acne products that contain essential oils such as chamomile and sandalwood oils to reduce the swelling and irritation, help prevent infection, and heal your skin. Tea tree, cedarwood, lemon, eucalyptus, lavender, and sage not only do all of this, they also help oily skin that is prone to breaking out. Any eucalyptus will do, although the variety called *dives* or broad leaf eucalyptus, which is high in the compound cineole, is considered the very best type for acne. Likewise, any lavender will do, but the species called Spanish

lavender is especially effective on acne. To understand more about the chemistry of different essential oils, see Chapter 15. Clary sage, fennel, frankincense, rosemary, and patchouli reduce inflammation, rejuvenate your skin, encourage oil production, and balance your hormones in case you have acne that is combined with dry or mature skin. Dermatologists say don't pop pimples, but if you do, use the following compress on the spot before and afterwards.

Essential oil formula: *To make an acne compress:* Pour 1/4 cup boiling water over 1 teaspoon Epsom salts (also called magnesium sulfate — buy this muscle-relaxing salt in the grocery store). When the salts dissolve, add 4 drops each lavender and tea tree oils. Soak a small absorbent cloth in the solution, wring out, and press it directly on your pimples for a minute or two. Place the cloth back in the hot solution and then reapply it several times. To make an acne paste: Stir 12 drops tea tree oil into 1/2 teaspoon comfrey root powder and add enough distilled water to make a paste (about 1 tablespoon). Mix well, then dab the paste directly on your acne spots. Let it dry into a mask for 10 to 20 minutes before rinsing it off. Store any leftover paste in the refrigerator for the next treatment. Also read up on general skin care in Chapter 7.

Healthy habits: Taking evening primrose oil capsules may help prevent recurring acne. Try taking vitex seeds and herbs that improve liver like burdock root, milk thistle seed, or turmeric.

Appetite loss

Medical description: You can lose your appetite for many reasons; stress or depression are common culprits. Losing your desire to eat is also a side effect of some pharmaceutical drugs. Because loss of appetite can be a symptom of a far more serious physical or emotional disorder, be sure to check with a doctor if your appetite doesn't perk up after a couple of weeks. It can be a sign of the eating disorder known as anorexia nervosa, which deals with psychological issues.

Essential oil remedies: Just smelling an aromatic herb or its essential oil stimulates your appetite and results in good digestion. Some of the best herbs to sniff are the culinary spices, such as anise, cardamom, cumin, coriander, and especially fennel and ginger. Conveniently, when you use herbs like these to flavor your food, both their direct action on the digestive tract and their scent help you digest your meal. They also aid anorexia nervosa, but only as a secondary treatment to psychological therapy. If your appetite decline is associated with stress or depression, then see my suggestions in those sections. I find that the scents of bergamot and rose can help you deal with compulsive behavior, and that geranium's fragrance encourages emotional stability. Also see information on digestion in Chapter 10.

Healthy habits: Exercise and eating a good, wholesome diet keep your appetite on an even keel.

Arthritis and rheumatism

Medical description: Swollen, painful, and stiff joints are the uncomfortable symptoms of arthritis or rheumatism. Doctors and aromatherapists alike treat the symptoms: inflammation and the resulting pain.

Essential oil remedies: Essential oils such as rosemary and marjoram may not cure arthritis or rheumatism, but they penetrate deep into your joints to lessen inflammation, and thus pain, so they're used in many liniments. (See Chapter 11.) Clove oil, and to some degree ginger and peppermint oils, directly numb arthritic and rheumatic discomfort. They also bring blood and heat to the area to further dull the pain. The scents alone of these oils also stimulate energy to encourage you to keep moving your stiff joints. Birch oil (usually sold as wintergreen because the two oils are almost identical) can be slightly toxic as an essential oil, but small amounts provide aspirin-like pain relief in a liniment. Other essential oils that you'll find in liniments for arthritis and rheumatism to reduce swelling are German chamomile, lavender, helichrysum, lavender, and sage. The scent alone of these oils helps to calm irritation you may feel from your discomfort. Another anti-inflammatory is frankincense, which helps arthritis sufferers by improving blood flow to the affected areas, repairing damaged blood vessels, and shrinking swollen tissue around painful and stiff joints. After that impressive list of accomplishments, it's no wonder the pharmacy sells tubes of frankincense cream, although it's identified by its botanical name, Boswellia. A liniment that contains these essential oils and the herb St. John's wort or arnica is especially effective to ease swollen joint areas. Besides using a liniment to reduce pain, take a warm bath that contains a few drops of these same essential oils now and then. Also see essential oils under "Circulation, poor" for more ideas that help relieve symptoms.

Essential oil formula: *To make a homemade liniment:* See the recipes and information in Chapter 11. *For a hot bath:* Use 3 drops each of rosemary and marjoram oil and 2 drops ginger oil in your tub. If your pain is localized in just your hands or feet, try soaking them in a pan or small basin of hot water that contains 1 drop of each of these oils.

Healthy habits: Work on arthritis and rheumatism with an herbal formula that contains devil's club root and the supplement glutamate to reduce inflammation Meadowsweet or willow leaves reduce pain.

Asthma

Medical description: This allergic condition is characterized by wheezing and shortness of breath, especially during an attack. The reaction intensifies if you're under emotional or physical stress. Likewise, having an asthmatic attack greatly ups your stress level. If you have asthma, chances are that you constantly battle a low-level lung congestion, which invites coughing and lung infection.

Essential oil remedies: Some aromatherapists advise asthmatics to completely avoid essential oils. What you can do is to rub your feet with aromatic salve, do a foot bath, or hover over steam in between asthmatic attacks to reduce their frequency and intensity. These techniques aren't for use during a full-blown asthma attack, but rather for in between attacks. Frankincense, lavender, chamomile, helichrysum, rose, geranium, marjoram, mandarin, and neroli (orange blossom) are especially effective antihistamines. Asthmatics rarely have a bad reaction to them. These oils sedate the bronchial passages in your lungs yet are gentle enough to use with small children. And, the scent of these oils does double duty by reducing stress. Eucalyptus, rosemary, and tea tree oils are sometimes used but aren't particularly recommended because some asthmatics react adversely to them. (When they are used, aromatherapists generally prefer the radiata species of eucalyptus for asthmatics because it's gentler but more effective. The softer, sweeter verbenone type is the best rosemary to use.) Between attacks, also use essential oils in a chest rub. Avoid essential oils like hyssop that contain potent compounds called ketones, which may bring on an asthmatic attack. Chapter 4 discusses

the potential problems with essential oils that contain ketone compounds. See more ideas under "Lung/bronchial congestion."

Essential oil formula: *For a foot or chest rub:* Use 3 drops frankincense, lavender, or chamomile oils (or make a blend using 1 drop of each) diluted in a tablespoon of vegetable oil. Rub on your chest or feet. *For a foot bath:* Put the same oils and the same amounts in a basin of hot water and soak your feet. *To make an asthma steam:* Add 3 to 5 drops lavender oil to a 2- to 3-cup pot of water that is just hot enough to produce steam and inhale the steam. (If you have asthma, steam that is too hot can be irritating. Also, pass on the typical technique of putting a towel over your head to capture the steam, which can make the steam too intense.) For a small child or baby, turn on the hot water in your bathtub and add about 10 drops lavender oil. Then hold them in the steam over the bathtub. The sooner this is done during an impending attack, the better it works to lessen the symptoms. *To make a simple chest rub oil:* Dilute 5 drops lavender oil (or 2 drops for a child) into a tablespoon of vegetable oil and rub this on your chest.

Healthy habits: Aromatherapy relieves the symptoms of asthma, but mullein leaf and elecampane root are herbs that strengthen and improve the general health of your lungs. Immune enhancers such as echinacea root, Chinese schizandra berry, and vitamin C help you to ward off further asthma attacks.

Athlete's foot/ringworm

Medical description: The most common fungal skin infection is ringworm. It's certainly not really a worm. What it does do is grow in a red, ringlike formation of itchy, peeling skin. Ringworm thrives in moist conditions, so it loves sweaty feet — your most likely spot to get the fungus. This is called athlete's foot, although everyone, even couch potatoes, can get it.

Essential oil remedies: Lavender, geranium, patchouli, lemongrass, cedarwood, fennel oils, and especially tea tree, eucalyptus, myrrh, and clove oils do an excellent job of fighting fungal infections. Of these, lavender, geranium, tea tree, eucalyptus, and myrrh oils also heal injured skin. Sage oil decreases excessive perspiration, and small amounts of peppermint oil relieve itching. Look for an antifungal product that contains at least some of these essential oils and dab it directly on the infection at least twice a day. A powder or vinegar-based product dries out the area and discourages fungal growth unless the infected skin is cracked and dry. In that case, look for a salve or cream-based product. You can also wash with an aromatherapy soap that contains any of the antifungal oils that I just recommended. Also see the general information on infections in Chapter 10.

Essential oil formula: *To make a foot powder:* Place ¼ cup cornstarch in a plastic sandwich bag. Drop in 25 drops (¼ teaspoon) tea tree oil or eucalyptus oil, 8 drops clove oil, 8 drops sage oil, and 3 drops peppermint oils. Close the bag and mix well with your fingers (through the outside of the bag). *For a liquid antifungal:* Add the same amounts of these essential oils to ¼ cup apple cider vinegar. Dab either of these preparations directly on the infected area 3 to 5 times a day.

Healthy habits: If the fungus persists, take an immune and infection-fighting herbal combination, such as pau d'arco bark, echinacea root, and black walnut hull, in tincture or pills.

Baldness

Medical description: Hair falls out all the time, but don't be alarmed because then it grows back. Baldness occurs when hair follicles in your scalp take a rest and never get going again. Hair typically thins with advancing years. Often the scalp tightens and blood flow decreases, both of which cut off the supply of nutrients to hair follicles. The most common type of baldness is male-pattern baldness, which is hereditary and spurred on by the presence of the male hormone testosterone and enzymes that discourage hair growth. Baldness can also be caused by hormonal disorders, drug treatments (especially including some types of antibiotics and cancer chemotherapy), radiation therapy, serious illness (especially nervous system disease), stress, malnutrition, and scalp disease.

Essential oil remedies: Essential oils can help re-establish hair growth, but don't look to them for a miracle. In the case of male-pattern baldness, it usually can only slow further hair loss. Stimulate circulation with a scalp formula that contains vitamin E and essential oils that improve circulation to your scalp. Rosemary oil is the age-old favorite. Other circulation stimulants are basil, eucalyptus, ginger, lemongrass, juniper, cypress, fennel, peppermint, and geranium oils. Avoid citrus essential oils if your balding head is exposed to the sun because they are photosensitizing agents that can cause skin reactions when the area is exposed to the sun. Cedarwood and ylang ylang are also sometimes recommended. Aloe vera is another good ingredient because it may promote hair growth. Ideally, look for a product that you can leave on your hair. Massaging it on your head further is a great way to enhance your circulation and stimulates hair follicles. Find a hair conditioner that also contains these essential oils and try to leave it on your head for longer than the typical few seconds before you rinse it off. Hair conditioners that contain balsams may not make your hair grow fuller, but they do give the illusion it's thicker.

Essential oil formula: *To make a hair-loss conditioner:* Combine ½ cup aloe vera gel, 2 tablespoons apple cider vinegar, 1 capsule 500 units vitamin E oil, and ½ teaspoon (25 drops) rosemary essential oil. Shake well and massage into scalp for 10 minutes nightly.

Healthy habits: Take vitamin E supplements and ginkgo leaves to increase the blood flow to your scalp and nettles for scalp health.

Bladder infection/cystitis

Medical description: Cystitis, or an inflammation of your bladder, is often caused by an infection, which is most often due to *E. coli* bacteria. If you don't already know the extent of your bladder infection, head straight for your doctor to make sure that you don't have the far more serious kidney infection.

Essential oil remedies: Many essential oils both promote urination and kill germs, a perfect combination to counter a simple bladder infection. These include sandalwood, pine, chamomile, cedarwood, juniper, tea tree, bergamot, and fennel oils. Studies show that bay laurel, thyme, clove, and cinnamon are some of the strongest essential oils to fight *E. coli*. See the general information on infection-fighting essential oils in Chapter 10. Find a massage or body oil that contains several of these oils (or make one yourself) and rub it directly over your bladder area, which is in your lower abdomen, above your pubic bone.

Essential oil formula: *To make a cystitis massage oil:* Add 14 drops tea tree oil, 5 drops fennel oil, and 5 drops bergamot oil in 2 ounces vegetable oil or a lotion. Rub this on twice a day. To help prevent the infection's return, stir a tablespoon of this same oil in your bath once a week.

Healthy habits: To treat a bladder infection, take antiseptic and anti-inflammatory herbs for the urinary tract, such as uva ursi and marshmallow.

Blood pressure, high

Medical description: Because high blood pressure — when your blood pressure level is consistently high — may be a life-threatening situation, be sure to consult your doctor.

Essential oil remedies: Simply smelling the citrusy scents of neroli (orange blossom), orange, melissa (lemon balm), and tangerine oils, as well as rose, ylang ylang, and geranium oils, can relax you enough to drop your blood pressure a couple of points. That may not be much, but it's a sign of that your stress level's dropping. Marjoram, and clary sage oils also slightly lower your blood pressure. You can sniff either the essential oils or the herbs themselves. Fortunately, this doesn't interfere with any blood pressure medication you take. Purchase a massage or bath oil that contains these oils or carry around smelling salts that contain them to inhale throughout the day.

Essential oil formula: *For a blood pressure-reducing massage oil:* Combine 8 drops geranium oil, 3 drops orange oil, and 1 drop cinnamon oil in 2 ounces of any vegetable oil or in a lotion. *To make a bath oil:* Place 4 drops geranium oil in the water. (Avoid using cinnamon orange essential oils because either one can redden and even burn the skin if you use too much.)

Healthy habits: Herbs to regulate your blood pressure include garlic, hawthorn, ginseng, and Siberian ginseng. If you're taking heart medication to treat high blood pressure, read up on these herbs before you take them on a regular basis. Taking hawthorn with heart meds sometimes boosts their activity so this may need to be regulated by your doctor. Also, see my suggestions in the section on "Stress."

Blood pressure, low

Medical description: When your blood pressure falls too low, you can feel dizzy, weak, and disoriented. Even worse, that means that not enough blood and oxygen reach your cells. Also known as hypotension, low blood pressure can be due to many things. Because it can signal a serious problem like internal bleeding or a heart condition — and it can be serious in itself — make sure that you see your doctor.

Essential oil remedies: The scents of cypress and rosemary essential oils slightly increase blood pressure. Geranium is used to regulate both high and low blood pressure, depending upon what you need. For even more of an effect, use massage or body oils that contain them. German pharmacies sell a rosemary ointment designed to rub over your heart to increase blood pressure, improve poor circulation, and ease the headaches and dizziness that often accompany low blood pressure. The ointment is based on an old European formula that infused rosemary leaves in white wine for the same purpose. Note that while cypress and rosemary can both increase blood pressure, it's only a slight increase. If you have high blood pressure and are taking medication to lower it, smelling the aroma of a cypress tree or a little rosemary herb flavoring a dish won't be a problem for you. Even using small amounts of these essential oils shouldn't be any problem.

Essential oil formula: *To make a chest rub:* Add 12 drops rosemary oil, 5 drops geranium oil, and 4 drops cypress oil to ¼ cup olive or other vegetable oil. Rub this solution on your chest every day. This same formula can double as an oil to increase your circulation if low blood pressure is giving you cold hands and feet.

Healthy habits: Herbs that keep your blood pressure regulated are hawthorn, ginger, ginseng, and Siberian ginseng.

Bowel disorders

Medical description: Bowel problems represent any number of conditions that are caused by infection or irritation in your intestines. There are usually problems with indigestion, diarrhea, or constipation. Examples are *colitis*, which is an ulceration of your large intestine, and *irritable bowel syndrome*. Many bowel disorders are tied in to emotional or nervous system problems.

Essential oil remedies: When used in abdominal massage, Roman chamomile and peppermint oils ease all sorts of stress-related bowel problems in two ways. They directly relax your intestine muscles, and at the same time, their fragrances ease your mind and your worries. To relieve intestinal gas, try an herb tea of peppermint, or anise, cardamom, cinnamon, coriander, cumin, ginger, and caraway instead of essential oil. (You'll still get any essential oils that are in the tea because hot water draws them out.) Peppermint is a specific treatment for irritable bowel syndrome. European doctors treat it with *enteric* capsules of peppermint oil that are specially coated to not release their contents until they reach the large intestine. Otherwise, the essential oil is absorbed in your mouth and throat and never reaches its destination. The safest and most enjoyable way to take tasty herbs like these is in food or as a tea, tincture, or in pills.

Essential oil formula: *To make tea:* Pour 2 cups boiling water over a teaspoon each chamomile flowers and peppermint leaves. Steep about 5 minutes, strain, and drink at least 1 cup a couple hours after each meal. *To make a massage oil:* Add 7 drops fennel, 4 drops teaspoon Roman chamomile, and 3 drops ginger oils to 1 ounce vegetable oil or a lotion and massage over your abdomen.

Healthy habits: Herbs that help your bowels include chamomile flowers, wild yam root, licorice root, marshmallow root, and fenugreek seed. Include fermented foods, such as yogurt, sauerkraut, kimchi, and miso in your diet.

Burns and sunburn

Medical description: Burns from heat, fire, the sun, or radiation redden your skin and cause it to swell and blister. You can treat a minor burn at home, but have a doctor tend to any serious or extensive burns.

Essential oil remedies: The first step after you get burned is to quickly cool off the burn to stop its progress. A fast way is to hold the burned area under cold water. You can also immerse the burned area in a cold-water bath that contains a few drops of skin-healing essential oils. The essential oils will mostly rise to the surface, so you'll need to pull out of the water to dose the area. Follow this with any of the numerous natural burn remedies that contain aloe vera and the essential oils of lavender, chamomile, geranium, or neroli (orange blossom) to reduce inflammation, pain, and the possibility of infection. These essential oils also speed new cell growth and healing. Convenient if you have a sunburn, these same oils cool down your body if you feel overheated. You probably won't find a burn remedy containing helichrysum or rose oils unless you make your own because they're quite expensive, but both essential oils have similar properties. Tiny amounts of peppermint may not seem an obvious choice because this is a hot oil, but they do help relieve the pain. Having your burn remedy in a spray bottle is handy so that you don't have to touch the painful area. Keep the bottle or tube containing the burn remedy refrigerated to provide extra cold relief on a burn.

Essential oil formula: *For a cold water burn bath:* Plunge the burn into a basin that contains 5 drops chamomile oil or 8 drops lavender oil for every cup of very cold water. (If ice cubes are available, they're a quick solution to chilling the water.) *To make a homemade burn remedy:* Add ¼ teaspoon (25 drops) lavender oil, 2 drops peppermint oil to 2 ounces aloe vera juice. Shake well before using and apply as often as needed. I keep this in a handy spray bottle. You can also add 1 teaspoon vitamin E oil to the preceding formula, although it doesn't mix with aloe vera, so you'll need to shake the bottle first.

Healthy habits:

Candida

Medical description: Candida is a yeastlike fungus that occurs naturally in most people's digestive tract. However, it can multiply so much that you end up with gas, indigestion, fatigue, and feelings of fuzzy headedness. It's the same fungus that is responsible for thrush, a patchy white infection inside your mouth, and for the vaginal yeast infections that many women experience. Candida can also grow under your nails, making them cracked and discolored. It's especially prevalent after taking antibiotics, which encourage it to multiply. If the problem doesn't begin to clear up within a week, it may be time for you to consult a health practitioner.

Essential oil remedies: The essential oils of chamomile, lavender, bergamot, tea tree, and thyme inhibit about 70 percent of candida growth, at least in their lab experiments. Studies also find a long list of other essential oils that slow the growth of candida infections. These include clove, cinnamon, lavender, eucalyptus, lemongrass, lemon verbena, and garlic oils. So does thyme oil, although in this case, the gentler variety called geraniol is more effective than regular thyme oil because it doesn't tend to burn sensitive skin. Depending upon where you have candida, look for a mouthwash, nail soak, or douche formula that includes some of these oils or the same herbs. For a vaginal yeast infection, douching is very effective, but has met with recent criticism because some gynecologists fear it upsets the normal vaginal balance and may spread infection into the uterus. If you douche, suspend the bag no higher than shoulder level so that the flow of water isn't too strong. As an alternative, you can buy tea tree suppositories — yes, they're available!

Essential oil formula: *To make a candida remedy:* To 1-ounce black walnut husk tincture, add 5 drops lavender oil and 8 drops tea tree oil.

Shake very well before using and take 30 drops internally twice a day. Studies show that black walnut husk destroys candida better than a commonly prescribed antifungal drug. However, I'll forewarn you that it does produce a brown stain. You can also swab this formula directly on thrush a couple times a day. *To treat nail fungus:* Add 12 drops tea tree oil to 2 tablespoons castor oil. Soak your nails in this solution for 5 to 15 minutes a day. *To prepare an aromatherapy douche:* Add 2 drops each of lavender and 1 drop tea tree oil to 3 cups warm water. (You can also add 2 tablespoons yogurt to restore the vagina's natural flora and 1 tablespoon vinegar to restore acidic environment.) Mix well, put in a douche bag, and use once a day.

Healthy habits: Build up your resistance to candida by taking immune herbs that address fungal infections, such as pau d'arco and echinacea and avoid eating sweets.

Canker sores

Medical description: Canker sores are tiny, but painful, ulcerations with white patches that occur in your mouth. They make the inside of your mouth red and swollen. You can get them when your defenses are down from emotional or physical stress, or if you have a poor diet, an infection, or a chronic disease. Sometimes the use of antibiotics brings them on. These sores generally take a couple weeks to heal. If they remain longer than that, see your doctor as they may be something more serious.

Essential oil remedies: Use one of the natural mouth washes that contains tea tree oil, or the tastier fennel, chamomile, sage, or peppermint oils to promote healing and discourage further infection.

Essential oil formula: *For a homemade mouth wash:* Combine 3 drops tea tree oil, 2 drops fennel, and 1 drop peppermint oil in ½ cup warm water. Stir well and slosh around the mouth for a few minutes before spitting out. (If there's any left over, it will keep in the refrigerator for a couple days.) Once a day, you can also put a drop of tea tree oil on your toothbrush before adding the toothpaste.

Healthy habits: If you keep getting canker sores, build up your immune system with immune-boosting herbs like echinacea.

Carpal tunnel syndrome and repetitive strain injury

Medical description: You can get a repetitive strain injury from doing lots of the same work that repeatedly uses the same movement. Carpal tunnel is an example. In this case, the meridian nerve in your wrist (which runs through a narrow opening called the carpal tunnel) can become compressed from an activity such as typing, massage, or hammering. This makes your wrist feel numb with sharp, shooting pain so that it's difficult or impossible to use it.

Essential oil remedies: Look for a product that contains lavender, rosemary, and/or marjoram oils that you can rub over the injured area to ease the inflammation and pain. Although not proven, I've observed that these oils seem to help heal damaged nerves. These essential oils also help to prevent you from developing the strain in the first place if applied when you're doing a lot of computer work, playing a musical instrument, or some other activity that puts strain on your connective tissues.

Essential oil formula: *To make your own remedy:* Combine 15 drops lavender oil, 5 drops marjoram oil, and 4 drops rosemary oil with 1 ounce St. John's wort tincture. (It counters inflammation and nerve damage and is sold in natural-food stores.) If you prefer a remedy with an oily base, use St. John's wort oil instead of the tincture. The other benefit of using these essential oils is their feel-good scents that can help you overcome pain and counter the frustrations that come with how this injury restricts your activity.

Healthy habits: Take herbal nerve tonics such as St. John's wort flower/leaf and skullcap leaf.

Cholesterol, high

Medical description: Cholesterol is a type of fat that can accumulate in your blood stream. It can be measured in your blood to determine whether the level is too high. When an excessive amount builds up inside your arteries, it can cause you to have heart and circulation problems. Eating a high-fat diet is often blamed, but that's only part of the problem. It's beginning to look like not just what you eat, but also your level of stress may be one of the major culprits.

Essential oil remedies: The essential oils in onion, garlic, cayenne, rosemary leaf, fenugreek seed, and ginger root reduce high cholesterol, but it's best to eat all of these as foods rather than using them as pure essential oils. You only need to eat three onions or five cloves of garlic a week for results. If you find garlic good for your heart, but not your social life, try deodorized garlic capsules. Lavender helps normalize cholesterol and can be used in a massage oil. The amount that any massage oil directly lowers cholesterol is questionable, but it certainly decreases stress so helps in that way. Cayenne and ginger essential oils help your body break down cholesterol into bile acids, which is an important step in eliminating cholesterol. The best way to utilize them is to season your food with these spices rather than ingesting essential oil.

Essential oil formula: *To make a cholesterol-lowering massage oil:* Add 8 drops lavender oil, 3 drops ginger oil, and 2 drops rosemary oil in 2 ounces vegetable oil.

Healthy habits: Eat a balanced diet of vegetables and grains that includes onion, garlic, cayenne, rosemary, fenugreek seed, and ginger root.

Circulation, poor

Medical description: If you tend to have cold hands and feet, you may have poor blood circulation. Because poor circulation is a symptom of some other disorder — often low blood pressure (which I also cover in this guide) — look for the source of your problem and treat it as well. It can signal a serious condition, so get a doctor's evaluation. If you have the circulation disorder called Raynaud's disease, the small blood vessels, particularly those in your hands and feet, are so sensitive that they go into spasm. This decreases the flow of blood to these areas and can eventually lead to the damage of your cells, including nerves.

Essential oil remedies: Plenty of essential oils can get your blood moving. These include eucalyptus, ginger, lemongrass, juniper, cypress, rosemary, fennel, and geranium oils. Chamomile, frankincense, bergamot, grapefruit, lemon, and cedarwood oils are effective. They do improve the integrity of the blood vessels themselves. Frankincense also improves blood circulation. All these oils decrease swelling and bloating. One of the best ways to encourage circulation is to combine aromatherapy with *hydrotherapy*. This is the therapeutic use of water (*hydro* means water). Alternating between hot and cold water increases circulation. (If you have a circulation disorder, such as Raynaud's syndrome, stick to using only hot water because cold water can lead to spasms.) Essential oils that increase circulation can be incorporated into a massage oil. You can also drink a tea made from ginger, lemongrass, rosemary, fennel, or geranium. (The hot water pulls the essential oils from the plants).

Essential oil formula: *To do a hand or foot bath:* Stir 1 drop each ginger, rosemary, cypress, and juniper essential oils into a basin or pan of hot water and soak your hands or feet for at least five minutes. Or, use 4 drops of any one of these oils. To increase circulation and water elimination even more, also have a pan or basin of cold water and go back and forth several times between the hot and cold. *To make a circulation oil:* Combine 8 drops lemon, 3 drops rosemary, 3 drops geranium, and 2 drops cypress oils in 1 ounce vegetable oil or a skin lotion and rub on your hands, feet, back of neck, or legs. *To make a tea:* Take 2 teaspoons total of your choice of these herbs and cover them with 2 cups boiling water to steep 5 to 10 minutes. Then strain the herbs and drink.

Healthy habits: Take herbal antioxidant supplements to improve the integrity of your blood vessel walls.

Cellulite and fat

Medical description: Cellulite is just fat, but what gives it a distinction from just any fat is the lumpy, orange peel texture of the skin that covers it. Really a fancy word for puckered fat, it occurs in women more than men and most often in the thighs and buttocks. The likelihood of having it depends on the number of fat cells you have (although thin people do develop it), how good your circulation is, and if it runs in your family. Hormones may also play a role.

Essential oil remedies: You can easily find cellulite massage and body oils for sale. Essential oils of geranium, fennel, and grapefruit are used to facilitate weight loss. I suspect that they increase metabolism along the way. Even their scent conveniently encourages you to eat less. (This may be hard to believe, but researchers have found that the scent of chocolate can lower your appetite. So, you can sniff a chocolate bar, but you'll need iron willpower to keep from putting *it* in your mouth!)

Use the scent of bergamot to sniff if you have trouble with compulsive eating. Cypress and juniper are good adjuncts because they stimulate your circulation and ease fluid retention, problems that are often associated with cellulite. The massage itself treats cellulite. Perhaps not as enjoyable, but the massage oil is still helpful if you forgo the massage and rub it on yourself.

Essential oil formula: *To make a massage or bath oil:* Add 5 drops each cypress, geranium, grapefruit, and bergamot oils and 2 drops each juniper and fennel oils in 2 ounces vegetable oil. You can add the same number of drops (240 of essential oils to 2 ounces body lotion) to get the same results. The concentration of this oil or lotion is too strong to use as a total massage, but you can rub it directly on cellulite areas. Do that once a day, if possible. (I'd also better warn you that this formula doesn't smell as appealing as the other essential oil combos that you'll see in this book. I do find that people who want to work on their cellulite usually don't care a bit.) *In your bath:* Add 2 tablespoons of this blend to the water or add 3 drops of your choice of the essential oils that are suggested previously.

Healthy habits: A deep, rolling massage on the cellulite area (with an aromatherapy oil, of course!) seems to stimulate fat reduction. If you're trying to lose fat, aromatherapy is much more effective when you combine it with a total weight-loss plan.

Colds/sinus infection

Medical description: Colds and sinus congestion go hand in hand because a cold virus is the most common type of sinus infection. The symptoms include inflamed and congested sinuses and a runny nose, which makes it uncomfortable for you to breathe. Smoking cigarettes, irritation from environmental sources, and some medications can also make your nose stuffy.

Essential oil remedies: Eucalyptus, lavender, tea tree, lemon, thyme, marjoram, rosemary, basil, and peppermint oils inhibit a cold virus. These same oils also clear your sinuses by relieving inflammation and congestion. In addition, they fight the bacterial infection that often follows a cold (as well as staph, strep, and pneumonia infections). Plus, if your cold is leaving you down in the dumps, the scents of lavender, lemon, and marjoram will lift your spirits. Peppermint, ginger, anise, and chamomile stop inflammation by slowing the release of the body's *histamine* (which causes allergic-related inflammation). Use an aromatherapy steam to carry the therapeutic oils into your sinuses where it can counter the infection and inflammation. (The steam alone makes it easier for you to breathe when you're congested.) When steaming is impractical, get a nasal inhaler that contains some of these same essential oils. Eating hot herbs that contain essential oils, such as cayenne, horseradish, garlic, and onions, drains your sinuses and can even stop a cold in its tracks if you catch it soon enough.

Essential oil formula: *To prepare a steam:* Put 3–5 drops eucalyptus oil (or another of the oils listed) in 3 cups simmering water. Turn off the heat, place your face over the steam, and drape a towel over the back of your head to collect the steam in a mini sauna. Take deep breaths through your nose, coming out for fresh air as needed at about 2-minute intervals. Repeat this for at least three rounds. If possible, do this routine a few times a day. *As an alternative method:* You can steep 2 tablespoons of these same herbs (fresh or dried) in 3 cups simmering water for a few minutes so that the heat releases the essential oils and the steam carries it up into the air. You can also take a hot, steamy bath that has 1 drop each of eucalyptus, lavender, and ginger essential oils added to the bath water. *For a nasal inhaler:* Combine 2 drops eucalyptus (or other) oil and ¼ teaspoon coarse salt in a small glass vial that has a tight lid. (Salt absorbs the oil and is convenient

to carry without danger of spilling it.) Throughout the day, open the vial and inhale the scent.

Healthy habits: Treat a sinus infection with a tea or nasal purge that contains goldenseal root (buy only cultivated roots, please, because the wild plant is endangered), the Chinese herb coptis, yarrow flowers, and/or elder flowers. A hot tea of elder flower, peppermint leaf, and yarrow flower helps clear your sinuses (and lowers a fever). Get extra rest because sleep, along with herbs like echinacea root and baptisia root, amp up your immune system so that you get well sooner.

Coughs, sore throat, and laryngitis

Medical description: You typically get a sore throat — an inflammation of your throat — if you have a cold, have a cough, smoke, strain your voice, or are exposed to air pollution or some other type of irritation. If you have a persistent cough and can't figure out why, have your doctor check it out.

Essential oil remedies: Anise, eucalyptus, tea tree, fennel, myrrh, ginger, peppermint, and thyme oils are ingredients in all sorts of cough drops, syrups, gargles, and sprays for sore throats. They make these products tasty, but more importantly, most of these essential oils tend to stop coughing, possibly by suppressing the brain's cough reflex. Sage, thyme, and marjoram oils relieve laryngitis and tonsillitis. You can follow the example of European singers who traditionally preserve their voices by drinking marjoram or sage tea sweetened with a little honey! (The tea pulls the essential oils from the herb into the water.) I give a lot of weekend seminars, and I find that a steam of lavender, tea tree, or eucalyptus is particularly good to keep my throat from being strained and to fend off laryngitis. (See the directions for making steams under "Colds/sinus congestion.") Other germ-fighting and soothing essential oils to treat a sore throat are cardamom, clary sage, benzoin, rose, rosemary, sandalwood, and bergamot.

Essential oil formula: *To make a gargle:* Add 2 drops tea tree oil (or your choice of another of the preceding oils) to ¼ cup cold water or apple cider vinegar with ¼ teaspoon salt dissolved in it. Several times a day, gargle with this solution and then spit it out. Or, make a strong tea by pouring a cup of boiling water over a teaspoon each of marjoram and sage herbs, let this steep about 5 minutes in a covered pan and then strain out the herbs. Add ½ teaspoon salt. When the salt is dissolved, gargle with this solution. If your neck is stiff or if your tonsils or the lymph glands on the side of your neck are swollen, you can make a neck wrap: Add 4 drops ginger oil to about 1 cup hot water. Soak a soft cloth, preferably of absorbent flannel, in the water. Then wring it out well and wrap it completely around your neck. To retain the heat, you can also wrap a thin towel around this. Remove the wrap when it cools. Repeat this treatment as many times as needed to reduce the swollen glands and ease the discomfort.

Healthy habits: Herbal cough syrups that contain herbs such as marshmallow root and horehound leaf and maybe some essential oils are excellent. Take immune stimulating herbs like echinacea in tea, tincture, or pills.

Cuts

Medical description: Broken skin is usually the result of injuring your skin or having a skin disorder in which the skin breaks open. Get medical treatment if you get a serious wound.

Essential oil remedies: Treat superficial cuts and scrapes with a spray or salve that contains antiseptic and wound-healing essential oils. A lot of antiseptic essential oils are available. The most popular ones for cuts are eucalyptus, lavender, lemon, thyme, marjoram, rosemary, and tea tree. Most of the salves on the market contain antiseptic and skin-healing essential oils. A spray container is a convenient way to spritz antiseptic essential oils on a cut. In fact, spraying eucalyptus or lemon oils increases their antiseptic properties as the oils combine with the oxygen in the air. The germ-fighting abilities of tea tree oil also improves when it's in the presence of blood or the pus from an infection, so it works best when it's needed. Use the same highly antiseptic essential oils to treat an infected wound. Surround the infected wound with a diluted antiseptic oil, applying it directly to the reddened area around the wound. When dealing with a deep or dirty cut, first thoroughly clean the wound with an antiseptic like hydrogen peroxide to counter any initial infection before applying the aromatherapy antiseptic.

Essential oil formula: *To make an antiseptic spray:* Add 12 drops tea tree oil and 6 drops lemon oil to ½ ounce distilled water and ½ ounce vinegar (which is also antiseptic). This is convenient to use if you put it in a spray bottle. (For extra action, instead of water, you can use ½ ounce of an herb vinegar such as oregano, garlic, or calendula.) Shake well to disperse the oils before spraying it on minor cuts, burns, and abrasions to prevent infection.

Healthy habits: Keeping in good general health reduces your risk of developing a serious infection. You can build up your immune system by periodically taking herbs that aid the immune system.

Dandruff

Medical description: This scalp condition is characterized by flaking skin on your scalp that often causes itching. If you have dry skin in general, you're more likely to also have dandruff.

Essential oil remedies: Look for a hair conditioner that contains geranium, lavender, clary sage, and bergamot oil and especially rosemary, sandalwood, and/or tea tree oils. Cedar, juniper, and patchouli oils are good additions if your dandruff is a result of an overly oily scalp. If you have a flakey head due to a dry scalp, chamomile, myrrh, and sandalwood are good essential oil choices. Also see the essential oils that are suggested for dry skin and oily skin in this guide for more ideas and general hair information in Chapter 7. Once a day, you can dab a couple drops of rosemary or sandalwood oil on your fingertips and massage your head or put a couple drops on your comb before combing your hair.

Essential oil formula: *For a quick, homemade hair rinse:* Combine 4 drops rosemary oil, 4 drops lavender oil, 2 drops tea tree oil, ⅓ cup vinegar, and ⅔ cup water. Shake this mixture well before using it to rinse your hair. Vinegar itself is an excellent hair rinse. You can rinse it out in a few minutes, but it's even better to leave it on. (Don't worry; I promise that the smell of vinegar will dissipate within a few minutes after applying this rinse.) *For another hair rinse technique:* Use super-strong rosemary tea. (The hot water draws out the rosemary's essential oils.) Prepare the tea by pouring 2 cups boiling water over 3 teaspoons rosemary leaves (dried or fresh). Steep for 10 minutes and then strain. Add ⅓ cup vinegar and use the mixture to rinse your hair. Keep any leftover rinse in the refrigerator.

Healthy habits: Include flaxseed in your diet. A supplement that's high in essential fatty acids may help.

Depression/anxiety

Medical description: Depression is a mental state in which you feel emotions that can range from chronic sadness to despair. It often makes you unable to feel joy. Anxiety is another emotional condition that is closely related to depression. Unjustified fear, insomnia, and difficulty concentrating can accompany either problem.

Physical imbalances in brain chemistry are most often the cause, so you may need professional advice to help you deal with it.

Essential oil remedies: The citrus scents of orange, bergamot, rose, lavender, lemon, lemon verbena, melissa (lemon balm), chamomile, petitgrain, and neroli (orange blossom) oils are some of the favored essential oils that can lift your mood. The scents of orange, according to research, and of fir and juniper reduce anxiety. In India, basil's fragrance is used to prevent agitation and nightmares. In addition, aromatherapists find that the scents of cedarwood, cypress, clary sage, marjoram, and geranium oils ease emotional upset. I find that any of these oils also help anyone undergoing a major life transition. If you get heart palpitations and chest pains or dizziness along with your anxiety attack, also use a relaxing scent. Ylang ylang, sandalwood, frankincense, and marjoram are particularly effective. Look at the fragrances that I mention under "Stress" for more ideas. Choose any aromatherapy method described in Chapter 6, such as an aromatherapy diffuser that dispenses scent into the air. If you're on the go a lot, carry them with you in an aromatherapy inhaler (easy to purchase) or as smelling salts that you make yourself. If you are already taking anti-depressive or anti-anxiety drugs, it's safe to use aromatherapy with them.

Essential oil formula: *To make anti-depressive or anti-anxiety smelling salts:* Add 3 drops bergamot oil, 2 drops geranium oil, and 3 drops petitgrain oil, to 1 tablespoon rock or other coarse salt. Carry in a closed container and sniff as needed. *To make massage oil:* Add the same essential oils (in the same amount) to 4 ounces vegetable oil. If you can't get a massage, then add a couple teaspoons of this massage oil to your bath water and enjoy!

Healthy habits: Aromatherapy helps you deal with depression and anxiety, but for a permanent solution, seek a complete and holistic approach. Herbal antidepressants, such as a tincture or pills of St. John's wort leaf/flower, help ease many kinds of depression. Have a knowledgeable health professional help you select anti-depressive herbs if you're already on medication to treat depression or anxiety.

Dermatitis, psoriasis, and eczema

Medical description: If you suffer from any of these skin conditions, your skin may be inflamed, red, itchy, and flaky, develop unsightly skin lesions that ooze, and then crust over. Secondary skin infections can occur if your skin is rough or broken. If you're under stress, allergies and exposure to environmental toxins worsen and can even cause the problem.

Essential oil remedies: Turn to products containing skin-healing and anti-inflammatory essential oils that also kill any bacterial or fungal infections to treat a wide range of skin problems. Lavender, chamomile, tea tree, melissa (lemon balm), neroli (orange blossom), and spikenard oils all fit the bill. If you can't find an herbal salve that contains these essential oils, then add essential oils to a store-bought salve following the recipe in the next paragraph. Use your salve directly on your skin condition a few times a day. If you also have dry skin, which is often associated with these skin conditions, look at my suggestions under "Dry skin." For healthy skin care, also see Chapter 7.

Essential oil formula: *To custom-make a dermatitis salve:* Using a toothpick, stir 10 drops tea tree oil, 8 drops lavender oil, and 5 drops chamomile oils into a ready-made 2-ounce jar of skin salve. (A salve containing the herb calendula flowers and perhaps comfrey is a good choice.)

Healthy habits: Follow the advice of herbalists and some progressive dermatologists and clear up your skin condition by improving the functioning of your liver — the primary organ of detoxification. Your liver also helps keep your hormones in balance. Other herbs that aid your liver so they are especially good for skin conditions are burdock root, Oregon grape root, turmeric, dandelion root, red clover flower, milk thistle seed, and yellow dock root. Take them as a tea or in pills. You can cook burdock as a vegetable. (It's sold fresh in Asian markets and some natural-food stores; prepare it like a carrot.) You can grind up milk thistle seeds and even sprinkle them on your oatmeal or soup. Taking supplements of evening primrose oil often helps.

Diaper rash

Medical description: Skin irritation from diapers chafing baby's delicate skin causes a rash, reddening, and inflammation. Moisture from wet diapers makes it worse.

Essential oil remedies: Using a baby powder and an herbal salve with every diaper change protects your baby from diaper rash by absorbing moisture and preventing chafing. Better yet, select a baby powder that contains essential oils that reduce inflammation, soothe irritated skin, and promote skin healing. Two gentle essential oils that do this are lavender and chamomile. Baby powder that is made with white (or China) clay, cornstarch, or arrowroot powder is much better than talc, which is sometimes contaminated with harmful substances like asbestos. Be sure to choose a diaper salve that is made with vegetable oil rather than mineral (petroleum) oil.

Essential oil formula: *To make your own baby powder:* Put ½ pound cornstarch (sold in grocery stores) in a plastic bag and add 25 drops lavender essential oil, drop by drop. Distribute the drops throughout the starch. (It clumps if you pour it all in one spot.) Seal the bag. Break up any clumps with your fingers on the outside of the sealed bag. Let the bag sit for four days to evenly distribute the scent. Spice or salt shakers with large perforations in their lids make handy containers to keep and dispense your powder.

Healthy habits: An herbal salve designed especially for babies further protects baby's skin from moisture and chafing. Find baby salves and powders that are made with herbs and essential oils at natural-food or herbs stores and online.

Dry skin

Medical description: Dry skin is obviously dry, containing very little water. It doesn't have any luster and chafes and peels easily.

Essential oil remedies: Increase your skin's oil production and rejuvenate it by encouraging the growth of new cells with a cream that contains essential oils such as lavender, geranium, neroli (orange blossom), rosemary, sandalwood, chamomile, jasmine, and rose. Less common essential oils that you may encounter in dry skin creams are spikenard, carrot seed, and vetiver. Lavender, chamomile, geranium, jasmine, rose, and carrot seed are especially good on skin that is mature or very sensitive or cracked. Tea tree or the variety of thyme called geraniol (which is much less harsh on skin than regular thyme) make good additions to dry skin products if you're prone to any type of skin infection. A small amount of peppermint activates your skin's glands to produce more oil. Avoid the use of bar or liquid soaps, which are very drying and can irritate dry skin, except when you're super dirty. At other times, you can wash with a soap substitute such as powdered oatmeal tied in a loose-weave cotton bag. Also read about dry skin care in Chapter 7.

Essential oil formula: *To make a skin moisturizer:* Combine 6 drops geranium, 4 drops sandalwood, 1 drop chamomile, and 1 drop jasmine or rose oil (expensive so these are optional), 2 ounces aloe vera gel, 2 ounces orange blossom water (often

sold as neroli hydrosol), and 800 IUs vitamin E oil (use liquid E oil or pop open a couple of 400 IU vitamin E capsules) in a blender and mix. If you don't object to its smell, 1 teaspoon vinegar helps retain skin health by maintaining natural acidity. About that vinegar smell, it's not so bad. Vinegar helps balance the pH of dry skin to turn it to a healthy acidic state and then the smell dissipates quickly. Shake before each use and apply as a daily dry-skin conditioner. *To make a soap substitute for your complexion or sensitive skin:* Add the same essential oils in the same quantities to ¼ cup ground oatmeal. (Make your own ground oatmeal by putting it in your blender or coffee grinder or purchasing oatmeal flour.) Place the ground oatmeal in a piece of loose-weave cotton fabric that is about 8 inches square. Tie the ends of the cloth to make a bag. Use this in place of bar soap at the sink or in the tub or shower. It lasts for at least a couple washings. Then empty the bag and replace it with a new mixture.

Healthy habits: Drink water and be sure to get plenty of vitamin C in your diet or to take supplements. For excessively dry skin, try taking supplements of evening primrose capsules.

Ear infection

Medical description: A bacterial or fungal infection in the ear causes inflammation that can be very painful, as you already know if you've ever had one. Simple ear infections of the external ear canal can be self-treated, but infections in the middle ear need a doctor's care. Don't hesitate to see your doctor if you're unsure of the source of your infection because it can eventually damage your eardrum and lead to other, more serious consequences.

Essential oil remedies: To treat an ear infection, choose antiseptic oils that also relieve inflammation and pain. You can use diluted lavender, tee tree, and chamomile essential oils to massage around the outside of your ear. The essential oils pass through your skin to go into the infected area. A clove of garlic cut in half also works if you don't mind smelling like pizza! A few drops of garlic-mullein flower oil several times a day often takes care of an ear problem. You can find a selection of herbal ear oils readily available. Never drop undiluted essential oil directly into your ear, although you can put one drop on a piece of cotton and place this in your ear. If your eardrum is injured, see your doctor before using ear drops. Always treat both of your ears, even if only one hurts, because when one ear is infected, it's likely the other is on its way. Continue the treatment several days after your pain disappears to make sure that the condition doesn't return.

Essential oil formula: *For an ear oil:* Add 8 drops each lavender and tea tree oils to ½ ounce olive oil. Rub a little of this oil around the outside of your ear and down the side of your neck. If your child comes down with an ear infection, use the same formula, but half the number of essential oils (4 drops each) and remember to use this around, not in their ears.

Healthy habits: If you get ear problems often, several conditions can be causing this. One of these is that you may have a food allergy. Many foods cause allergies, and dairy and wheat are common culprits in ear infections. Immune herbs help fend off allergic reactions, so see "Immune System Problems" for more suggestions.

Eye inflammation/strain

Medical description: If your eyes are red, swollen, and sore from eye strain or lack of sleep, aromatherapy remedies can help. See a doctor if your eye problem continues for more than a few days, your eyes start oozing, your vision is affected, or they're very painful. Also get checked if you have an eye infection.

Essential oil remedies: Sties, eye inflammations, and strained eyes respond well to placing a compress over your eyes. Lavender or chamomile are good choices because both ease inflammation and sore muscles. As an added plus, they have a relaxing effect on your brain, and they smell great! It probably goes without saying, but don't ever put essential oils in your eyes, even when they're diluted. Don't even touch your hands around your eyes if they have essential oil on them. If you accidentally do so, flush your eyes immediately with eye drops. If necessary, you can use a vegetable oil instead of water because essential oils go into oil but not water. However, hydrosols of rose and other gentle herbs like chamomile make excellent eye washes if they're pure without any harmful ingredients added. Because they're water-based, only use hydrosols that aren't contaminated with bacteria — unfortunately, these are two things that you can't always be sure about.

Essential oil formula: *To make an eye compress:* Put 4 drops lavender oil in about a cup of water and slosh a soft cloth around in it. Stir well before dipping the cloth in the solution. You don't want undiluted drops on the cloth, then on the eyelid (Use cool or hot water depending upon which feels best to you. Swollen eyes usually respond better to cold because it reduces inflammation. Hot often feels better if you have eye strain.) Wring out the cloth and place it over your closed eyes and leave on this compress at least three minutes. *Another compress method:* Use herbs instead of essential oils by first preparing a strong tea of chamomile or lavender. Pour boiling water over 2 heaping teaspoons of the herbs and steep for five minutes. Strain out the herbs and soak the cloth in the tea. *For a quick compress:* While you're traveling or at work, steep two tea bags of chamomile or regular black tea for a few minutes in hot water. Then squeeze the excess water from the bag and place a tea bag over both of your closed eyes. If convenient, also put a small, folded cloth over the tea bags to hold them in place and block out any light. Keep the mini compress on for at least three minutes.

Healthy habits: If you do much close work with your eyes — say, you stare at a computer screen all day — be sure to look away now and then at an object in the distance. If you're stuck in a cubicle at work, at least pretend to look out to the horizon. Supplements that increase blood circulation and increase the oxygen flow to your eyes include vitamin E and antioxidants derived from herbs like bilberries, grape seed, and pine bark.

Fatigue

Medical description: Whatever causes your chronic tiredness, remember that it's just a symptom of another disorder. Try to determine its source and treat that.

Essential oil remedies: The sharp scents of eucalyptus, cypress, pine, and rosemary oils and the spicy scents of clove, basil, black pepper, cinnamon, and ginger oils all pep you up and reduce drowsiness, irritability, and headaches. To a lesser degree, the aromas of orange, bergamot, patchouli, and sage are also stimulating. Sniffing any of these scents helps counter fatigue that involves muscle weakness. For chronic fatigue syndrome, specific oils are ginger, and a cultivar of rosemary oil called cineole. Sniff these oils or, better yet, incorporate them into a muscle massage oil. Other oils for chronic fatigue are those that have a combination of both stimulating and focusing effects, such as lavender, petitgrain, and lemon eucalyptus. One thing about aromatherapy stimulants is that they don't over-amp your adrenal glands and then leave them flat the way coffee, cola, black tea, mate, and other caffeinated drinks can. In fact, these oils counter an adrenaline rush and prevent the sharp drop in attention that typically

occurs after working about 30 minutes. Some even offer specific treatments for adrenal problems. Along with other aromatherapists, I suggest that you use the scents of clary sage, spruce, and pine (particularly the species of pine called *sylvestris)* to help counter adrenal insufficiency in massage and body oils. When you're trying to stay awake, sniff your choice of these aromas every five minutes or so. Use the methods that I describe in Chapter 6, such as a few drops of essential oil in a diffuser. Or, use a commercial aromatherapy inhaler or smelling salts or carry a sprig of the herb itself when you're on the run.

Essential oil formula: *A good anti-fatigue combination:* Combine 6 drops bergamot oil, 4 drops lemon oil, 2 drops eucalyptus oil, 1 drop cinnamon oil, and 2 drops peppermint oil (and 1 drop cardamom oil, if you have it). Use this combination in a diffuser or add it to 2 ounces vegetable oil to create a massage or body oil. You can also add the same blend of essential oils to a hand or body lotion.

Healthy habits: Take herbs that help you sustain your energy, such as Siberian ginseng root.

Fever

Medical description: A fever increases your body temperature to burn off a viral or bacterial infection. Until a fever gets near a dangerous level of 104°F, do yourself a favor and let it cook (unless you're generally in poor health, very weak, or treating a baby or small child). Because a fever is only a symptom of something else, try to figure out the sources and then treat the problem directly.

Essential oil formula: *To make the fever wash:* Add 5 drops lavender oil to every cup of cold water and use this to wash off or sponge down the hands and feet or the entire body.

Healthy habits: In addition to the wash, drink a hot cup of my favorite fever tea: Equal parts of yarrow flower, peppermint leaf, and elder flower.

Fever blisters (cold sores)

Medical description: Cold sores are an infection that is caused by the herpes virus. It manifests as small, painful blisters around your mouth that inflame nerve endings. The virus stays dormant in your nervous system until it's triggered by stress, low immunity, or sunlight. These same suggestions work to treat genital herpes and another herpes infection, shingles.

Essential oil remedies: Several commercial herpes ointments, including a capsaicin cream, are available for sale, even in drugstores. Some of these remedies are sold in handy lip balm sticks in containers that roll up like lipstick. They make application easy. The natural fever blister products generally contain the essential oils of tea tree, eucalyptus, or myrrh. These oils, along with geranium and lavender oils, are effective treatments. (Lemon eucalyptus is the preferred species of eucalyptus in this case.) Studies on melissa (lemon balm) oil show that it's a strong deterrent to herpes, although it's also quite expensive, and these other oils work fine. (Any tea tree will do, although the type called niaouli is especially effective.) Small amounts of peppermint oil or capsaicin, the hot essential oil compound in cayenne, may be included to deaden the nerve-tingling pain. Also see the general information on dealing with viral infections in Chapter 10.

Essential oil formula: *To make a cold sore remedy:* Add 10 drops tea tree oil, 5 drops myrrh oil, and 5 drops geranium oil (and 1 drop peppermint oil is optional) to ½ ounce of echinacea tincture. (If using the tincture stings too much, then add it to an infused calendula oil instead.) Apply directly on blisters several times a day. This recipe

contains a high percentage of essential oils, so apply it carefully only to the blistering area. This is for external use only so do not take this formula internally.

Healthy habits: Increase your immunity with echinacea root and heal your nerves with St. John's wort flower. In addition, seek ways, including aromatherapy, to reduce your emotional and physical stress levels.

Fibrocystic breasts

Medical description: Breast lumps or cysts that are nonmalignant are common in women. They're associated with hormones, especially an overabundance of estrogen and associated hormonal compounds. Exactly why they form in the first place is not completely understood, although ingesting caffeine is partially responsible because it blocks the pathway that prevents them from forming. Make sure that you have the lump checked out by a doctor instead of self-diagnosing.

Essential oil remedies: To ease inflamed and painful breasts, use a compress made from chamomile, ginger, or lavender oils and place it directly over the cyst. Estrogenic herbs, due to the complex way that plants work on your physiology, often are beneficial in conditions like this that are associated with too much estrogen. However, no one knows yet if these essential oils help or hinder the situation. The current advice is to go easy on your use of cypress, angelica, and coriander oils, and especially anise, clary sage, fennel, and sage oils because they have light estrogenic properties. It's just essential oils that are restricted because they're so concentrated. It's fine to eat a curry flavored with coriander or have fennel sauce on your fish.

Essential oil formula: *To make the compress:* Add 4 drops lavender oil, 2 drops ginger oil, and

1 drop chamomile oil to 1 cup strong calendula tea. (Make the tea double strength by pouring 1 cup boiling water over 2 teaspoons calendula flowers, steep about 10 minutes, and then strain.) Soak a small, soft cloth in the solution. Wring the cloth out, fold it into several layers, and place it over your swollen breast. Run another cloth under cold water and wring out. After 5 to 10 minutes, exchange the hot compress for the cold cloth, and leave it on about 2 minutes. Repeat this procedure several times a day if possible.

Healthy habits: Herbal formulas that contain vitex berry, which helps balance women's hormones, reduce the size of breast cysts. For more detailed herbal information on fibrocystic breasts, see my book *Women's Herbs, Women's Health,* co-authored by Christopher Hobbs (Botanica Press).

Fluid retention

Medical description: Swelling from fluid buildup can occur just about anywhere in your body, but the most common location is your extremities — in your hands, feet, ankles, and legs. The problem is often twofold: The body isn't moving water out of your cells fast enough, and your kidneys are not eliminating enough of it. General *edema* (a fancy name for fluid retention) is a symptom of some other disorder, such as high blood pressure, varicose veins, constipation, PMS, arthritis, kidney problems, or heart disorders. Seek your doctor's evaluation to make sure that you don't have a serious heart or kidney condition. Find the source of your problem so that you can treat it. (Then look in this guide for more of my treatment suggestions.) Many women also experience fluid retention in the last trimester of their pregnancy. If you're pregnant, be sure that you read the safety precautions for pregnancy in Chapter 4. Essential oils may help you with this symptom, but not necessarily cure whatever condition is causing it.

Essential oil remedies: Quite a few essential oils reduce fluid retention, including grapefruit, lemon, lemongrass, juniper, cypress, rosemary, eucalyptus, fennel, sandalwood, and geranium oils. Chamomile, frankincense, and cedar wood oils are also effective. All these essential oils encourage general circulation and the elimination of excess water through sweating and via your kidneys. They also decrease swelling and bloating. Carrot seed oil (although it smells rather strongly of carrot) also aids water elimination. Use these essential oils in a compress or massage oil that is used directly over the bloated area or in a full or foot bath. You can also ingest one or a combination of the herbs as a tea. (The hot water pulls the essential oils from the plants in minute amounts suitable for ingestion.)

Essential oil formula: *To make a massage oil:* Combine 5 drops grapefruit oil, 3 drops rosemary oil, 3 drops cypress oil, and 1 drop fennel oil in 1 ounce vegetable oil or a lotion. (Be forewarned that this is one of the few blends in this book that doesn't smell great.) *For a compress:* Use these same oils in about ½ cup hot water. Soak a soft cloth in the solution, wring it out, then fold it, and apply it over the area that you want to treat. To increase circulation and water elimination even more, alternate this cloth with one soaked in cold water and go back and forth several times. *Prepare a hand or foot bath:* If your hands, ankles, or feet swell, stir 2 drops each grapefruit, rosemary, cypress, and fennel oils into a basin or pan of hot water and soak your hands or feet in the water for at least five minutes. You can get immediate results if every couple of minutes, you place your hands or feet in a cold-water soak for about 30 seconds and then return them to the hot, scented water. *Make a tea:* Cover 1 teaspoon each fennel and chamomile with 2 cups boiling water and steep for 5 to 10 minutes. Then strain the herbs and drink.

Healthy habits: Limit how much salty foods you eat so that you don't retain as much water.

Forgetfulness

Medical description: If you have a poor memory, chances are there's some reason for it. Depending on what is causing your forgetfulness, there may be a fix. The problem is often that there's too little blood, and therefore not enough oxygen, reaching your brain. A common reason is hardening of the arteries due to aging, but other things can be responsible, such as continual stress, which affects brain chemistry so that you can't think properly.

Essential oil remedies: Sniffing spicy scents such as cinnamon, bay leaf, basil, pimento bay, clove, rosemary, and sage perk your memory. These same essential oils also stimulate blood circulation when used in a massage oil. Sniff the essential oil or the plant throughout the day whenever you need to remember something or use any of the aromatherapy techniques that I describe in Chapter 9.

Essential oil formula: *For a nice-smelling blend:* Combine 10 drops lemon oil, 5 drops rosemary oil, 3 drops sage oil, and 1 drop cinnamon oil. If stress affects your memory, use these essential oils with the calming oils that I recommend under "Stress."

Healthy habits: The herbs ginkgo leaf, gotu kola leaf, ginseng root, and Siberian ginseng root as a tincture or in pills can improve your memory, but only if you're already experiencing memory problems. (Sorry, this combination won't make you smarter.)

Gum problems

Medical description: The gum problem that you're most likely to face is an infection, which can lead to inflammation and bleeding, a problem known as gingivitis. Plaque buildup, smoking or chewing tobacco, a severe nutritional deficiency, and even overzealous tooth brushing can also promote this condition.

Essential oil remedies: Many of the toothpastes and mouthwashes sold in both natural-food stores and drugstores rely on essential oils such as myrrh, eucalyptus, peppermint, and thyme, which studies show fight bacteria and reduce the buildup of plaque on your teeth. Other oils that effectively reduce bleeding gums are sage and rosemary. Toothpicks and dental floss that are soaked in antiseptic tea tree oil are also available. Many of the sticks from various bushes and trees that are traditionally used throughout the world to clean the teeth contain essential oils that help to prevent gum disease.

Essential oil formula: If you'd rather make your own *herbal gum treatment:* Add 20 drops tea tree oil and 8 drops myrrh oil to 1 ounce tincture of echinacea root. Shake very well and then put about ¼ teaspoon of the solution in ⅛ cup water and swish in your mouth for at least one minute. Spit it out. You can add a couple drops of this same mixture to your toothbrush before adding toothpaste and then brush your teeth as usual.

Healthy habits: Be diligent with your dental hygiene.

Headache

Medical description: Your headache may be related to allergies, stress, and immune system imbalances. Vascular headaches such as migraines are caused by constrictive blood vessels in the head. If you get chronic headaches, get an examination by a medical doctor because they sometimes result from an injury, a tumor, or other serious disorders. Stress or a tight neck or shoulders increase the intensity of a headache.

Essential oil remedies: Inhale lavender or melissa (lemon balm) or a combination of peppermint and eucalyptus to reduce your headache. Studies show that it can also be effective to rub a balm made with these essential oils on your temples. Take a hot bath if it eases your headache pain. (Some people, especially if they have a migraine, find that heat only makes it worse.) One innovative way to stop a migraine is to place your hands in a basin of very hot (around 110°F or 43.3°C) water with 5 drops of lavender oil. Relieve the pain of a cluster headache with capsaicin cream. It blocks a neurotransmitter called substance P (the P stands for pain!) to stop the brain from registering pain impulses. Be patient. You may need to use this cream four to five times a day for several weeks before it is totally effective. Other essential oils to sniff when you develop a headache are basil, chamomile, lemongrass, and marjoram. Even coriander and cumin can ease your headache woes and are especially good if your headache has to do with digestive upset. If problems such as insomnia, indigestion, or sinus congestion prompt your headache, then see the suggestions that I give under those headings. Everyone is unique, especially when it comes to headaches. You may need to experiment with different essential oils or combinations of oils to find what works best for you. Also, go easy at first on the sniffing. Sometimes essential oils, such as eucalyptus and bay laurel, trigger headaches in a few people rather than relieve them.

Essential oil formula: *To make a headache compress:* Add 5 drops lavender oil to 1 cup cold water and swish a soft cloth in the solution. Wring out the cloth and place it over your forehead and eyes as often as you like. If it feels better, use hot water instead of the cold or alternate cold and hot water. If your headache is prompted by muscle or emotional stress, it often helps to place a second hot compress under your neck. If you don't have time for using a compress, dab a small dot of lavender oil, eucalyptus oil, or

peppermint essential oil on each temple instead. Studies back the use of all three oils to relieve headaches.

Healthy habits: Feverfew leaves help migraine headaches, especially if taken on a regular basis. Ginkgo leaves, and ginger root increase circulation in your head to relieve even migraines. Valerian root or skullcap soothe muscle tension and pain.

Heartburn

Medical description: The heat and pain produced by heartburn may make you feel like you're experiencing a heart problem, but this complaint is caused by a spasm in the stomach or esophagus as gas and acid from your stomach move up the throat. Severe heartburn may be the result of a hiatal hernia, a condition in which the top of the stomach bulges into the diaphragm. See your doctor to get a correct diagnosis of any chronic stomach pain before you embark on self-treatment.

Essential oil remedies: Chamomile, lemon, melissa (lemon balm), and fennel oils reduce stomach acid, inflammation, and infection and even help protect your stomach lining from its own acid. The best way to take them is as a tea made with your choice of these herbs. (The hot water draws the essential oils out of the herbs.) Fortunately, they're all quite tasty. Drink a cup with each meal. Rubbing a massage oil that contains these essential oils over the chest area also helps relieve this condition.

Essential oil formula: *To make a heartburn massage oil:* Combine 4 drops each chamomile, fennel seed, and lemon oils in 1 ounce vegetable oil. Rub on as a daily belly massage or whenever heartburn strikes. This oil will ease your symptoms, although not necessarily cure the problem.

Healthy habits: At mealtimes, choose grains and steamed vegetables instead of fried, spicy, or high protein foods. An herb tea that soothes heartburn is marshmallow root and licorice root.

Hives

Medical description: Hives are rash-like skin bumps that can itch like crazy. They often result from a food allergy, although not always.

Essential oil remedies: Use a skin wash or compress, or poultice to stop the itching, decrease inflammation and sensitivity, and to slow the allergic reaction. Good essential oils to choose are lavender and especially chamomile, which helps counter allergic reactions. A cool bath with essential oils and oats also helps relieve your itching.

Essential oil formula: *To make either remedy:* Start off by adding 10 drops chamomile oil, 3 drops peppermint oil, and 3 tablespoons baking soda to ½ cup cool water (or elder flower tea). *To make a compress:* Soak a soft cloth in this solution and wring out the excess water. Apply to irritated skin. Reapply every 10 minutes or so until itching is alleviated. *To make a poultice (paste):* Stir 3 to 4 tablespoons ground oats into the solution. Allow it to thicken for a few minutes and then apply the paste with your fingers directly on the hives. Leave the paste on the skin for 20 minutes before washing it off. This poultice is an effective treatment, but if you want to avoid the mess, you can use the same liquid solution without the oats as a rinse for your skin. *For a bath:* Add 5 drops lavender oil and 2 drops peppermint oil and a cup of ground oatmeal to a cool bath water and soak in it. (Be sure to place a strainer over the tub drain to prevent the oatmeal from clogging the drain.)

Healthy habits: Investigate why you get hives in the first place. They're often caused by food allergies.

Immune system problems

Medical description: If you have allergies or come down with frequent infections, even colds or sinus trouble, it signals that you have a weakness in your immune system. Lymph nodes located in the throat, groin, breasts, under the arms, and in other areas of the body, act as filtering centers for cleansing the blood of waste residues that are produced by the body's metabolic functions or infection.

Essential oil remedies: Many antiseptic essential oils, such as lemon, myrrh, lavender, thyme, eucalyptus, and tea tree, also support your immune system. These same oils promote faster healing by encouraging new cell growth. Some of the best essential oils to use are tea tree, bay, lavender, and melissa (lemon balm). Eucalyptus, thyme, and the more camphorous spike lavender seem to help to bring up low immune cell counts. It's handy that all these essential oils double as a strong antibacterial and antiviral in case your immune system is dealing with an infection. Any eucalyptus will do, but the three species called dives, polybractea, and radiata are especially potent allies for the immune system. So are the linalool and thuyamol types of thyme oil. I know that the names of some of these special types of essential oils can be a mouthful. To understand more about the different specialty essential oils that you'll see for sale and why you might consider using them, check out Chapter 15. Other good immune essential oils are myrtle and peppermint. A good choice to increase immunity is to use at least one of these essential oils in a castor oil pack treatment. Clean out the infection with your choice of lemon, rosemary, grapefruit, and bay oils, which stimulate the drainage of your lymph system throughout your body to better collect toxins. One of the best ways to use these aromatic immune-regulating essential oils is in massage oil that you rub on lymph areas, such as the sides of your neck, armpits, or groin to move out the garbage. Even better if this remedy is accompanied by a lymphatic massage. My favorite oils base for essential oils to treat the immune system is castor oil, which has been shown to up immune response when applied to the skin. If you find castor oil is too thick, you can always mix it with another oil like olive oil to thin it out.

Essential oil formula: *To make a lymphatic massage oil:* Put 12 drops each lemon, rosemary, and grapefruit oils in 4 ounces vegetable oil (preferably castor oil). If available, also add 6 drops true bay oil. *To make a castor oil pack:* Soak a cotton flannel cloth in 2 to 4 cups warm castor oil that contains 3 drops lavender oil per cup. (The size of the area treated determines the size of the cloth and the amount of oil needed to thoroughly soak it.) Fold the cloth and place it over the afflicted area. Cover the oily cloth with a towel (protected by a sheet of plastic wrap if you want to avoid getting the towel oily). Then place a heating pad, hot water bottle, or heated flaxseed pillow on the towel to retain the warmth. Remove everything when it cools in about half an hour. If this sounds a little messy, you're right, but at least one study found that these packs increase immunity.

Healthy habits: Lymphatic massage uses deep strokes that move toxins out of your body. Herbs that improve your immunity include echinacea root, and the Chinese herb astragalus. Mullein leaf, red root, cleavers leaf, and prickly ash bark facilitate lymph drainage.

Indigestion

Medical description: Indigestion encompasses many disorders, including gas pains, stomachache, nausea, and stomach ulcers. Frayed nerves, anxiety, and overexcitability restrict your digestive juices and digestive tract muscles. If you don't have enough hydrochloric acid in your stomach to properly break down protein, you can develop a food allergy.

Essential oil remedies: The same aromatic herbs that make food tasty — rosemary, sage, fennel, cumin, anise, basil, caraway, cardamom, cumin, dill, thyme, and coriander — also improve digestion. You can sniff them directly from the spice rack or use them in cooking. They stimulate the release of digestive juices to relieve belching, stomach pains, and intestinal gas. Some essential oils have specialty jobs for digestion. These oils are best taken by adding the aromatic herbs themselves to food or as teas. (The essential oils are extracted into the hot water.) You can also put them into massage oils to rub directly over the area. Rosemary improves poor food absorption; lemongrass, chamomile, fennel, and melissa (lemon balm) oils relieve nervous indigestion and inflammation; and black pepper and juniper berry increase stomach acid. All these oils, but especially peppermint, ginger, fennel, coriander, and dill oils, relieve gas pains. One clinical study showed that irritable bowel syndrome or general stomach upsets, such as belching, nausea, heartburn, spasms, and loss of appetite, responds better to one herbal combination than the indigestion drug metoclopramide. That combination contains mostly peppermint, caraway, and some fennel. If you have a problem digesting fatty foods, then rosemary, peppermint, lavender, and black pepper stimulate bile production. Use them as herbs in your meals and as essential oils for abdominal massage. Studies show that bay laurel, thyme, clove, and cinnamon are some of the strongest essential oils to fight *E. coli*, an infection responsible for most intestinal infections (and even many vaginal infections). They'll help if you add the herbs themselves to your meals. Also read the general digestive information Chapter 10.

Essential oil formula: *To make a massage oil:* Add 12 drops peppermint oil, 12 drops orange oil, 8 drops ginger rhizome oil, and 5 drops fennel oil in 4 ounces vegetable oil or a lotion. *To make tea:* Select one of the herbs mentioned and pour boiling water over 1 teaspoon of the herb. Let steep 5 to 10 minutes and then strain and drink.

Healthy habits: Indigestion is a symptom of an underlying problem. If you're not digesting food properly, take an herbal bitter formula with herbs such as gentian before each meal to promote your digestive juices.

Insect bites and stings

Medical description: A bite or sting from an insect. If you get bit by a poisonous insect or experience any allergic reaction, be sure to see a doctor.

Essential oil remedies: Chamomile, cedarwood, eucalyptus, tea tree, and lavender oils reduce the swelling, itching, and inflammation and help stop allergic responses when you're bitten or stung by an insect. For mosquito or other tiny insect bites that don't demand much attention, a simple dab of one of these essential oils provides relief. If you're bitten by spiders or stung by a bee, use a clay paste that contains essential oils. As the clay dries, it pulls toxins from the bite or sting to the skin's surface to keep them from spreading. This method is also good to draw out pus (or splinters that are imbedded in your skin). Lots of natural bug repellents are available in all sorts of stores. The most effective ones contain citronella or some other lemon-scented essential oil.

Essential oil formula: *To make a bite oil:* Put 5 drops lavender oil and 3 drops German chamomile oil into a teaspoon of vegetable oil or alcohol (either vodka or rubbing alcohol). Dab this directly on insect bites.

Healthy habits: Eat garlic and nutritional yeast so that bugs don't bother you as much.

Insomnia

Medical description: Lack of sleep leaves you tired the next day. If you don't get adequate

sleep for days, you may begin developing symptoms of sleep deprivation, such as dizziness, confusion, agitation, and depression.

Essential oil remedies: For insomnia due to mental agitation or overwork, try sniffing several scents: bergamot, chamomile, lavender, clary sage, frankincense, sandalwood, or rose. Other relaxing scents come from the essential oils of neroli (orange blossom), melissa (lemon balm), bergamot, tangerine or mandarin, and geranium. Even better, get a massage with a massage oil that contains these essential oils. One of the most relaxing treatments before bedtime — or anytime — is a warm aromatherapy bath. An old-fashioned, but effective, treatment is to stuff a small pillow with dried hops. Its scent has sedative effects.

Essential oil formula: *For a general insomnia massage:* Put 6 drops bergamot oil, 5 drops lavender oil, 5 drops sandalwood oil, 2 drops chamomile oil, 1 drop frankincense oil, and 1 drop rose oil (expensive and optional) in 2 ounces vegetable oil or a lotion. *For a bath oil:* Add 1 teaspoon of this massage oil to your bath. You can also add a total of 5 drops of any of these essential oils directly to the water. If you don't have time for a bath, rub a little of the blend on your temples or under your nose. This blend can also be applied to your wrists so you can sniff away. To make a sleep pillow or to scent your bedroom, see Chapter 6.

Healthy habits: Take teas, tinctures, or pills of sedative herbs like valerian root, kava root, catnip leaf, hops strobiles, skullcap leaf, and passion flower leaf. All these common herbs will be easy for you to find. Sip these teas or take an herbal tincture or pills not just before going to bed, but whenever the day becomes stressful. If you suspect that your insomnia is related to stress, depression, or other problems, see those sections in this guide.

Lung/bronchial congestion

Medical description: General congestion or inflammation of your *bronchioles* (the small air tubes in your lungs) can make it difficult for you to take a deep breath. If you have almost constant lung congestion, it may be due to an allergy such as asthma or food allergies.

Essential oil remedies: Decongestant essential oils that clear lung congestion include eucalyptus, peppermint, lavender, and frankincense. Use any of these essential oils as a steam or in a vaporizer to bring these antibiotic oils directly into your lungs. The steam also opens your bronchial passages and makes it easier for you to breathe. You can also use these same essential oils in a massage oil. Rosemary, tea tree, thyme, or ginger oils are recommended when congestion is due to an infection in your lungs. A good way to use them is to rub a salve that is loaded with essential oils (called a *vapor balm*) over your chest and throat to increase circulation and warmth in these areas to help fight infection. This way, the essential oils are both absorbed through your skin and inhaled into your lungs. A piece of flannel fabric on your chest after rubbing in the balm holds in the heat to increase absorption of the essential oils. Vapor balm made with a vegetable oil and beeswax base (a healthier solution to the drugstore variety that has a petroleum oil base) are available in natural food stores.

Essential oil formula: *For a homemade vapor balm:* Add 12 drops eucalyptus oil, 5 drops peppermint oil, and 5 drops thyme oil to 1 ounce vegetable oil (such as olive oil). Shake well before using. Gently massage onto your chest and throat several times a day.

Healthy habits: Build up your immune system and lungs with herbal tonics such as mullein leaf, elecampane root, horehound leaf, echinacea root and the Chinese herb schisandra.

Menstrual cramps

Medical description: Painful uterine muscle cramping during menstruation. Either emotional or physical stress can worsen your cramping.

Essential oil remedies: Muscle relaxants that reduce menstrual (and other muscle) cramps are chamomile, ginger, lavender, marjoram, and melissa (lemon balm) oils. These same essential oils also ease cramps resulting from disorders such as endometriosis and uterine fibroids. For general information on pain-relieving essential oils, turn to Chapter 11. If you have a uterine problem, also see my advice in this section.

Essential oil formula: *To make a muscle-relaxing massage oil:* Combine 12 drops lavender, 8 drops ginger, 4 drops marjoram, 4 drops chamomile in 1 ounce vegetable oil. Rub over the cramping area as needed to relieve the pain. Use St. John's wort infused oil instead of plain oil for an even more effective remedy. For severe cramping, after you rub on the oil, cover the area with a thin cloth and then with a hot water bottle, heating pad, or a flax-filled pillow that has been heated in a microwave oven to provide long-lasting heat. *For your bath:* Add a total of 6 drops essential oil to a hot bath. (Choose one oil or a combination of those suggested.)

Healthy habits: Herbs that ease cramping are cramp bark, wild yam root, and valerian root. Some women report relief by taking evening primrose capsules, flaxseed, and olive oil throughout their cycle to adjust hormone-like substances that cause cramping. For herbal and nutritional information on relieving menstrual cramps, see my book *Women's Herbs, Women's Health* (Botanica Press) written with Christopher Hobbs.

Menopause

Medical description: Menopause is when the menstrual cycle slows down and then ceases. This happens as your ovaries slow down their release of eggs. The average age is 52, but menopause can occur earlier or later. The many symptoms, which include hot flashes, bone fragility, confusion, depression, and a dry, less elastic vagina due to a thinner lining, are apparently caused by the reduced and erratic hormonal activity.

Essential oil remedies: Several essential oils can help you through menopause. Use essential oils that include clary sage, sage, anise, fennel, and to some degree, cypress, angelica, and coriander, in your bath and as body lotion or cream. These oils seem to have hormonelike activity to promote estrogen in the body. Geranium, neroli (orange blossom), rose, and lavender help balance hormones and are useful not only in facial creams to reduce aging and wrinkles, but to counter vaginal dryness. Hot flashes are partially relieved by peppermint, sage, and lemon oils.

Essential oil formula: *To enhance a body lotion or cream:* Purchase your favorite cream or lotion or buy a basic, unscented lotion at a natural-food store or body shop. Stir in 6 drops geranium oil, 6 drops lavender oil, 2 drops neroli oil (orange blossom), 1 drop rose oil, and 1,500 units vitamin E oil to a 2-ounce jar (or into 2 ounces pure vegetable oil). Use daily. (Vitamin E oil improves the strength and flexibility of the vaginal lining and heals abrasions. Buy the liquid or pop several vitamin E capsules and squeeze out the oil.) *To cool hot flashes:* Add 10 drops lemon oil, 5 drops peppermint oil, and 2 drops clary sage oil to 1 ounce aloe vera juice. (Be sure to use aloe juice

rather than the gel so the solution is thin enough to go through the sprayer.) Put in a spray bottle that's small enough to be convenient to carry around. Shake the bottle blend to mix it all together before spraying. Spray this in the air around your head, on your wrists, face, or neck whenever a hot flash threatens to hit. You can also get a clary sage hydrosol (created while distilling the essential oil) to use as a hot flash spray. *To make a hot flashes tea:* Cover a teaspoon of sage leaves with a cup of boiling water and steep about 5 minutes. Then strain and drink a cup or two every day or at the first sign of a hot flash. (The water pulls out sage's essential oil.)

Healthy habits: Herbs like black cohosh root and natural treatments can get you through menopause smoothly.

Muscle cramps and back pain

Medical description: Pain in your muscles. Pain is the red flag your body puts up to alert you there's a problem. If it's persistent and you don't know why you're hurting, get it checked out by your doctor to make sure that you don't have a kidney, lung, heart, or bowel problem or that your discomfort is not the result of some injury of which you weren't aware.

Essential oil remedies: Rub a massage oil that contains muscle-relaxing essential oils like lavender, chamomile, and marjoram on sore muscles, and they relax twice as quickly than with just rubbing alone. (And, the scent of these same oils helps you destress, just in case stress is adding to your aches and pains.) Juniper, rosemary, and peppermint oils are deep muscle pain relievers that penetrate the discomfort. For the ultimate relaxation, enjoy a massage with pain-relieving massage oils. If you can, take a hot bath before your massage with the same essential oil formula, or at least take the bath. To help alleviate pain, alternate hot and cold compresses on the area. If you have pinched nerves from a recent injury, apply only cold compresses for the first 12 hours after the injury to reduce the inflammation. If you plan to exercise enough to strain your muscles, think ahead and limber up beforehand with warmups and rub on a liniment. (See Chapter 11 for information on liniments.)

Essential oil formula: *To make a muscle cramp massage oil:* Combine 8 drops lavender oil, 4 drops marjoram oil, 6 drops German chamomile oil, and 4 drops peppermint oil in 2 ounces vegetable oil. For an even more effective massage oil, use St. John's wort oil or arnica oil instead of plain vegetable oil. You can buy these oils or make your own. (The herbs are infused into vegetable oil.) *In your bath:* Add 2 drops each of these same essential oils to the hot water, along with ¼ cup Epsom salts to further relax tight muscles. *For a compress:* Add 3 drops ginger oil and 2 drops lavender oil to ½ cup hot water. Soak a soft cloth in the solution and wring out the excess. Fold the cloth and lay it on the painful area. To hold in the heat, cover the cloth with a towel, a hot water bottle, or a flaxseed pillow that has been heated in the microwave. Before it cools, replace the hot cloth with another one that has been soaked in plain cold water. Leave the compress on 5 to 10 minutes, or until it starts to cool, and then replace it with another hot one. Repeat this procedure several times.

Healthy habits: Muscle relaxant herbs include chamomile, valerian, skullcap, and kava. Many formulas contain these herbs.

Nausea and motion sickness

Medical description: Feeling sick to your stomach and nauseous is common. This can be due to an illness, eating spoiled food, drinking bad water, the flu, emotional distress, hormonal imbalance (as in pregnancy), or motion sickness.

Chronic bouts of nausea can also signal something even more serious, so be sure to see your doctor about it.

Essential oil remedies: Basil, ginger, chamomile, and peppermint oils relieve nausea. The best way to take these oils is in a breath freshener, mint, natural ginger ale, or as herb tea. (The hot water pulls essential oils out of the plant into the water.) You can also rub a massage oil that contains any of these oils over your stomach. This approach is good for children who refuse to drink the tea or take other medications. Sometimes, you'll find that just inhaling a little of peppermint's aroma is all you need. See the general discussion on oils for digestion in Chapter 10.

Essential oil formula: *To make an antinausea tea:* Pour 2 cups boiling water over 2 teaspoons of the herb or herbs of your choice listed in the preceding bullet. Cover and steep for 5 to 10 minutes and then strain and drink. *For a massage belly oil:* Mix 8 drops chamomile and 4 drops ginger into 1 ounce vegetable oil and rub as needed over the stomach area. This blend is also good for general digestive tract upset, and the massage that goes along with rubbing on the oil also helps to ease digestive distress.

Healthy habits: Nausea can be due to poor eating habits and poor food choices. If so, you know what to do. If you're subject to motion sickness, watch a stationary object outside the vehicle.

Nerve pain

Medical description: Pain that is caused by injured or pinched nerves.

Essential oil remedies: The essential oils of lavender, chamomile, marjoram, and helichrysum relieve nerve pain. To some degree so do sandalwood, caraway, and lemongrass oils. Use these oils in a massage oil to reduce the pain of any condition related to nerves, such as a pinched nerve, sciatica, carpal tunnel syndrome, and shingles (a painful skin eruption related to herpes). These essential oils can even give you some relief if you suffer from nervous system conditions like multiple sclerosis and chronic fatigue syndrome. General information on essential oils and pain is in Chapter 11.

Essential oil formula: *To make a massage oil for your nerves:* Combine 8 drops lavender oil, 4 drops chamomile oil, 4 drops helichrysum oil (if available), and 3 drops marjoram oil in 2 ounces of an infused oil of St. John's wort. Apply as needed for relief.

Healthy habits: Relaxation helps to calm nerve conditions. See Chapter 9 to find more relaxation techniques that incorporate essential oils.

Oily skin

Medical description: Oily skin has luster and may even be slightly shiny from all the oil. It also tends to have a coarser texture, with large pores, and is prone to acne because the excess oil attracts dirt and clogs your pores with dead cells, which can breed bacteria and infection.

Essential oil remedies: Basil, eucalyptus, tea tree, cedarwood, cypress, lemongrass, spike lavender, and ylang ylang oils help to normalize skin that has overactive oil glands. Sage and lemongrass slow down oil production. (They also reduce sweating.) Use these essential oils in aromatherapy steams and facial masks, which help unclog your pores and encourage the release of excess oil. Citrus, such as lemon or orange, is appropriate for use on oily skin. Keep in mind that citrus oils have a photosensitizing effect that causes a rash on some people if you're in the sun after using them. A skin lotion is more moisturizing for your oily skin than a cream. A little oil is fine but look for products that are based more on aloe vera or aromatherapy

hydrosols. (See the explanation of hydrosols in Chapter 14.) Vinegar is good to use on oily skin. Most products don't contain it due to its strong smell, even though the smell dissipates within in a few minutes once you apply it to your skin. Some witch hazel and grain alcohol also dry your skin. Just don't overdo it. Putting too much drying substance on your skin only encourages more oil production. Find more on oily skin in Chapter 7.

Essential oil formula: *To make a skin toner:* Combine 5 drops cedarwood oil, 3 drops lemongrass oil, 1 drop ylang ylang oil, ¼ cup aloe vera, and 1 ounce witch hazel distillate. Shake well before applying to your skin.

Healthy habits: Cleanse your oily skin a couple times a day with an aromatherapy soap to remove excess oil.

PMS (premenstrual syndrome)

Medical description: Irritability, mood swings, depression, headaches, bloating, and swollen breasts are a few of the symptoms that can occur just before menstruation. Known as premenstrual syndrome, or PMS, the condition is related to the rise and fall of hormones just before menstruation. They disappear after menstruation begins. PMS is mildly unpleasant for some women and temporarily debilitating for others.

Essential oil remedies: Try to begin your PMS treatment a couple of days before you expect the symptoms to hit. Essential oils that help are angelica, chamomile, lavender, marjoram, and especially geranium and clary sage. Several of these essential oils appear to help balance hormones. For problems with water retention, a massage oil that contains grapefruit, carrot seed, and/or juniper can offer some relief. For depression associated with PMS, switch that to clary sage, neroli (orange blossom), jasmine, or ylang ylang. If you experience fatigue, acne, fluid retention, headaches, or other symptoms, refer to these specific sections in this guide for more advice on how to deal with these conditions.

Essential oil formula: *For a PMS massage/body oil:* Add 10 drops geranium oil, 6 drops chamomile oil, 3 drops clary sage oil, 3 drops angelica oil, and 2 drops marjoram oil to 2 ounces of vegetable oil. Use as a body oil — or better yet, have someone give you a massage with it.

Healthy habits: Vitex berries balance PMS hormones. Dandelion root tea or tincture treats water retention and evening primrose capsules help relieve symptoms. For more information, see my book *Women's Herbs, Women's Health* (Botanica Press), co-authored by Christopher Hobbs. Go easy on salt and sugar at least a week before menstruation.

Poison oak/ivy/sumac rash

Medical description: An allergic reaction from contact with any one of three plants causes a rash with extreme itching.

Essential oil remedies: Look for a remedy that combines herbs with essential oils. Chamomile and helichrysum are examples of essential oils that help ease the painful rash and heal the skin, while cypress dries it up. The menthol in peppermint relieves the painful burning and itching. You can wash with a liquid peppermint soap. Stay away from oil-based products during the first stages. Later, you can use a lotion containing these essential oils during the subsequent dry stage of a poison oak, ivy, or sumac rash.

Essential oil formula: *For a homemade poison oak, ivy, or sumac remedy:* Add 3 drops lavender oil, 3 drops cypress oil, and 2 drops peppermint oil to a solution of 1 tablespoon apple cider vinegar or distilled witch hazel (from the drugstore) and

2 tablespoons water. Dissolve ½ teaspoon Epsom salts into this and use it as a skin wash. *For a paste to dry up an oozing rash:* Stir 1 teaspoon ground oatmeal into this solution to make a paste. Dab the paste on your rash as often as needed. *For a bath to relieve itching:* Pour 1 tablespoon of the solution, ½ cup Epsom salts, and 4 cups quick-cooking oats (they dissolve best) into a tepid bath and bathe in it. (When you let out the water, put one of the screens designed to catch hair over your drain to prevent the oats from cogging your drain.)

Healthy habits: Echinacea root and chamomile flower reduce inflammation. Good external washes include mugwort leaf, manzanita leaf, and jewelweed leaf. And, try not to itch.

Sprains and bruises

Medical description: When you injure a *ligament* — springy tissue that holds your muscles to your bones — that's a sprain. You get bruised when soft tissue is damaged. In either case, the result is pain and often discoloration as the area swells. If this happens to you often without apparent reason, it's wise to get a doctor's checkup to make sure that your bruising isn't the result of an even more serious, underlying disorder, such as a kidney problem.

Essential oil remedies: Both sprains and bruises are treated similarly with essential oils like lavender, chamomile, or helichrysum as a liniment in an oil or alcohol base. These oils reduce swelling and bruising and help relieve the pain. General information on essential oils to reduce swelling is in Chapter 11. You'll also find more information on making and using liniments in this same chapter.

Essential oil formula: *To make a sprain and bruise oil:* Add 12 drops lavender oil to ½ ounce St. John's wort tincture or arnica flower tincture. This oil is a great item to carry in your aromatherapy first-aid kit.

Healthy habits: If you do warmups, such as slow stretching exercises, you're not as likely to develop a sprain. If you bruise or get sprains easily, get plenty of vitamin C that includes bioflavonoids in your diet.

Stress

Medical description: Emotional stress occurs when you feel overly pressured, nervous, or anxious. It takes a toll on your adrenals and the rest of your hormonal system, your nervous system, and your brain.

Essential oil remedies: Fragrance alone can make you less tense. Lavender, bergamot, marjoram, sandalwood, lemon, and chamomile (in that order) have a relaxing effect on brain waves. You'll find the citrusy scents of neroli (orange blossom), petitgrain, and tangerine or mandarin oils very relaxing. Aromas of ylang ylang and chamomile essential oils also have a sedating effect. Anise's aroma is for stress that develops from working too hard. Any of these essential oils can be sniffed by themselves or in whatever combination you like. Just be sure to avoid any scent you dislike. You can purchase nasal inhalers that contain blends of these essential oils. Or, how about adding a few drops of any of the individual oils (or the blend described in the next paragraph) to a vial that you can carry with you. Empty nasal inhaler containers that you can fill yourself are also available. You can find more on stress in Chapter 9.

Essential oil formula: *For an antistress scent:* Combine 10 drops lavender oil, 4 drops sandalwood oil, 4 drops bergamot oil, 4 drops chamomile oil, 4 drops ylang ylang oil in 4 ounces vegetable oil. Use as a body oil or, better yet, as a massage oil. Add 1 to 2 teaspoons massage oil to your bath. You can use 5 drops of any of the suggested oils individually in a bath or hot tub.

Healthy habits: Sure, I know that it's easier said than done, but do try to relax! Herbs, such as valerian root, kava root, catnip leaf, scullcap leaf, and passion flower leaf, relax your mind. Siberian ginseng, ginseng, licorice, fresh oats, and the Ayurvedic herb ashwagandha help to balance your nervous system. Also, if appropriate for you, refer to the sections in this guide on depression and nervous system problems.

Toothache and teething

Medical description: Painful teeth due to disease or, in babies and young children, from new teeth emerging.

Essential oil remedies: Dull your tooth pain with a diluted essential oil such as clove bud. Clove works great to numb tooth pain, but it's hot stuff so dilute it before sticking it in your mouth. It's also one of the potentially toxic essential oils so use even small amounts with care if you have liver of kidney problems. Although it's an old teething remedy for babies, it's probably too strong to use on them. I'm actually hesitant about putting any essential oil, even small amounts, into a baby's mouth, but especially clove oil. Instead, an alternative pain reliever that's safer for baby is chamomile oil, but only tiny amounts that are well diluted, please.

Essential oil formula: *To make a toothache oil:* Dilute 4 drops clove bud oil in 1 teaspoon vegetable oil and rub this on your gums just in the area where the tooth hurts. Repeat this as needed. If it is too hot, dilute it with more vegetable oil. *To make a teething oil:* Mix 1 drop chamomile oil in 1 teaspoon vegetable oil and rub a small amount on your baby's sore gum up to six times a day. This can also be rubbed externally along baby's gum line.

Healthy habits: Practice good oral hygiene by brushing your teeth and flossing. To ease teething pains, give your baby a teething biscuit.

Uterine problems

Medical description: Uterine problems include endometriosis, uterine fibroids, and cervical dysplasia. Causes of these disorders are varied, complicated, and not well understood. It's likely that hormones are involved, especially estrogen. These disorders are difficult to treat either naturally or with drugs, so aromatherapy is only an adjunct therapy to use along with herbal medicine and other treatments.

Essential oil remedies: A sitz bath with rosemary, lavender, and chamomile oils promotes circulation and eases inflammation.

Essential oil formula: *To make a sitz bath:* Fill your bathtub with just enough hot water to reach your navel when you're sitting in the tub. Add 2 drops each of rosemary, lavender, and chamomile oils. Fill a plastic washing basin (like the kind sold in hardware stores to wash your dog) half full of cold water. Switch back and forth, staying in the hot bath about 5 minutes and the cold one for a minute or so. If you have the time, do this about four times. Also see "Immune system problems" in this guide for instructions on how to do a castor oil pack.

Healthy habits: Turn to a health professional to help you deal with uterine problems and refer to my book, *Women's Herbs, Women's Health,* co-authored by Christopher Hobbs (Botanica Press), which devotes entire chapters to these conditions. What you can do on your own is to take herbs such as red raspberry leaf to tone your uterus.

Varicose veins and hemorrhoids

Medical description: Believe it or not, these two conditions are closely related. In fact, hemorrhoids are a type of varicose vein. Because your circulation relies on leg and pelvic muscles to push the blood back up to the heart, varicose veins and hemorrhoids occur when the flow bogs down. The extra load stretches out your veins. If you sit or stand for long periods of time, are overweight, pregnant, constipated, or wear skintight pants or a girdle, blood flow through your pelvic area is especially restricted and encourages their development.

Essential oil remedies: Because they're so similar, use these remedies on either varicose veins or hemorrhoids. Chamomile, lavender, myrtle, juniper oils, and especially neroli (orange blossom), frankincense, and cypress oils diminish the inflammation, pain, and size of your varicose veins or hemorrhoids. Look for a product that contains these essential oils or make your own with the formula below. Add myrrh and carrot seed essential oils to the massage oil if the problem is so bad that your veins are beginning to distend or leak. I'm calling this a massage oil, but you should apply it lightly because massaging it in vigorously could encourage already damaged veins to break.

Essential oil formula: *To make a varicose vein compress:* Add 3 drops each of chamomile, lavender, and helichrysum oil and 1 drop neroli (orange blossom) oils to 1-ounce distilled witch hazel (from the drugstore). Soak a soft cloth in the solution, wring out, fold the cloth, and apply externally. *For seriously extended or broken varicose veins:* Add 3 drops each of myrrh and carrot seed oils to this solution. For hemorrhoids, pour 2 tablespoons of this solution into a jar of the witch hazel or aloe vera cotton wipes that are available in drug and natural food stores. Apply as a compress directly to your hemorrhoids.

Healthy habits: The antioxidants found in bilberry, blueberry, pine bark, and other herbs have similar properties.

Warts

Medical description: Warts are small, hard growths on the skin caused by a viral infection. There are several types of warts. If you have genital warts, see a doctor to have them removed because this virus (the human papilloma virus, or HPV) is passed to sexual partners and can lead to cervical dysplasia in women.

Essential oil remedies: Several essential oils help get rid of warts. Which one works the best depends on the type of wart you're treating. Tea tree and oils fight wart viruses. Thuja oil has a reputation for diminishing warts, but this isn't my first choice because it can burn sensitive skin and adversely affect the nervous system. Use thuja only in very small amounts in a less toxic form as a tincture (the herb extracted into alcohol and water). For warts that may be cancerous, of course visit a doctor first for a proper diagnosis. You may be able to decrease the size of a pre-cancerous wart while you're waiting for

an appointment. I've found carrot seed and helichrysum essential oils the most effective. One thing to consider about treating warts is that they have a "root." They may disappear on the surface with that underlying root still ready to grow back so follow your doctor's advice.

Essential oil formula: *To make a wart oil:* Add 12 drops tea tree oil to ¼ ounce castor oil, along with 800 IU vitamin E oil (use a liquid vitamin E oil or pop open a vitamin E capsule and squeeze it in). Apply two to four times a day with a glass rod applicator, rounded toothpick, or extra-small dropper directly — and only — to the warts. Keep it away from your eyes. A little trick to help reduce it is to cover the wart with a piece of tape or a waterproof bandage after applying the oil to seal it from air exposure.

Healthy habits: Build up your immune system so that you're better able to fight the virus by taking immune herbs.

Essential Oil Guide

I|n this Essential Oil Guide, I offer a quick reference to more than 40 fragrant plants that produce the most popular essential oils. This guide provides a description of the plant and its scent — an important factor when discussing essential oils and aromatherapy. I explain the healing properties that the essential oils have on the body and the mind. I tell you the most common method of producing each oil.

In this guide, I list each plant by its *common name* (the name it commonly goes by), followed by the *botanical name* (scientific name). The two-part botanical name has the genus first, which is capitalized, followed by the species. It's better to know oils by their botanical names so that you can properly identify the plant and its essential oil. For more details on how botany plays a role in essential oil usage, check out Chapter 1.

WARNING

Essential oils are very concentrated and can be toxic if used improperly. You'll want to almost always dilute an essential oil before applying it to the skin or hair. Do not ingest them unless it's in something like sore throat lozenges, which contain only tiny amounts of essential oils. For more information on essential oil safety, see Chapter 4.

In general, many essential oils tend to reduce inflammation and are very good at fending off all sorts of infections. Many essential oils are wound healers and improve skin conditions and the complexion and hair. Almost all essential oils help with digestion problems, although these are more likely to be treated with an herb tea. Most essential oils have scents that impact your mood or emotions positively.

The fun facts in this section come from scientific studies, history, folklore, and my experience as a clinical aromatherapist.

TECHNICAL STUFF

The medicinal uses for treating physical and emotional conditions that I discuss in this chapter are for the essential oils only. These essential oils come from herbs that can contain other medicinal compounds with additional healing properties. When you read an herb book instead of a book like this one that's specifically about essential oils, it will cover attributes not found in the essential oil. For example, chamomile tea works much better to aid digestive problems than the chamomile essential oil.

Fragrant plants and the essential oils they contain offer tremendous health and healing benefits. I hope that this guide provides you with a ready reference to an exciting and healthful exploration of aromatherapy.

Basil

Latin name: *Ocimum basilicum*

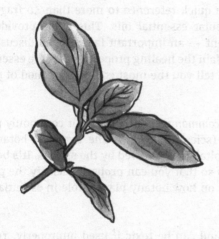

Description: Basil, originally from India, seasons culinary delights like pizza and pesto. Mediterranean peoples have cultivated the fragrant, compact bush for thousands of years. In fact, the name *Ocimum* is probably derived from the Greek word "to smell." The essential oil is distilled from the leaves and flowering tops. Surprisingly, it serves as an inexpensive substitute for the very floral scent of *mignonette* (lily-of-the-valley) in perfume and soap.

Several different basils are steam distilled into essential oil. The most common one you'll find is tulsi basil (*Ocimum tenuiflorum* or *Ocimum*

sanctum*). Originally from India, it has similar actions on the mind and body, plus it represents devotion when used in Hindu ceremonies.

Scent: The scent is sweet and spicy and smells just like basil from the spice rack.

Uses: Sixteenth-century herbalist John Gerard said that basil's scent "taketh away sorrowfulness." Modern aromatherapists agree, recommending it to overcome emotional negativity and mental fatigue and whenever you simply need a lift. Researchers found that sniffing basil increases the brain's beta waves to cause attentiveness. Basil also aids in memory recall and stimulates blood circulation. Using an aromatherapy inhaler (a tube that's designed to be held up to your nostrils) or an aromatherapy steam relieves a headache or sinus congestion. Basil is excellent to treat nausea — even when due to chemotherapy. Plus, it can help fight off viral fungal infections. All this makes basil an obvious choice when you have a cold or flu. A salve containing basil treats herpes blisters and shingles. A basil body oil eases the pain of sore muscles and menstrual cramps. It is sometimes used in body-care products for oily skin and hair.

Caution: Large amounts of basil essential oil may overstimulate the nervous system. It relieves nausea but don't use the oil if you're pregnant.

Bay

Latin name: *Laurus nobilis*

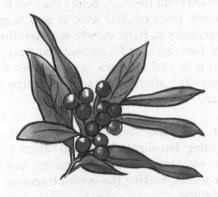

Description: The ancient Greeks loved the bay laurel tree and placed its leaves on the heads of scholars. Greek soothsayers at Delphi sniffed the smoke from burning bay leaves to increase their prophetic visions. The essential oil is distilled from the leaf and occasionally the berry.

The source of most present-day bay, including the oil used in the men's cologne Bay Rum and bay soap, is really from berries of the Bay Rum (*Pimenta racemosa*) tree which grows in the Virgin Islands. I refer to true bay as bay laurel and call the pimento bay from the Virgin Islands tree bay rum.

Scent: The strong, spicy, and pungent aroma may remind you of cooking because this is the same bay laurel that is used to flavor food.

Uses: Bay laurel's most popular aromatherapy use is in a liniment or massage oil to stimulate lymph and blood circulation. The oil also produces a heat sensation, which alleviates muscle tension when rubbed on the body. Studies prove what the Greeks already knew that bay laurel's aroma improves the memory. Inhaling it also relieves headaches, as well as sinus and lung congestion. A massage oil made with bay laurel is perfect to rub on swollen lymph glands (tonsils, for example) due to an infection. It boosts the immune system and helps ward off viral and bacterial infections. It even shows signs in lab tests of helping to counter Covid-19. In the future, researchers say that bay may help with some neurodegenerative diseases that affect memory, such as Alzheimer's disease. The smell deters insects like grain weevils and moths, so many cooks place a few bay leaves in their stored grains to keep insects "at bay."

Caution: Sniff this essential oil lightly because too much produces the reverse effect; you end up with a headache instead of curing one! Undiluted, the oil causes irritation when applied to skin.

Benzoin

Latin name: *Styrax benzoin*

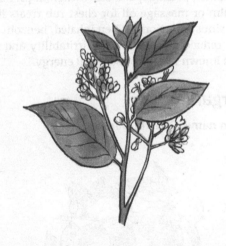

Description: The trunk of this tall Southeast Asian tree, when cut, exudes a gum resin. The Arabic name for benzoin, *luban jawi*, means "incense of Java." Tongue-tied European traders shortened this to *banjawi* and then changed it to "Benjamin," and eventually to benzoin. An absolute is made, but is so thick, it is usually thinned for use with the chemical solvent ethyl glycol. I prefer buying the resin and thinning it myself with alcohol because it won't dissolve into vegetable oil. This limits its use because it only mixes into water-soluble ingredients.

Scent: With its sweet, warm, vanilla-like odor, benzoin is sometimes used in place of the much more expensive true vanilla.

Uses: The essential oil of benzoin in a cream or salve protects chapped skin. It also improves skin elasticity and heals redness, irritation, and itching. If you've worked in a hospital, you're probably already familiar with tincture of benzoin that's used in adhesive dressings. It is antibacterial, even penetrating through the protective biofilm layer that surrounds some forms of bacteria. As an added benefit, benzoin is a natural preservative that delays spoiling in creams and lotions. As a "fixative," it retains the scent of potpourri, perfume, and other fragrant products. A balm or massage oil for chest rub treats lung and sinus infections. When inhaled, benzoin can also reduce drowsiness and irritability and has been known to improve mental energy.

Bergamot

Latin name: *Citrus bergamia*

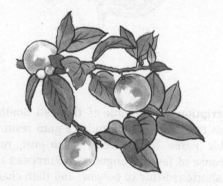

Description: This small citrus tree produces an attractive round, green fruit, but one that tastes too bitter to eat. The green-tinted bergamot oil is pressed from the rinds before the fruit is ripe. Originally from tropical Asia, it now is grown commercially in Italy, mostly as a flavoring for many beverages and candies. You may have tasted it in Earl Gray tea. It also scents men's colognes and aftershaves, so is a familiar scent to many.

Scent: The fragrance is fresh, citrus, and refreshing, but slightly spicy and balsamic compared with other citruses. It mixes well with other scents, making the overall fragrance rich, but mellow.

Uses: Bergamot destroys bacteria, viruses, and fungi, so it's used to treat infections like flu. It increases the production of white blood cells, which helps the body rid itself of the residues of infection. Diluted in a salve or massage oil, bergamot can be applied on a variety of skin problems that include eczema. The antiviral actions work against herpes blisters, shingles, and chicken pox. It also makes a pleasantly scented, natural deodorant that kills odor-causing bacteria. The aroma is second only to lavender in its ability to relax brain waves when sniffed and, thus, is very calming. The sedative properties can relax you right to sleep! Just sniffing the aroma acts as an antidepressant.

Caution: Bergaptene, a compound in the essential oil, can make your skin sensitive to light. (See Chapter 4 for more info about safety issues.) A bergaptene-free essential oil is available and is a safer choice.

Birch

Latin name: *Betula lenta*

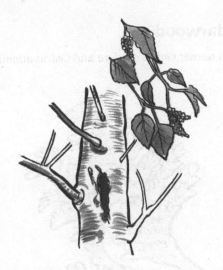

Description: North American birch is a large tree with a fragrant inner bark. When chewing gum, breath mints, and medicines have a wintergreen flavor, it's actually coming from the less expensive birch essential oil. The two oils share a similar chemistry and the same properties and fragrance. Birch essential oil is the main ingredient in the men's fragrance "Russian Leather" (so named because the Russians used birch oil to keep their leather book bindings soft and free of insects).

Scent: The aroma is of wintergreen chewing gum or candy: Clean, sweet, sharp, invigorating, and minty. Many people say that birch smells medicinal, probably because it flavors so many over-the-counter drugs.

Uses: A birch salve or lotion softens roughness caused by skin problems, such as eczema. Muscular and arthritic pain and stiffness are relieved when a birch massage oil or liniment is rubbed over painful areas. A few drops of the essential oil can also be added to your bath to ease pain. Birch delays "pain" messages from reaching your central nervous system. What your brain doesn't know won't hurt! The oil also increases blood circulation and menstruation when delayed by physical or emotional stress. I like to use birch in tingling, pain-relieving, circulation-promoting foot baths and foot massage oils for tired feet because it also softens calluses. It helps prevent dandruff when added to hair conditioners.

Caution: Birch may smell like candy, but high doses can be toxic. Store it away from the reach of children.

Cardamom

Latin name: *Elettaria cardamomum*

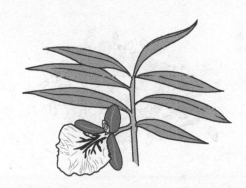

Description: Cardamom is a relative of the common ginger root. It's native to the Middle and Far East where it's used as a condiment in sweet dishes. If you're a fan of Turkish coffee or East Indian chai tea, that warm, spicy flavor is partially due to cardamom seed. The essential oil is distilled from the seed.

Scent: The best quality essential oil has a warm, sweet, and spicy scent, while the inferior oil is harsher, with a slight hint of eucalyptus. A little of this potent fragrance goes a long way, so it's mainly used in a blend to accent other essential oils.

Uses: Almost everyone who inhales the aroma falls in love with the aroma of cardamom. I always think of it as a warm and happy aroma. East

Indians have long considered the aroma invigorating, warmly romantic, and an aphrodisiac — a good combination! The essential oil also treats digestive problems, such as poor appetite and upset stomach, and it eases coughs and muscle spasms. It is a bacteria and virus fighter. It relieves inflammation and pain of headaches, menstrual cramps, bruises, insect bites, and so on. This multipurpose oil also improves your concentration by reducing drowsiness and irritability.

Carrot Seed

Latin name: *Daucus carota*

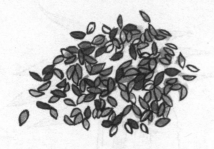

Description: Carrot essential oil is distilled from the seeds of wild Queen Anne's lace, the ancestor of the common vegetable carrot. Indeed, the flowering, lacey plant closely resembles the carrot leaves growing in my vegetable garden.

Scent: Not surprisingly, this essential oil has a carrotlike fragrance, which makes it pungent, so use it in only small quantities. Despite its strong aroma, it finds its way into expensive perfumes as a contrasting note to sweeter fragrances.

Uses: Carrot seed's best claim to fame is the care of dry or damaged skin and hair, dermatitis, eczema, rashes, and even precancerous skin conditions. It's used in complexion creams to improve skin tone, elasticity, and general skin health. It may even slow the progression of wrinkles. It reduces sun damage and may even

slow the growth of precancerous cells. The essential oil in a massage oil treats blood circulation, liver function, and digestive complaints.

Cedarwood

Latin name: *Cedrus deodara* and *Cedrus atlantica*

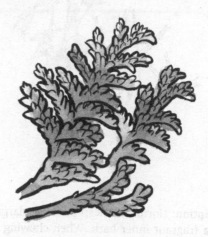

Description: The majestic Himalayan and Atlas cedar trees grow to 100 feet tall and live more than 1,000 years.

There are also North American and European cedars that are steam distilled into essential oils. All of the cedars have similar properties as germ-fighters and bug repellants.

Scent: The scent is similar to camphor, but with a richer, woodsy, balsamic undertone, especially the Himalayan cedarwood.

Uses: An aromatherapy steam with cedar essential oil treats respiratory infections and clears sinus and lung congestion. A few drops in a *sitz* bath, in which you sit in a shallow tub of warm water, reduces the pain and irritation of a bladder infection. The essential oil is also an astringent that dries oily or blemished skin when used in a facial wash or spritzer. Added to a salve or hair conditioner, it relieves eczema, psoriasis, skin inflammation, and dandruff, especially when these conditions are related to excessively oily skin. Cedarwood is good for dry hair because it increases the ability of your skin and scalp to hold in water. You can also put it on itchy bug bites. Although I have no proof, it is reported to slow hair loss. Cedar's fragrance is a well-known deterrent of clothes moths and bugs in general. I've followed the family tradition of storing woolens in a cedar chest. The fragrant wood of cedar trees has been burned as incense. Himalayan cedarwood (*Cedrus deodora*) is a sacred tree in India where it can be found growing in protected groves.

Caution: Cedar essential oil contains strong compounds that are best avoided during pregnancy.

Chamomile, German

Latin name: *Matricaria recutita*, formerly *Matricaria chamomilla*

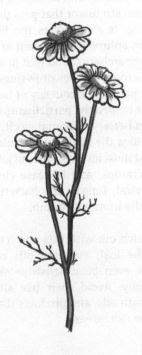

Description: Chamomile resembles tiny daisies with its miniature white-petaled flowers and yellow centers. A chemical reaction during distillation, which creates the compound chamazulene, seems like a real magic act. It makes the essential oil turn bluegreen (azulene means "blue"). This increases its already potent anti-inflammatory properties.

Buying chamomile can be confusing because there are several other essential oils called chamomile. This is a good time to rely on botanical names, although some confusion exists because botanists have changed some of the botanical names. Roman chamomile (*Chamaemelum nobile*) is the other chamomile that is most often available. The closely related Moroccan chamomile (*Cladanthus mixtus*) is sometimes identified by older names: *Chamaemelum mixtum*, *Anthemis mixta*, *Ormenis mixta*, and *Ormensis multicaulis*. The same aroma of both oils is similar to German chamomile and has the same calming action on the mind. However, they do have different chemistry so do not reduce inflammation as well. Cape or African chamomile (*Eriocephalus punctulatus*) from South Africa is a shrub that bears aromatic, chamomile-like flowers. When steam distilled, it produces the same anti-inflammatory azulene as German chamomile and has the same uses. It is strongly antiseptic and anti-inflammatory and treats respiratory, skin, and digestive disorders. Traditionally it has been used for depression. To help you sort out species and botanical names, see Chapter 1.

Scent: Sweet and herbaceous, the chamomile scent is so apple-like that the Spanish call it manzanilla, or "little apple," and the Greeks know it as "earth-apples."

Uses: Research shows that it relaxes the mind and body, soothing those who feel stressed, anxious, depressed, or can't sleep. As a result, a massage oil, aromatherapy bath, or compress are popular treatments for insomnia, depression, PMS, menopause, headaches, hyperactivity, and nervous indigestion. The aroma relaxes stimulating brain waves. It works in a similar way to pharmaceutical antidepressants to balance brain transmitters. Both chamomile massage oil and sniffing the aroma have reduced anxiety, stress, and insomnia for hospital patients. I often use the essential oil when the skin — as well as the emotions — are oversensitive, inflamed, or bruised. Just smelling it has quelled the hurt during painful procedures. Chamomile on the skin also reduces the inflammation of burns, eczema, skin rashes, allergic reactions, and numbs the pain of stiff joints and cramping muscles. It also helps the body fight off infection by increasing the production of white blood cells. A cream, compress, or salve is suitable for all complexion types, enlarged capillaries, varicose veins, and acne. Added to shampoos, the essential oil brightens the hair and brings out highlights.

Cinnamon

Latin name: *Cinnamomum verum*, previously *Cinnamomum zeylanicum*

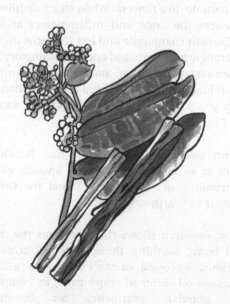

Description: Cinnamon is a large, subtropical tree with fragrant bark that can be harvested twice a year for 30 years. A reddish-brown essential oil is distilled from both leaf and bark. Yardley's famous Brown Windsor soaps are based on cinnamon and, of course, you know the spice!

Cassia (*Cinnamomum cassia*) is usually a less expensive essential oil that is used as a cinnamon substitute. It is considered inferior because its aroma (and taste) is a little less robust, but it is still very similar.

Scent: Chances are you are already familiar with cinnamon's sweet, spicy-hot fragrance. It is so potent, only small amounts can be used, but that's all you need to perk up any essential oil blend. The scent is well known because cinnamon flavors candies, cookies, oatmeal, and, of course, baked goods like cinnamon rolls.

Uses: The essential oil of cinnamon is best described as a mover and shaker. It is a physical and emotional stimulant that gets the blood and mind moving. It also affects the libido and is known as an aphrodisiac, as well as an antidepressant. Researchers found that just having the aroma in the room reduces drowsiness, irritability, and the pain and frequency of headaches. In one study, it helped the participants concentrate and perform better on mental work. The essential oil provides the heat in a warming liniment to relax tight muscles, ease painful joints, relieve menstrual cramps, and increase circulation. It also fights viral, fungal, and bacterial illnesses and boosts the immune system.

Caution: Watch out with this one. The bark and especially the leaf, essential oils can irritate, redden, and even burn sensitive skin, so use them carefully. Avoid their use altogether in cosmetics, bath oils, and products that will contact sensitive skin areas.

Citronella

Latin name: *Citronella nardus*

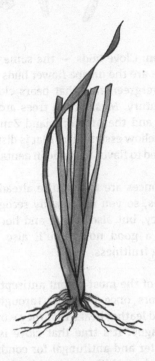

Description: This tropical grass releases an intense odor when broken. A story from 332 B.C. says that Alexander the Great, while riding an elephant near the Egyptian border, became intoxicated when he smelled "nard" (the old nickname for citronella) as it was crushed underfoot. That must have been quite the aromatherapy experience! However, intoxication is an unlikely scenario these days because most everyone associates the scent with bug spray. The deep yellow essential oil is distilled from the grassy leaves. Intoxication is an unlikely scenario these days because most everyone now associates the scent with bug spray.

Scent: Distinctly lemony, the scent is sharp and camphorlike.

Uses: Citronella essential oil treats colds, infections, and oily complexions, but its main use is in insect repellents — flea collars, bug sprays, and candles — to keep away mosquitoes, ticks, fleas, and other pesky insects. The scent is very relaxing and can help relieve insomnia. That seems the perfect rection because it's so often used during picnics and on vacation to keep bugs away. It often is used to adulterate the far more expensive and more mellow-scented oils, lemon verbena and melissa (lemon balm).

Caution: The essential oil is safe to use, but it can irritate skin so it's rarely used in cosmetics.

Clary Sage

Latin name: *Salvia sclarea*

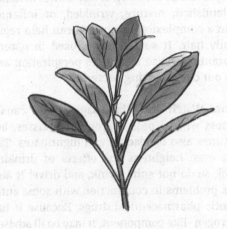

Description: Distilled from the flowering tops and leaves of a three-foot tall perennial, clary sage is produced mostly for flavoring foods. It is related to common garden sage, but it has a different fragrance.

Scent: The scent of culinary sage is obvious, but there is also a nutty, wine-like aroma that I can only describe as heady. Perhaps heady is an understatement. Every time I stick my nose into the plant to describe it, I'm at a loss for words. In fact, this scent is so relaxing that it becomes difficult to think at all.

Uses: Added to a massage oil or used in a compress, clary sage essential oil eases muscle and nervous tension, pain, and indigestion. It slightly promotes the action of the female hormone estrogen, so it is used to help balance hormones. It's good for female conditions, such as easing menstrual cramps and PMS symptoms. I often recommend a clary sage spray during menopausal hot flashes. Researchers found the fragrance works as well as lavender or chamomile to relieve depression, probably by acting on receptors in the brain. It rejuvenates tired adrenal glands, which are responsible for controlling anxiety levels in the body. It also comes in handy for blemished, mature, wrinkled, or inflamed skin in a complexion cream and can help regulate oily hair. It sometimes is used in natural deodorants because it reduces perspiration and wipes out odor-causing bacteria.

Caution: Watch out! Clary sage always causes giddiness when I pass it around in classes, but sometimes also headaches and nightmares. The aroma even heightens the effects of drinking alcohol, so do not sniff, drink, and drive! It also causes problems in conjunction with some antipsychotic pharmaceutical drugs. Because it has an estrogen-like component, it may be ill advised in disorders that involve too much estrogen (but there is no research on this).

Clove Bud

Latin name: *Syzygium aromaticum*, previously *Eugenia caryophyllata*

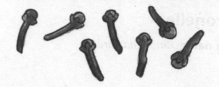

Description: Clove buds — the same as used in cooking — are the unripe flower buds of a short, slender evergreen tree that bears cloves for at least a century. Most of the trees are grown in Indonesia and the African island Zanzibar, and the pale-yellow essential oil that is distilled from them is used to flavor food and in dental products.

Scent: Chances are that you're already familiar with cloves, so you will readily recognize their sweet-spicy, but also strong and hot aroma. If you have a good nose, you'll also detect an underlying fruitiness.

Uses: One of the most potent antiseptics, European doctors once breathed through strange, clove-filled leather beaks that they wore to ward off the plague. It's true that clove is a potent germ-fighter and antifungal for conditions like flu, colds, bronchitis, and athlete's foot. The essential oil gives heat to a liniment, helping relieve muscle and arthritic pain. Dental preparations contain clove essential oil, or its eugenol compound to numb toothache. Researchers found that sniffing the spicy aroma reduces drowsiness, irritability, and headaches, assists memory recall, and increases blood circulation. This powerful essential oil also can abate depression.

Caution: The essential oil is irritating to skin and especially to mucous membranes. Although clove bud smells stronger, the leaf contains almost pure eugenol — a very irritating compound. Don't put clove oil undiluted on a teething baby's gums or you will have a screaming baby.

Cypress

Latin name: *Cupressus sempervirens*

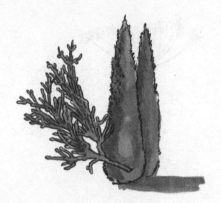

Description: The essential oil is distilled from the needles or twigs and sometimes the cones of this statuesque evergreen. Most of the oil is used in men's colognes and aftershaves. You'd probably recognize it after you smelled it.

Scent: The scent is fresh, woody, and pinelike, but more pungent and almost smoky compared to the fragrance of a pine tree.

Uses: A massage oil or compress of cypress essential oil treats circulation problems, such as low blood pressure, poor circulation, varicose veins, and hemorrhoids. The same technique works well to diminish excessive menstruation, urinary infection, or water retention. A drop of the essential oil on your pillow or a steam will lessen laryngitis, spasmodic coughing, and sinus congestion. In cosmetics, it reduces excessive sweating and an overly oily complexion as well as controls oily hair. Smoke from the burning resin was inhaled in southern Europe to relieve sinus congestion, and the Chinese chewed its small cones to reduce gum infection and inflammation. Long associated with death, French and Northern Americans plant the tall, narrow cypress in their graveyards. Aromatherapists use the scent to comfort those who are grieving. It is not surprising that the oil is also an antidepressant. Cypress can increase mental energy and attentiveness by reducing drowsiness and irritability. In Japan, they have the right idea. Inhaling cypress is suggested for reducing fatigue and tiredness, but not at work. This is done after a long workday to have the energy to enjoy the weekend.

Eucalyptus

Latin name: *Eucalyptus globulus*

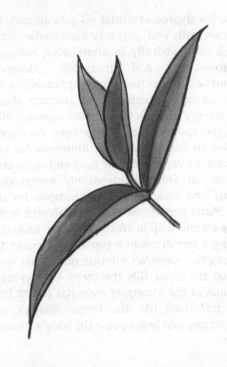

Description: Eucalyptus trees hail from Australia and Tasmania but are now found in subtropical regions all over the globe. They are one of the tallest and fastest growing trees. Out of the more than 600 species, the blue gum is the most widely cultivated variety and provides most of the essential oil.

Aromatherapists also use several other eucalyptus oils. All are highly antiseptic. The most popular of these are the potent infection-fighting Blue Malle *(Eucalyptus polybracta)* and Grey Eucalyptus *(Eucalyptus radiata)*, a specific for upper respiratory and herpes infections. There is also a lemon eucalyptus *(Eucalyptus citriodora)* with relaxing qualities and a pleasant, lemony scent.

Scent: Pungent and camphor-like, the scent of eucalyptus is so sharp, it seems to hit the top of your nose when inhaled.

Uses: Eucalyptus essential oil gets around. It's quite versatile and, yet, very inexpensive. You'll find it used liberally in aftershaves, colognes, mouthwashes, and household cleansers. Researchers found that the scent provides a real wake-up call, so using these products should help you get through the day. The essential oil of eucalyptus, or its main component, eucalyptol, is used in many drugstore liniments for sore muscles, in vapor rubs for lung and sinus congestion, in skin blemishes/oily complexions lotions and creams, and in shampoo for oily hair. Many people use either eucalyptus leaves or the essential oil in steam baths and saunas by placing a few drops in a cup or so of water and pouring the water/oil mixture on the hot rocks so that the scent fills the room. Eucalyptus is also one of the strongest essential oils to fight viral infections like flu, herpes blisters, and chicken pox and helps boost the body's immune system.

Caution: Do not use eucalyptus during an asthma attack. Some people are sensitive to the smell, and their eyes water just from inhaling the aroma, so be cautious using it in a public sauna.

Fennel

Latin name: *Foeniculum vulgare*

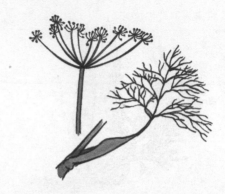

Description: This tall, featherlike Mediterranean herb is often referred to as "licorice" plant or anise because it tastes and smells so much like licorice, even though it's not either one. The essential oil is distilled from the seed.

Scent: The scent is herbaceous, sweet, and very licorice-like.

Uses: Both the aroma and a fennel massage oil are said to be good for weight loss and to reduce water retention. I suspect that it promotes the body's metabolism and slightly stimulates the adrenal glands. Aromatherapists use fennel's scent to improve self-motivation, including the ability to diet, although it's known to both reduce and stimulate the appetite. The essential oil heals bruises and is especially useful for rejuvenating mature skin, as well as dry skin prone to acne. In previous centuries, a fennel cream was said to remove complexion wrinkles. It increases mother's milk, but a nursing mom should drink the tea instead because the dose is much safer.

Caution: Because large amounts of fennel can overexcite the nervous system and essential oils are so concentrated, individuals with nervous system problems like epilepsy should completely avoiding the essential oil.

Fir

Latin name: *Abies alba* and other species

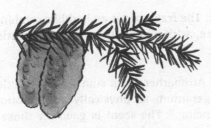

Description: A native of northern Europe, the fir is well known as the source of the Christmas tree aroma. It produces a clear essential oil that is distilled from the needles.

Several different species of firs are distilled. All have similar properties. Pine (*Pinus* species) needles have similar properties, but their aroma is sharper and harsher.

Scent: Fresh, softly balsamic, invigorating, and forest-like, the essential oil is the fragrance of walks through the woods.

Uses: The essential oil of fir soothes muscle and rheumatic pain and increases poor circulation when used in a massage oil, liniment, or bath. It reduces coughing from lung congestion, bronchitis, or asthma when used in a steam or a chest rub. Research has found that the scent of fir increases energy. All this makes it a good winter remedy. The woodsy smell makes people happy and may be one reason the traditional European Christmas trees were brought into the home at

the time of year when short daylight hours make some people depressed. The essential oil is occasionally added to a salve or other skin preparation as an antiseptic for skin infections.

Caution: Fir is good to treat asthma, but only use it in between attacks as a preventative rather than while an attack is happening.

Frankincense

Latin name: *Boswellia carteri and Boswellia serrata*

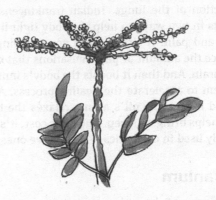

Description: This small tree grows on rocky, dry ground in Yemen, Oman, North Africa, Somalia, China, and India. The yellow oil is distilled from hard "tears" of gum resin that ooze from the tree when the trunk is cut. Arabian frankincense (*Boswellia carteri*) is one of the three priceless gifts that the Magi brought to the Christ child, and its fragrance still fills Greek Orthodox churches and Roman Catholic churches during high Mass. The fragrance has long been valued to inspire one to prayer and meditation. Indian frankincense (Boswellia serrata) smells less like a quality perfume. Most of the studies on medicinal use have been done with it. See Chapter 3, "On the Scented Trail: Shopping" for more on environmental concern with buying trees that are harvested in the wild.

Scent: Soft and balsamic, the heady fragrance can seem slightly lemony or camphor-like.

Uses: Frankincense may be an expensive essential oil, but it's also an important healer. It rejuvenates skin, so it's used on mature and aging complexions and to fade old scars, reduce inflammation and acne, and moisturize dry skin and hair. Skin products containing frankincense have been shown to reduce skin damage, such as from sun exposure. Its antiseptic properties fight bacterial and fungal skin infections as a salve, lotion, or as a compress. It also treats infection of the lungs. Indian frankincense oil works in two ways to help the body fight infection and pain. It first numbs nerve endings to reduce the amount of pain sensations that reach the brain. And then it boosts the body's immune system to accelerate the healing process. As an added bonus, the oil's aroma relaxes the brain and helps bring on sleep. Due to its cost, it's primarily used in cosmetics — expensive ones.

Geranium

Latin name: *Pelargonium graveoloens*

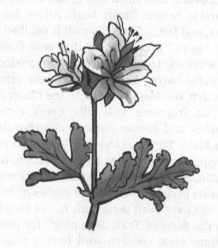

Description: Also known as rose geranium to herbalists, this small, South African perennial is one of 600 varieties of scented geraniums that have been hybridized. Most of the geranium essential oil is steam distilled from the leaves. Its deep green essential oil was not distilled until the 19th century. The main chemical compound, geraniol, is used as the base to make synthetic rose oil and added to true rose oil to adulterate it and bring down the price.

Scent: The fragrance is an herblike combination of rose, with some citrus and a suggestion of wood.

Uses: Aromatherapists sum up the reaction to rose geranium as physically and emotionally "balancing." The scent is good for those who experience mood swings to anger and want more stability. It has been combined with lavender to relax anxiety associated with personality disorders. Experimental clinics in Azbajian had patients smell it to stabilize blood pressure. While it is a sedative that induces sleep, it can also energize you when you feel fatigued. In one hospital, it took geranium about 20 minutes of having to relax anxious women during childbirth. In cosmetics, it's suitable for all complexion types and is said to slow the skin's aging process. As a salve, cream, lotion, or massage oil, geranium essential oil treats a long list of skin problems and fights bacteria, viruses, and fungi. As a result, it is known to relieve inflammation, eczema, acne, burns, infected wounds, ringworm, and lice. It also works against the virus that causes shingles and herpes. It helps decrease scarring and stretch marks. It's excellent for treating hormonally related problems, such as PMS, menopause, and fluid retention.

Ginger

Latin name: *Zingiber officinale*

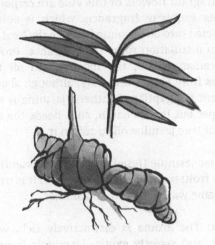

Description: Ginger grows in the tropics with tall, narrow leaves and a knotty root (botanically speaking, a *rhizome*). The root is used in cooking around the world and also distilled into a pale yellow essential oil that is used extensively in the food industry.

Scent: The scent is best described as peppery, sharp, pungent, aromatic, and warm, sometimes with a hint of camphor or lemon. You already know the aroma well if you have had ginger ale or ginger snap cookies or dined on Asian food containing it.

Uses: Ginger is a multipurpose essential oil with a special knack for reducing inflammation. In a massage oil or liniment, its heating action relieves pain from arthritis or sore muscles, menstrual cramps, and headache. It also combats pain by delaying pain sensations from registering in the brain. Ginger stimulates both appetite and poor blood circulation when used in massage oil and relieves nausea and motion sickness just by sniffing its aroma. It's been used in hospitals to help prevent nausea, including for those undergoing chemotherapy. It also acts as a sexual stimulant. For a sore throat, laryngitis, or lung and sinus congestion, try wrapping a warm ginger compress around the neck. Ginger also reduces drowsiness and irritability and jump-starts the brain to keep concentration and mental energy high.

Helichrysum

Latin name: *Helichrysum angustifolium* or *Helichrysum italicum*

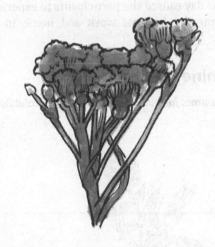

Description: This everlasting flower is a Mediterranean and North African native. You may not be familiar with this plant, but it is certainly worth getting to know. You may know its unscented relative straw flower, which is used in dried floral arrangements.

Scent: The pleasant fragrance is spicy, sweet, almost fruity, and a little reminiscent of curry powder. In fact, the common name is curry plant.

Uses: Helichrysum has many of the same properties as lavender, yet it may be superior in stimulating the production of new cells. It is used in skin-care products to treat acne, scar tissue, bruising, mature skin, and burns. It is in some commercial creams to help prevent sunburn. It treats bacterial infection and inflammation and helps to boost the body's immune system. Its healing properties can quell a chronic cough, bronchitis, or fever. Helichrysum slightly alleviates pain by numbing nerve endings. It lessens muscle pain, arthritis, enlarged veins, and liver problems and counters allergic reactions like asthma. Its scent relieves depression, nervous exhaustion, and stress. Using an inhaler of helichrysum, peppermint, and basil throughout the day caused the participants to experience less burnout both at work and home in one study.

Jasmine

Latin name: *Jasminum officinalis* and *J. grandiflorum*

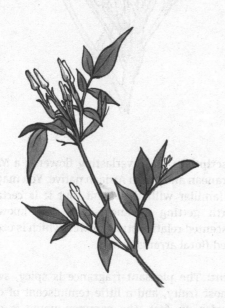

Description: Jasmine captured the imagination of poets as a symbol of beauty. It has been the mainstay of expensive perfumers for centuries. The fragrant flowers of this vine are responsible for its exquisite fragrance, which is solvent-extracted into an absolute because the heat from steam distillation ruins the fragrance. Probably an Iranian native, the most prized oil today comes from France and Italy, although about 80 percent is Egyptian. Synthetic jasmine is much cheaper but is also harsh, so it needs the addition of true jasmine oil to soften it.

Sambac jasmine (*Jasminum sambac*) essential oil has a fruitier and sweeter fragrance. It is used in the same way as the other jasmines.

Scent: The aroma is distinctively rich, warm, floral, and sweetly exotic. Jasmine's fragrance sometimes has a fruity-tea undertone.

Uses: The scent sedates the nervous system, so it's good for jangled nerves, headaches, insomnia, and depression and for taking the emotional edge off PMS and menopause. Seventeenth century herbalist Nicholas Culpeper recommended rubbing the oil into "contracted limbs," and indeed, a massage oil eases muscle cramping, including menstrual cramps. The essential oil is used in cosmetics for sensitive or mature, aging skin. In India, jasmine flowers are applied to difficult-to-heal sores. The scent does stimulate energizing beta brain waves and sharpens mental awareness. Researchers have compared the scent's ability to increase mental accuracy, vigilance, visual awareness, and feel-good emotions with peppermint. In one study with jasmine's scent, computer operators were able to reduce the number of mistakes they made by one-third. Its age-old reputation is as a stimulating aphrodisiac.

Juniper Berry

Latin name: *Juniperus communis*

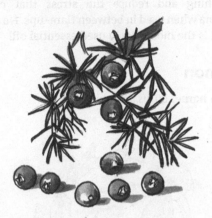

Description: The needles and berries from the prickly, evergreen bush or tree offer the highest quality essential oil. An inferior oil is made from berries that have already been distilled into gin.

Scent: Pungent, herbaceous, peppery, pinelike, and camphor-like describes the lively scent of juniper. If you've ever sharpened a pencil, you know this scent because they are made from juniper wood, which is often called "cedarwood."

Uses: Juniper oil is used in massage oils, liniments, and baths because of its ability to treat the pain and inflammation of arthritis and rheumatism, varicose veins, and hemorrhoids. It relieves muscle pain by warming and thereby relaxing tight muscles. It increases circulation and can also help release fluid retention during PMS. The essential oil is very antiseptic and seems to help the body eliminate metabolic waste. Inhale it as a steam to relieve bronchial congestion, infection, and spasms. Indigenous peoples in both Europe and North America have burned the branches as a *smudge* to purify sick individuals and sickrooms. Sniffing the oil serves as a pick-me-up to counter tiredness

and reduce anxiety, but at the same time, it produces a very relaxing effect. It is suitable in cosmetics for acne and eczema and in shampoos for greasy hair or dandruff. It repels wool moths.

Caution: Juniper is best avoided during pregnancy. There are some cautions of avoiding it when you have a kidney infection, but avoid most essential oils then. Refer to Chapter 4 for more information on using essential oils safely.

Lavender

Latin name: *Lavandula angustifolia*

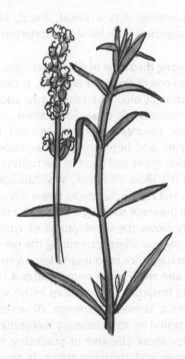

Description: The name of this well-loved Mediterranean herb comes from the Latin *lavandus*, meaning to wash because the Romans added it to their bathing water. Lavender still remains the most popular scent for soap and many other aromatherapy products.

The hybridized Lavandin (*Lavendula* x *intermedia*) dominates the market. It is what you'll find in most aromatherapy products, because it is easier to grow, has more flowers, and is produced in a greater quantity. All of this makes it slightly less expensive. Many versions of lavandin exist, each with a slightly different scent. It is sometimes considered an inferior lavender oil; when I talked to producers in France, they regarded their family's selection of lavandin like fine wines. They are sold under their family names, such as Grosso, Abrialis, and Super. A less expensive Spike Lavender (*Lavendula latifolia*) has a more camphor scent. It is used in liniments and acne formulas.

Scent: Lavender has a sweet, floral, but very herbal fragrance with balsamic undertones.

Uses: Among the safest of all essential oils, lavender is also one of the most antiviral, antibacterial, and antifungal oils. Just taking a lavender bath boosts immunity. It treats lung, sinus, and skin infections; reduces inflammation; and relieves muscle pain and headaches. It is suitable for all complexion types and hastens the healing of skin cells, so it's used on burns, sun-damaged skin, wounds, and rashes. Lavender treats oily skin and acne and prevents scarring and stretch marks and reputedly slows the development of wrinkles. It reduces pain by slightly numbing the nerve endings. The fragrance encourages deep sleep. Babies cry less and sleep more soundly after a lavender bath, and hospital patients sleep better with less pain after a lavender massage. Of several fragrances tested by aromatherapy researchers, lavender was most effective at producing relaxing brain waves and reducing stress. It also eliminated almost one-quarter of computer errors made by office workers. Lots of studies show that it only takes about ten minutes of inhaling lavender's aroma to ease a long list of problems. Lavender eases headaches, pain, depression, confusion, PMS, anxiety, and memory problems. It has also been successfully used when feelings of

dejection crop up or Alzheimer's patients become aggressive. It modulates the immune, nervous, and hormonal systems. Lavender can also improve breathing and reduce the stress that causes asthma when used in between flare-ups. No wonder it is the most widely used essential oil!

Lemon

Latin name: *Citrus limonum*

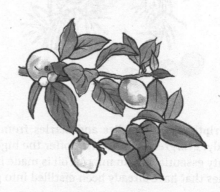

Description: Here's a plant and scent that everyone is sure to know. The lemon tree hails from Asia but has been cultivated in Italy because at least the 4th century. The essential oil is either steam distilled or pressed out of the peel. (For descriptions of forms of extracting essential oils, see Chapter 14.) Like other citruses, the oil keeps for only about a year unless you prolong its life by storing it in a cool place or even in the refrigerator.

Scent: Lemon carries a well-known citrus scent that is clean and sharp. The better the quality, the smoother the aroma.

Uses: Lemon is known throughout the world as a remedy that relieves fevers, sore throat, coughs, and indigestion. The essential oil counters a wide range of viral and bacterial infections. It increases immune system activity by stimulating the production of the white corpuscles that fight infection. The massage oil also relieves lymph glands congested from infection. It reduces bloating, and some say it promotes weight loss. It also reduces inflammation and relaxes stiff muscles. Incorporated into cosmetics, lemon is used on oily complexions, skin blemishes, and oily hair. The scent is diffused through the air systems of some Japanese offices and factories to increase worker's concentration and ability to memorize. Having lemon lingering in the air has cut the number of mistakes made by volunteers in studies by half. It relaxes brain waves, showing that it produces a relaxing effect. Inhaling the scent also slightly lowers blood pressure, a sign of relaxation. Studies support its use to relieve depression, anxiety, and pain.

Caution: Lemon can make your skin sensitive to light and irritated when the essential oil is pressed, but not if it's distilled.

Lemongrass

Latin name: *Cymbopogon citratus*

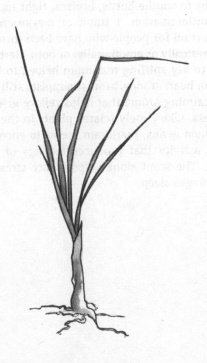

Description: This tall perennial grass is originally from India and Sri Lanka but has found its way into the traditional cuisines throughout Southeast Asia. An inexpensive essential oil, it is the source of much of the lemon scent found in cosmetics and hair preparations, soaps, perfumes, and deodorants. It also flavors processed foods. In fact, lemongrass is one of the bestselling essential oils in the world. The distilled oil is an amber-yellow color.

Lemongrass has a close relative, palmarosa (*Cymbopogon martini*), that is also a popular essential oil. It has the same lemony fragrance, but nicely combined with rose. It's not quite as lovely, but still is sometimes used to substitute for the more expensive geranium. Like lemongrass, palmarosa helps to reduce stress and nervous exhaustion. It's been used for a long time to treat pain and various nervous system problems, such as epilepsy. It's a skin cell regenerator that can be used on any type of complexion, but it's especially good for skin that's dry or has problems with acne or infections.

Scent: Rose and lemony, but herbal and slightly bitter. It gives Ivory soap its familiar scent.

Uses: Lemongrass essential oil is found in cosmetics such as hair conditioner, facial water, lotion, and vinegar for oily hair and skin. Added to water or vinegar and sprayed in the air, on a countertop, or along walls and floors (or on your pet!), it is an insect repellent and attacks fungi by discouraging mold growth. An antiseptic wash or compress is used on skin infections, especially ringworm and infected sores. According to researchers, it is more effective against staph infection than either penicillin or streptomycin. Lemongrass reduces pain sensations that reach the brain to ease headaches and rheumatic pain. It also slightly numbs nerve endings, which dulls the intensity of the pain. In India, the plant is infused into coconut oil to massage away pain and itching. In the Caribbean, a strong lemongrass tea is used as a medicinal wash. The scent alone decreases irritability, stress, nervous exhaustion, and drowsiness, acting much like a pharmaceutical drug to encourage the production of substances in the brain that cause relaxation, such as GABA. Similarly to lemon, the fragrance helps improve self-esteem.

Caution: The oil is nontoxic but it can cause skin sensitivity in some people.

Marjoram

Latin name: *Origanum majorana*, formerly *Majorana hortensis*

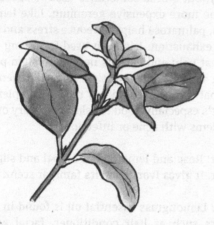

Description: The low, bushy perennial is native to Asia, but was naturalized in Europe where it was a favorite of the ancient Greeks, who named it "joy of the mountain." A species of marjoram was probably really the hyssop used in the Bible to make an aromatic ceremonial oil. The greenish-yellow oil is distilled from the plant's flowering tops. The scent and properties are milder than the closely related and potentially toxic essential oil of oregano (*Origanum vulgare*).

Scent: The sweet, herblike, pungent, sharp, and spicy scent has just a hint of camphor. It smells a lot like pizza, which contains marjoram as a seasoning.

Uses: Marjoram is a good sedative. Testing shows that it's one of the most effective fragrances to relax brain waves. A calming massage oil, the essential oil eases stiff joints and muscle spasms, including tics, excessive coughing, indigestion, menstrual cramps, and headaches, especially migraines. It's a sedative that slightly lowers high blood pressure and is known to relieve pain. In a steam, compress, or vapor rub, it fights the viruses and bacteria responsible for colds, flu, and laryngitis. It's used in salves and creams to soothe burns, bruises, tight muscles, and inflammation. I think of marjoram as a comfort oil for people who have been through a lot physically or emotionally, or both. Herbalists used to say sniffing marjoram helped to heal a broken heart. Today, aromatherapists still use it as a calming aroma that helps relieve grief and sadness. Like closely related plants in the same *Origanum* genus, marjoram seems to encourage brain activity that produces feelings of well-being. The scent alone helps reduce stress and encourages sleep.

Melissa (Lemon balm)

Latin name: *Melissa officinalis*

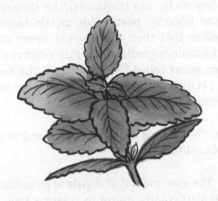

Description: Melissa, known to herbalists as lemon balm, is a southern European native. The essential oil is distilled from the leaves, but it's expensive because so little is produced. As a result, oil sold as melissa is often adulterated or replaced altogether with the far less costly lemon or citronella.

Scent: The sweet smell is soft and distinctly lemon with a dash of herbiness.

Uses: The 17th-century herbalist Gerard said that melissa "maketh the heart merry, joyful, strengtheneth the vital spirits." Even earlier, the 11th century herbalist Avicenna recommended it to elevate a bad mood. The scent is a sedative that helps reduce shock, distress, anger, depression, nervousness, and insomnia. It also helps relax stiff, sore muscles, as well as calms the mind. A medieval favorite, it was the main ingredient in the famous "Carmelite Water." Women splashed this combination of alcohol and essential oil on their faces to ease nervous headaches. At the same time, it improved their complexion. The essential oil of melissa treats indigestion and lung congestion and slightly lowers high blood pressure. It reduces inflammation and fights viral infections such as strep throat, herpes blisters, and chicken pox, as well as fungal diseases. Research centers are investigating how lemon balm acts on the brain's chemicals to improve moods.

Myrrh

Latin name: *Commiphora myrrha*

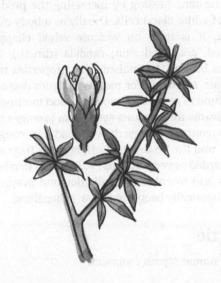

Description: Myrrh is a small, scrubby, spiny tree that is found in arid regions of the Middle East and Northeast Africa. For several thousand years, and still today, the valuable gum it exudes has been an important trade item for use in cosmetics and incense and to inspire prayer and meditation. Despite its bitter taste, this deep, amber-colored essential oil is used in toothpastes and in gum preparations to heal mouth ulcers, gum inflammation, and infection.

The fragrance of another myrrh called Opopanax or Indian Myrrh (*Commiphora erythraea*) has been shown to be a nervous system relaxant.

Scent: The aroma is warm, spicy, and bitter, with smoky and musky undertones.

Uses: Myrrh's essential oil is a strong antiseptic that fights viral and fungal infections like athlete's foot. A salve containing it effectively treats eczema, bruises, and difficult-to-heal wounds. Myrrh also reduces the swelling of infection and even hastens healing by increasing the production of white blood cells. Usually as a body oil or lotion, it is used on varicose veins; chapped, cracked, and aged skin; candida (thrush); and herpes blisters. Its moisturizing properties treat dry hair. A remedy for mouth and gum diseases, it's found in gargles, mouthwash, and toothpaste. It activates the immune system, so lozenges or a syrup containing myrrh are good for coughs, colds, and flu. To top it all off, myrrh's fragrance is regarded as very relaxing, so it is used to relieve stress and to enhance meditation and prayer. It has historically been used as an aphrodisiac.

Myrtle

Latin name: *Myrtus communis*

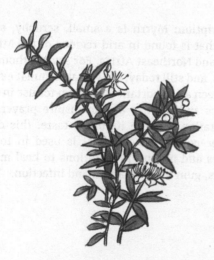

Description: This small, attractive North African tree now grows throughout the Mediterranean. It was a favorite in the ancient gardens of Baghdad, Grananda, and Damascus. The Greeks and Romans honored poets with myrtle leaves to symbolize that their fame would never die. It was the main ingredient in a 16th century complexion water called "Angel Water." The essential oil is distilled from the leaves and twigs and sometimes the flowers.

Scent: The scent is attractive, spicy, and slightly camphor-like.

Uses: The essential oil of myrtle is an antiseptic that is particularly useful in treating lung and respiratory infections. It relaxes muscle spasms and takes the inflammation out of hemorrhoids and enlarged surface veins. The aroma has the ability to calm and relax the mind, as well as increase the libido. It is useful in cosmetics for oily complexions and acne.

Neroli or Orange blossom

Latin name: *Citrus aurantium*

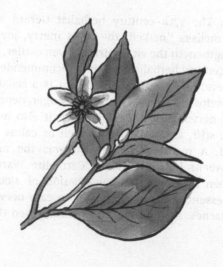

Description: The tree that produces flowers for this essential oil, the bitter orange, is a different species from the sweet orange. The name *neroli* is used for the blossoms of the bitter by perfumers and aromatherapists. It is said to have been named after a 16th-century princess from Nerola, Italy, who loved the scent of orange blossom. Petitgrain *(Citrus aurantium)*, which means "little fruit," is a less expensive essential oil that is made from the twigs, leaves, and small immature fruit of the same tree. Its scent is less elegant and more herblike, but it also costs much less than neroli.

Scent: The scent is bittersweet, floral, spicy, and quite strong until it is diluted.

Uses: Neroli's favored use is to regenerate skin cells and to tone mature, dry, and sensitive skin, although its healing properties are appropriate for all skin types. It helps circulation problems and hemorrhoids and reduces high blood pressure. It is one of the best of the essential oil antidepressants, although it is also one of the most expensive. It may seem contradictory, but this oil stimulates brain waves and relaxes the body at the same time. Along with orange essential oil, it appears to affect the brain's neurotransmitters and balance stress levels of cortisol. The cost of products that contain it reflect the oil's value. A byproduct of distilling orange blossoms, "orange flower water" is the main ingredient of the original eau de cologne, which was used both as a body fragrance and as a skin toner. Not surprisingly, this sweet-smelling aroma also doubles as an aphrodisiac.

Orange
Latin name: *Citrus sinensis*

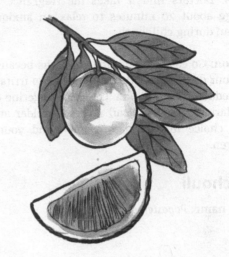

Description: The orange tree was brought to the Mediterranean from Asia by the Saracens during the Crusades. It now grows in Sicily, Israel, Spain, and the United States, with the essential oil having different characteristics depending upon the country of origin. The essential oil is cold pressed from the orange fruit peel from the sweet orange tree.

Scent: The perky, lively scent is distinctively the scent of the orange that is eaten as fruit — which this is.

Uses: Although not as antiseptic as lemon, orange essential oil still combats flu and colds. A massage oil eases indigestion and overcomes a light case of insomnia or depression. The scent of orange reduces anxiety and slightly lowers blood pressure that has been heightened by stress. Doctors find it takes the fragrance of orange about 20 minutes to relax an anxious woman during childbirth.

Caution: Go easy using orange in baths because just four drops in a bathtub is enough to irritate and redden sensitive skin. Oil from tangerine or mandarin *(Citrus reticulata)* makes a milder and safer choice for pregnant women and young children.

Patchouli

Latin name: *Pogostemon cablin*

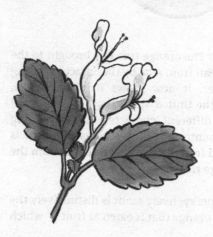

Description: The succulent leaves of this pretty, East Indian bush carry little indication of their potential, because the scent is developed by exposure to air while the leaves are drying and aged. Even after being distilled, the harsh, translucent yellow oil must age to a syrupy brown before it develops a rich patchouli scent.

Scent: Patchouli's scent is quite heavy, earthy, musty, and penetrating.

Uses: The oil rejuvenates skin cells, so it's used on mature, aging skin and treats dry skin prone to acne problems. It is also an antiseptic and antifungal on skin problems, such as eczema, inflamed or cracked skin, and athlete's foot. In India, it is even a traditional treatment for snakebite and poisonous insect stings. The aroma reduces appetite and relieves headaches. It helps to counter depression, nervousness, and insomnia. It slows down the nervous system and helps protect it from being damaged. As a hair conditioner, it helps eliminate dandruff. It repels wool moths and other insects. A "fixative," it retains the scent in potpourri, perfume, and other fragrant products. It is an aphrodisiac that is the fragrance in many famous perfumes, including Tabu and Shocking. However, if you're one of those people who dislikes patchouli, it will probably be a complete turn-off.

Pepper, Black

Latin name: *Piper nigrum*

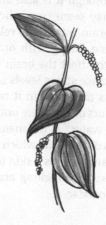

Description: This climbing shrub from India supplies the black (or white) pepper in your peppercorn shaker used for seasoning. The essential oil is distilled from the unripe fruits for extensive use in prepared foods and a pinch in perfumery.

Scent: Pepper's pungent and spicy scent is so well-known that we "pepper" our conversation with comparisons. Sniffing pepper is more likely to make you sneeze before you detect its warm, herbaceous aroma, but it's there.

Uses: Use pepper in a chest rub during a cold or flu to counter congestion and infection. It improves poor circulation and helps to heat up tight muscles and sore joints as a liniment. The scent has a reputation as an aphrodisiac. Inhaling a steam of black pepper essential oil relieves the symptoms of tobacco withdrawal.

Peppermint

Latin name: *Mentha piperita*

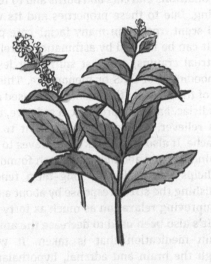

Description: Peppermint is a creeping herb with fragrant leaves that make a popular tea. It's probably a familiar scent to you because it flavors beverages, ice cream, sauces and jellies, liqueurs, medicines, dental preparations, cleaners, cosmetics, tobacco, desserts, and chewing gums.

Some prefer the scent of spearmint essential oil, which can be used as a substitute for peppermint if you don't mind that it doesn't produce the same heating sensation. It does pretty much the same as peppermint, although it's a little less effective.

Scent: The minty-fresh and slightly camphor-like scent of peppermint is familiar due to its use in gum, candy, and herbal tea.

Pine

Latin name: *Pinus* species

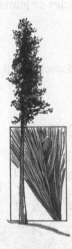

Description: Pine is a stately tree that graces many North American forests and is found throughout most of the world. Several of the many different species are distilled. Common species used to produce the oil are *palustris*, *abies*, and the Scotch pine, *sylvestris*. They all have similar scents, although you can detect the difference if you have a good nose.

Scent: Pine's fresh, pungent smell is easy to imagine if you've ever been in a pine forest. Perhaps unfortunately, if you're like most people today, you associate pine with cleaning solution or paint because pine is also used to make turpentine.

Uses: Pine is popular in cleaning solutions. It's also in European bath preparations to increase circulation and for its fresh, invigorating scent. The scent is stimulating to the senses, and the species of pine called sylvestris is used in massage and body oils to help counter adrenal gland insufficiency. Because pine is sharper and less sweet than the fir tree of Christmas tree fame, fir is usually preferred in an aromatherapy blend that needs a forest scent. However, as a disinfectant and an infection fighter, pine can't be beat. It's also very good in a penetrating liniment for sore muscles or joints.

Rose

Latin name: *Rosa damascena, R. gallica,* and other species

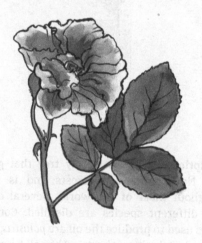

Description: Originally from Asia Minor, Turkish merchants brought rose bushes out of their regions. Bulgaria produces the most valued essential oil these days. Roses have a small yield of essential oil, and because of the care required to cultivate the bushes, the essential oil is expensive, so it's used in costly perfumes. It is either steam distilled or made into an absolute. Not all of the rose oil separates during steam distillation, so a highly scented rose water *hydrosol* is the byproduct. The oil congeals into a waxy thickness when the temperature is cool.

Scent: Intense, sweet, and floral, the fragrance of rose has inspired poets and lovers throughout history. The Greek poetess Sappho christened rose as the "queen of flowers."

Uses: Suitable for all complexion types, rose essential oil is a cell rejuvenator, an antiseptic, and an anti-inflammatory that is used in skin creams and lotions to soothe and heal various skin conditions and cuts and burns and to reduce swelling. Due to these properties and its wonderful scent, rose is in many facial-care products. It can be inhaled by asthmatics. It relieves menstrual cramps, and just sniffing it lessens the moodiness of PMS or menopause. This is a plant of the heart, with a scent that is used as an aphrodisiac, an antidepressant, a sedative, and a stress reliever. Aromatherapists use it to ease heartache. It also stimulates brain waves to keep the mind focused and alert. Research found that rose helps you deal with long-term tension, diminishing the stress response by about a third and improving relaxation as much as forty percent. It's also been used to decrease the amount of pain medication that is taken. It works through the brain and adrenal, hypothalamus, and pituitary glands. It also increases GABA activity, which results in a calming effect on the mind. Rose is also the plant of spiritual devotion in several cultures. Roseries, as their name implies, were originally made with rose beads that scented the prayers. Mohammed said the scent of roses is the closest thing to God's heart.

Rosemary

Latin name: *Salvia rosmarinus*

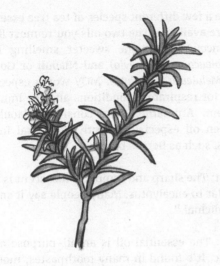

Description: Rosemary's name is derived from *rosmarinus*, which means "dew of the sea." It is cultivated worldwide, but France, Spain, and Tunisia are the main essential oil producers.

Scent: The scent is herbaceous, woody, sharp, and camphor-like.

Uses: Japanese researchers have preliminary evidence that rosemary improves memory; as Shakespeare's Ophelia says, "There's rosemary, that's for remembrance." At the same time, it is also a stimulant to the nervous system. Research finds that rosemary relieves tension, anxiety, confusion, and fatigue and increases energy. It enhances the brain's beta waves to make you feel more alert. People find that rosemary helps their memory and makes it easier to do mental work like math. Inhaling rosemary for just five minutes causes levels of stress hormones to drop. This helps prevent the damage caused by long-term stress. Smelling rosemary actually slows down the breakdown of the neurotransmitters your brain uses for memory. It is even being considered as a treatment for Alzheimer's disease. In a massage oil, liniment, compress, or bath, the essential oil improves poor circulation and eases muscle and rheumatic pain. Just smelling rosemary reduces pain as much as rose or lavender. Rubbing a rosemary vapor balm on the chest relieves lung and sinus congestion. Cosmetically, it encourages dry and mature complexion types to produce more oil. It also treats acne, especially for those who also have dry skin. It also helps get rid of bacterial infections, canker sores, and many other viruses. The bacteria it kills includes those that cause food to spoil. Add it to hair conditioners for dandruff and hair loss and to keep hair healthy.

Caution: Large amounts of rosemary essential oil can be stimulating and increase blood pressure in those already prone to high blood pressure.

Sandalwood

Latin name: *Santalum album*

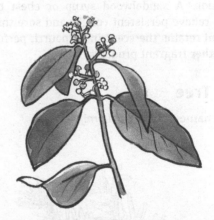

Description: One of the oldest perfume materials, sandalwood essential oil has been in use at least 2,000 years. Sandalwood is a parasite on surrounding trees. The oil is usually not distilled from the roots and heartwood until trees are about 30 years old. Mysore, India, produces a quality essential oil that is grown in plantations that is regulated by the government, although not well controlled by it. (See Chapter 3 for sustainability concerns.)

Sandalwood (*Santalum spicatum*) from Australia that is grown on plantations is usually a more environmentally friendly choice than that grown in India.

Scent: Soft, warm, woody, and balsamic.

Uses: Sandalwood is a major remedy in Ayurvedic medicine to reduce nervousness, anxiety, insomnia, and nerve pain. Researchers found that it even relaxes brain waves while increasing attentiveness and good mood at the same time. No wonder it has long been regarded as the perfect scent to use during meditation. Suitable for all complexion types, it repairs skin damage; encourages new cell growth; and is useful for acne, dry, oily, or chapped skin, rashes, and inflammation. This antifungal and bacteria-fighting oil also increases the production of white blood cells to help the body get rid of infection. A sandalwood syrup or chest balm helps relieve persistent coughs and sore throat. The oil retains the scent in potpourri, perfume, and other fragrant products.

Tea Tree

Latin name: *Melaleuca alternifolia*

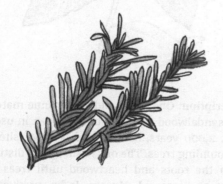

Description: This Australian tree has interesting bark that peels off the trunk, giving it the nickname "paper-bark" tree.

Quite a few different species of tea tree essential oil are available. The two oils you're most likely to encounter are the sweeter smelling MQV (*Melaleuca quinquenevia*) and Niaouli or Gomen oil (*Melaleuca viridiflora*). MQV works especially well for respiratory conditions and the immune system. Aromatherapists consider Niaouli or Gomen oil especially effective for viral infections, such as herpes blisters.

Scent: The sharp and camphor-like scent is very similar to eucalyptus. Many people say it smells "medicinal."

Uses: The essential oil is an all-purpose antiseptic. It's found in many toothpastes, mouthwashes, and dental picks; its use is strongly supported by medical studies. It's effective against bacteria, fungi, and viruses, including those causing flu and colds. A three-percent solution was found effective against herpes blisters. It's also helpful for treating related viral infections like shingles, candida, thrush, and chicken pox. It stimulates the immune system and increases white blood cell production. In one study, tea tree was able to suppress inflammatory skin disorders that are associated with immune system problems and skin cancer. It treats mouth infections and hastens the healing of wounds, diaper rash, acne, and insect bites. It helps to protect skin from radiation burns, encourages the regeneration of scar tissue, and reduces swelling. The presence of blood and pus from infection only increases its antiseptic properties. It's also one of the best essential oils to destroy head lice. Use it in compresses, salves, massage oil, and washes.

Thyme

Latin name: *Thymus vulgaris*

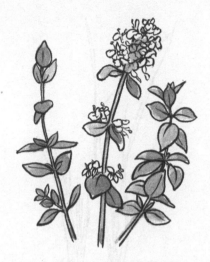

Description: This fragrant, culinary ground cover has at least a hundred varieties. Most thyme essential oil is produced from the common thyme that is used to season foods. The oil is red after it is distilled only once, but a second distillation yields a clear oil without the color or so much heat. Red thyme oil is available for use in hot liniments.

Not all thymes are available as essential oil but several different thymes are steam distilled. They can be more gentle or harsher and more or less antibiotic, depending upon which one is used. The "linalool" type is the most popular because it specifically treats bronchitis, acne, psoriasis, and fatigue with less toxicity than the regular essential oil. It is an offshoot of thyme called a chemotype. (To understand chemotypes, go to Chapter 15.)

Scent: The herbaceous, strong, hot, and sharp fragrance led Rudyard Kipling to write of the "wind-bit thyme that smells like the perfume of the dawn in paradise." Ancient Greeks complimented each other by saying that one smelled of thyme.

Uses: The essential oil is used in a compress, salve, or cream to fight or to prevent serious viral or fungal infection from a wound, gum, or mouth infection. The compound thymol, which is in the essential oil, is one of the strongest antiseptics known. It increases the production of white blood cells in the body, relieves indigestion and, when used in a liniment, can warm and relax sore muscles. It is an ingredient in numerous drugstore gargles, mouthwashes, cough drops, and vapor chest rubs. These products include Listerine mouthwash and Vick's VapoRub. Thyme influences the brain to increase feelings of well-being. Aromatherapists use it to counter memory loss, depression, and melancholy.

Caution: Thyme essential oil can irritate the skin and mucus membranes, so use it in low doses. "Red" thyme oil is so strong, it's rarely used. Thyme oil should not be used by pregnant women or children.

Vanilla

Latin name: *Vanilla planifolia*

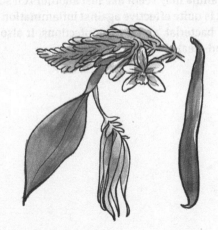

Description: This tropical orchid is a Mexican native that also is grown in Tahiti, Java, and Madagascar. The essential oil cannot be steam distilled, so it is extracted from the vanilla bean with solvents into a thick, dark brown absolute. If you're making your own essential oil product, working with this thick extract can be difficult. You can dilute it into alcohol but not so easily into vegetable oil. Most vanilla essential oil is already diluted into a chemical solvent to make it thin enough for use. If you're making a product that is water soluble or contains water, such as facial cream, one answer is to use vanilla extract instead of essential oil.

Scent: Vanilla's sweet, honeylike, and distinct scent is familiar to people worldwide from its popular use as a food flavoring.

Uses: This well-loved fragrance produces feelings of happiness and often evokes pleasant childhood memories. Children like it, perhaps because researchers found that the scent is the closest to mother's milk. It also doubles as an aphrodisiac, depending upon what other essential oils are blended with it. (I'd go with jasmine to make it sexy.) The aroma is considered stimulating but also has been used to subdue hysteria. Vanilla may seem like just another fun scent, but it is quite effective against inflammation and viral, bacterial, and fungal infections. It also is a wound-healer and an antioxidant.

Vetivert

Latin name: *Vetiveria zizaniodes*

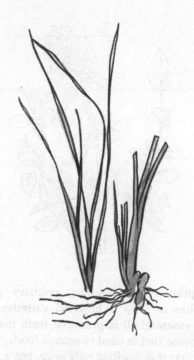

Description: Vetivert, also called vetiver, is a clump of thin, grassy leaves. Its roots are spindly, but intensely aromatic. In India, they are woven into fans and screens called *tatties* for doors and windows. These are sprinkled with water on hot days to cool the air and so that the breeze blows the scent through the room. (An inferior oil is made from the used screens!) India inspired the famous British vetivert colognes and perfumes of the 19th century.

Scent: Heavy, bitter, and very earthy, some people bluntly say that the smell of vetivert resembles dirt. Many find the scent unappealing, but the oil is a crucial ingredient in fine perfumes where its heaviness brings out the sweet smell of other essential oils.

Uses: Vetivert's essential oil is used to heal acne, wounds, and cracked and excessively dry skin. It is also helpful for notably dry hair and to regulate oily hair. It helps fight bacteria and other infections by increasing the production of the body's white blood cells. The scent is relaxing and acts as an antidepressant. It has been shown to cause faster visual reactions and to enhance the ability to work on a computer. The East Indians say that it cools the mind, as well as the body, of excessive heat. In a lotion or massage oil, it eases muscular pain, sprains, and stimulates circulation. In addition, it's used in conditions of liver congestion. A scent fixative, it retains its fragrance for a long time and is used in small amounts to keep the scent in perfumes and other aromatic products.

Ylang Ylang

Latin name: *Cananga odorata*

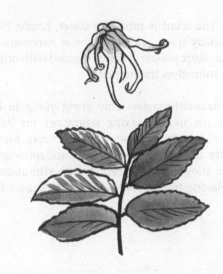

Description: The tall ylang ylang tree originated in the Philippines and is now grown throughout tropical Asia for the perfume trade and even used as a flavoring in beverages and desserts. The name, meaning "flower of flowers," describes the sweet, yellow blooms, which produce the essential oil. The oil varies greatly due to climatic and botanical differences. As a result, you can find several commercial grades with distinctly different smells.

Scent: The scent is intensely sweet, heady, floral, slightly spicy, with overtone of narcissus or banana. Most people prefer it blended with other scents to mellow its intensity.

Uses: Aromatherapists find ylang ylang to be one of the most relaxing fragrances for both mind and body. It also slightly lowers blood pressure and serves as a natural antidepressant. Studies show that the scent is both stimulating and relaxing to brain waves. It is also known for its aphrodisiac properties. Like many natural remedies, it seems to energize or relax you, depending upon your individual needs. Use it in a bath or massage oil or simply sniff it when you need to completely chill out or when you experience insomnia. It balances oil production when used as a hair conditioner, and people in the Philippines and tropical Asia use it to protect their hair from the damages of swimming in salt water. It's good for all skin types, but especially those with combination skin.

Caution: High concentrations of ylang ylang's fragrance give some people headaches.

Appendix

Essential Oils & Aromatherapy Resources

This bonus content is an additional resource that I hope you turn to again and again. This appendix contains information about places where you can find out more about essential oils.

Aromatherapy Organizations

Here are professional aromatherapy organizations in the United States. They recommend aromatherapists and offer ways that you can take online and in-person education.

> **» Alliance of International Aromatherapists (AIA)**
>
> 3758 E. 104th Ave #36, Thornton, CO 80233
>
> www.alliance-aromatherapists.org
>
> The AIA sponsors aromatherapy conferences.

>> **National Association for Holistic Aromatherapy (NAHA)**

6000 S. 5th Ave, Pocatello, ID 83204

www.naha.org

NAHA membership includes their journal. They sponsor aromatherapy conferences.

Herb Organizations

>> **American Herb Association (AHA)**

PO Box 2482, Nevada City, CA 95959

www.ahaherb.com

AHA covers herbalism and aromatherapy news, research, and book reviews in its *American Herb Association Quarterly Newsletter,* edited by author Kathi Keville.

>> **United Plant Savers (UpS)**

PO Box 420, E. Barre, VT 05649

www.unitedplantsavers.org

UpS is a valuable organization created by herbalists to save North American medicinal plants, including sandalwood and other aromatics. Membership includes their newsletter.

Worldwide Aromatherapy Organizations

These organizations are in the English-speaking parts of the world, but outside of the United States. They recommend aromatherapists in their regions and offer aromatherapy education.

>> **Aromatherapy Trade Council (ATC)**

www.a-t-s.org.uk

The ATC is the trade association for essential oil suppliers.

>> **Aromatherapy Organizations Council (AOC)**

www.aromatherapycouncil.org

The AOC is a registry to certify and locate aromatherapists and training in the UK.

>> **Canadian Federation of Aromatherapists (CFA)**

www.cfacanada

The CFA is a registry to certify and locate aromatherapists and training in Canada.

>> **International Federation of Aromatherapists (IFA)**

www.ifparoma.org

The IFA is a registry to certify and locate aromatherapists in the UK.

>> **New Zealand Register of Holistic Aromatherapists (NZRHA)**

www.nzroha

The NZRHA is a registry to certify and locate aromatherapists and training in New Zealand.

Aromatherapy Tours

>> **Aroma~Herbalism Tour**

PO Box 2482, Nevada City, CA 95959

www.ahaherb.com

Tours of Tuscany (Italy) and Hawaii with aromatherapist-herbalist Kathi Keville

>> **Aroma Tours**

4 Cootamundra Rd, Invermay VIC 3352, Australia

aroma-tours.com

Tours of France, Spain, Italy, and Turkey

Aromatherapy Publications

These publications will keep you up-to-date on news and happenings about aromatherapy, essential oils, and aromatic plants.

>> **American Herb Association Quarterly**

Herbs and essential oil news published by the American Herb Association

www.ahaherb.com

>> **Aromatherapy Times**

Published by the International Federation of Aromatherapists

www.ifparoma.org

>> **International Journal of Aromatherapy**

Published by Elsevier scientific publisher

www.Science.direct.com

>> **International Journal of Professional Holistic Aromatherapy**

www.ijpha.com

>> **Journal of Herbs, Spices & Medicinal Plants**

Taylor & Francis Group

www.taylorandfrancis.com and www.tandfonline.com

Aromatherapy Schools

These are some of the long-established schools that teach about aromatherapy, essential oils, and distillation. This is only a sampling of what you'll find available in the United States.

>> **Aromahead Institute**

Andrea Butje

www.aeomahead.com

>> **The Atlantic Institute of Aromatherapy**

Sylla Hanger

16018 Saddlestring Drive, Tampa, FL 33618

» **Australasian College of Herbal Studies**

PO Box 57, Lake Oswego, OR 97034

www.ACHS.edu

» **College of Botanical Healing Arts**

Elizabeth Jones

1821 17th Ave., Santa Cruz, CA 95062

» **Flora Medica**

Valerie Cooksley

PO Box 130166, The Woodlands, TX 77393

» **Green Medicine Herb School**

Kathi Keville

PO Box 2482, Nevada City, CA 95959

www.ahaherb.com

» **New York Institute of Aromatherapy**

Amy Galper

www.newyorkinstituteofaromatherapy.com

» **The Institute of Dynamic Aromatherapy**

Jade Shutes

Chapel Hill, NC 27516

» **Pacific Institute of Aromatherapy**

Kurt Schnaubelt

PO Box 6723, San Rafael, CA 94903

» **The Tisserand Institute**

Robert Tisserand

5119 Via San Lucas, Newbury Park, CA 91320

www.tisserandinstitute.org; www.roberttisserand.com

Websites

The web is indeed a web of information — some accurate, some not. Here are some sites you can depend upon for accurate information.

- » **Aromaweb.** This site is filled with aromatherapy information: www.aromaweb.com

- » **Frontier Herb Company.** This site provides aromatherapy research and links: www.fragrant.demon.co.uk

- » **Purdue University.** This is the university's horticulture site for research on the cultivation of aromatic and medicinal crops: https://hort.putdue.edu

- » **Somamath.** Christopher McMahon's website is devoted to India's aromatic traditions and fragrant plants: members.aol.com/somamath/fragrant.html

- » **World Herb Library.** This site offers thousands of herb and aromatherapy books and journals online for the first time. This collection includes antiquity volumes written by the great herbalists: www.worldherblibrary.org

Index

hives, 314
holy basil, 178, 263
horseradish, 64
household bug repellent spray recipe, 215
household cleaners, 217
household spray, 214–215
hydrodiffusion, 236
hydrosols, 136, 231, 239–241
  commonly available, 239
  defined, 56, 97, 121
  storing, 240–241
  uses for, 240
hydrotherapy, 207–208
hypothalamus, 14, 146
hyssop, 57–58, 64, 257

I

IFA (International Federation of Aromatherapists), 359
immune system and cell repair, 166, 183–186, 314–315
  faster healing, 185–186
  lymphatic system and metabolic waste, 186
  white blood cell production, 185
incense, 9–10, 101–102, 134, 154, 269
indigestion, 315–316
infection, 166, 173, 302–304. *See also names of specific infections*
  bacteria, 173–176
  fungus, 178–180
  viruses, 176–178
infused oils, 75, 79–81
ingesting oils, 53–54
inhalers, 146, 154, 158, 201, 208
insect and pest control, 211–227
  garden, 220–222
  home, 212–217
  outdoors, 217–220, 316
  pets, 223–227
insect bite solution recipe, 219–220
insect repellents, 217–219
insecticides, 217
insomnia, 144, 161–164, 316
  recipes, 162–164
  recommended oils, 161–162
International Federation of Aromatherapists (IFA), 359

J

jasmine, 17, 27–28
  alterations, 41
  compounds, 251, 256
  concentration levels, 73
  enfleurage, 237
  infused oils, 79
  intensity levels, 72
  as main scent, 72
  mood and emotions, 90, 152–153
  overview, 340
  pricing, 46
  sex, 131, 134–135, 137
  skin care, 116
jatamansi (spikenard), 18, 48, 273
jewelry, 100–101
Johnson, Virginia, 128
jojoba oil, 77
juniper, 10
  circulation, 203
  compounds, 257, 260
  digestion, 180
  hydrosols, 241
  immune system and cell repair, 186
  infection, 178
  oxidation, 66
  pain relief, 190, 194, 197
juniper berry, 119, 148, 181, 121, 341

K

Kajima Construction Company, 153
ketones, 58, 253, 256–258
kidneys, 55, 57
kukui nut oil, 77

L

labels, 29, 41, 45, 69–70, 217
lanolin, 110
laryngitis, 303–304
lavandin, 20, 33, 43
lavender, 10, 13, 16, 18, 27
  amount of oil yielded from, 234
  Bouffant Bouquet recipe, 84–85

lotions, 111, 202
    as carriers, 74
    diluting with essential oils, 112
    Lotion for Emotions recipe, 155
    at work, 154
Louis XIV, 135
lung congestion, 317
lymphatic system and metabolic waste, 186

M

macadamia nut oil, 78
Madras sandalwood, 47
mandarin, 16, 62, 162, 237
manuka. *See* tea tree
marigold, 61, 221
marjoram
    amount of oil yielded from, 234
    compounds, 251–252, 258
    growing, 285–286
    infection, 175, 177–179
    mood and emotions, 146, 148–149
    overview, 285–286, 344
    pain relief, 190, 192, 195, 197–198
Mark Anthony, 132, 135
massage
    circulation, 203–205
    digestion, 181
    lymphatic massage, 184, 252
    massage oil, 137, 147, 152, 171, 205, 276–277
    office massage, 155
    pain relief, 13, 193
    sex, 129, 135, 137
    sports, 206–207
    temperature and, 12
Massage Oil for Circulation recipe, 205
Masters, William, 128
mature skin, 116, 120
Mayo Clinic, 16
measuring cups, 69
measuring oils, 71–72, 82
measuring spoons, 69
medicated powders, 172
Meditative Mood recipe, 84
melissa (lemon balm)
    alterations, 41
    combining drugs and, 54

compounds, 249, 254
digestion, 180–182
GRAS status, 40
growing, 286
hydrosols, 241
infection, 178
mood and emotions, 146, 148–149
overview, 286, 345
pain relief, 193
sleep, 162
substituting, 44
Memorial Sloan-Kettering Cancer Center, 16
memory, 14, 155–158, 256, 273, 312
menopause, 318
menstrual cramps, 317–318
methyl salicylate, 256
mice, 213
Midnight at the Oasis Balls recipe, 138–139
milk thistle seed, 58
mint, 134, 136, 174, 206, 213. *See also* peppermint;
    spearmint
minty scent type, 25–26
mislabeled oils, 41
monoterpenes, 259–261
mood and emotions, 141–164. *See also names of
    specific conditions*
    adapting to needs, 142
    anxiety, 147–150
    balanced approach, 142–143
    benefits of essential oils for, 143
    foot baths, 160–161
    insomnia, 161–164
    memory, 156–158
    stress, 143–147
    travel, 158–160
    work life, 150–155
moth balls, 214–215
moths, 213–214
motion sickness, 319
mouthwashes, 174
MQV (*Melaleuca quinquenervia*), 19, 33
mugwort, 64, 164
mulled cider mix, 97
muscle cramps, 318–319
musky scents, 130, 134
mustard, 64
myrcene, 260

V

vacuum cleaners, 216
vacuum distillation, 236
valerian, 146
vanilla, 16, 27
  diffusers, 93
  overview, 353–354
  pricing, 46
  sex, 130, 132, 136–138
varicose veins, 323
vegetable (fixed) oils, 75–79
  as carriers, 75
  cold pressed, 76
  common, 76–77
  diffusers, 93
  diluting with, 42
  fancy/fixed, 77–78
  fixed nature of, 76
  herb seed oils, 78–79
  oil butters, 79
  in skin-care products, 108, 110
verbenone, 263
vetiver, 20, 121, 123
vetivert
  compounds, 261–262
  immune system and cell repair, 185
  infection, 175
  overview, 354–355
  sex, 133
vinegars
  as carriers, 75
  skin and hair care, 112, 121–122
violet, 46, 243
Virginian cedarwood, 261
viruses, 176–178
vodka, 69, 74
volatile oils, 8

W

wall plug-in diffusers, 94–95
walnut oil, 134

warts, 324
water, as a carrier, 75
water distillation, 235
websites, 362
weight loss, 302
wheat germ oil, 78
white blood cell production, 185
wild farming, 47
wintergreen. *See* birch
wisteria, 46, 79, 243
witch hazel distillate, 74, 111, 121
wood scent type, 25–27, 130
wool, 23
work life, 150–155
  focus, 150–151
  Gotta Go-Go-Go recipe, 152
  Lotion for Emotions recipe, 155
  mind-stimulating scents, 151–152
  office massage, 155
  productivity, 153
  taking scents to work, 153–154
wormwood, 40
  compounds, 257
  insect and pest control, 213
  safety issues, 57–58, 224

Y

Yale University, 16
yarrow, 226, 239
yawning, 145
yellow Borneo camphor, 269
ylang ylang
  compounds, 261–262
  intensity levels, 72
  mood and emotions, 91, 148–149, 152
  overview, 355–356
  quick pick-me-up blend, 73
  Relax Away recipe, 84
  sex, 132, 134
  skin care, 116

About the Author

Kathi Keville is an internationally known clinical herbalist and aromatherapist. She's director of the American Herb Association and editor of the *AHA Quarterly Newsletter*. Kathi has authored 15 herb and aromatherapy books and 150 articles for magazines such as *Prevention magazine*; she has consulted for *National Geographic*, *Newsweek*, and *Woman's Day*; and she was associate editor of *Well-Being Magazine*. She's an honorary, founding member of the American Herbalist's Guild and the National Association of Holistic Aromatherapy. She is a member of United Plant Savers. Kathi's Green Medicine Herb School is in Nevada City, California, with gardens of more than 500 species of medicinal and aromatic plants. She offers herb walks, garden tours, and programs in aromatherapy and herbalism. Kathi owns the mail-order herb and aromatherapy company Oak Valley Herb Farm. Kathi's KVMR radio show is "The Garden Forum." She gives aromatherapy seminars at herb symposiums, universities, herb farms, and garden clubs throughout North America. These include San Francisco State University, University of San Francisco, University of California at Davis, Sierra College, American College of Ayurveda, and Omega Institute. Kathi leads Aroma-Herbalism tours to Tuscany. She has also co-led tours to Greece, and Provence, France. Find her and the American Herb Association on social media and at www.ahaherb.com.

Dedication

I dedicate this book to you, the reader, for being interested enough to pick it up. I hope you find it a fun and lively way to discover aromatherapy and the fascinating world of fragrance. And, to all my aromatherapy and herb students who have graced my classes through the decades: It's you who carry on these healing traditions to make our world a better place.

Author's Acknowledgments

It's a big job writing a book. It means translating lots of ideas into words and then compiling them into the text you hold in your hand. None of us do it alone. Thanks to everyone behind the scenes. I greatly appreciate Mindy Green, a marvelous aromatherapist and herbalist, for adding her insights.

Learning about aromatherapy hasn't been a lonely road. So many people graciously shared their knowledge and friendships with me. I acknowledge aromatherapists Jeanne Rose, Shirley Price, Robert Tisserand, Kurt Schnaubelt, Marcel Lavabre, and John Steele for all they've contributed to modern aromatherapy and for inspiring me and so many others. Special thanks to my father, Jesse Keville, for teaching me so much about his passion and vocation — chemistry — and how that knowledge applies to essential oils.

Publisher's Acknowledgments

Acquisitions Editor: Jennifer Yee
Copy Editor: Kelly Henthorne
Technical Editor: Mindy Green
Managing Editor: Kristie Pyles

Production Editor: Tamilmani Varadharaj
Illustrator: Pam Tanzey
Cover Image: ©Iryna Veklich/Getty Images

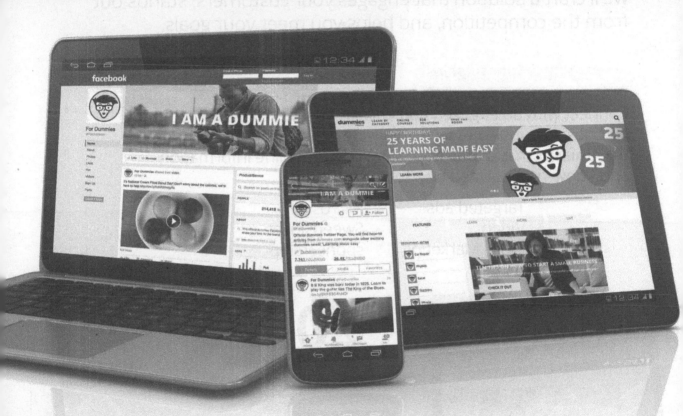
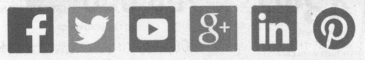
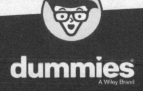

Leverage the power

Dummies is the global leader in the reference category and one of the most trusted and highly regarded brands in the world. No longer just focused on books, customers now have access to the dummies content they need in the format they want. Together we'll craft a solution that engages your customers, stands out from the competition, and helps you meet your goals.

Advertising & Sponsorships

Connect with an engaged audience on a powerful multimedia site, and position your message alongside expert how-to content. Dummies.com is a one-stop shop for free, online information and know-how curated by a team of experts.

- Targeted ads
- Video
- Email Marketing

- Microsites
- Sweepstakes sponsorship

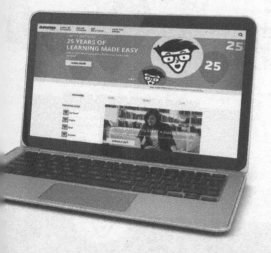

20 MILLION PAGE VIEWS **EVERY SINGLE MONTH**

15 MILLION UNIQUE VISITORS PER MONTH

43% OF ALL VISITORS ACCESS THE SITE VIA THEIR MOBILE DEVICES

700,000 NEWSLETTER SUBSCRIPTIONS TO THE INBOXES OF

300,000 UNIQUE INDIVIDUALS EVERY WEEK

# of dummies

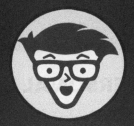

Custom Publishing

Reach a global audience in any language by creating a solution that will differentiate you from competitors, amplify your message, and encourage customers to make a buying decision.

- Apps
- Books
- eBooks
- Video
- Audio
- Webinars

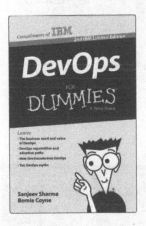

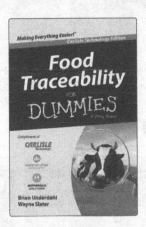

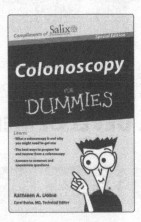

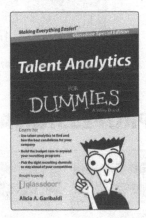

Brand Licensing & Content

Leverage the strength of the world's most popular reference brand to reach new audiences and channels of distribution.

For more information, visit dummies.com/biz

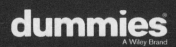

PERSONAL ENRICHMENT

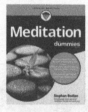 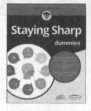 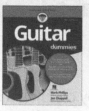 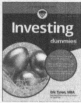 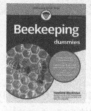 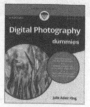

Staying Sharp	Facebook	Guitar	Investing	Beekeeping	Digital Photography
9781119187790	9781119179030	9781119293354	9781119293347	9781119310068	9781119235606
USA $26.00	USA $21.99	USA $24.99	USA $22.99	USA $22.99	USA $24.99
CAN $31.99	CAN $25.99	CAN $29.99	CAN $27.99	CAN $27.99	CAN $29.99
UK £19.99	UK £16.99	UK £17.99	UK £16.99	UK £16.99	UK £17.99

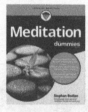 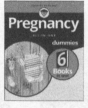 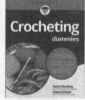 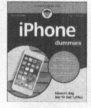 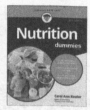

Meditation	Pregnancy	Samsung Galaxy S 7	iPhone	Crocheting	Nutrition
9781119251163	9781119235491	9781119279952	9781119283133	9781119287117	9781119130246
USA $24.99	USA $26.99	USA $24.99	USA $24.99	USA $24.99	USA $22.99
CAN $29.99	CAN $31.99	CAN $29.99	CAN $29.99	CAN $29.99	CAN $27.99
UK £17.99	UK £19.99	UK £17.99	UK £17.99	UK £16.99	UK £16.99

PROFESSIONAL DEVELOPMENT

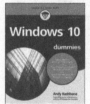 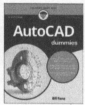 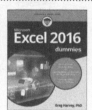 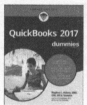 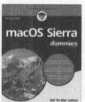 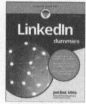

Windows 10	AutoCAD	Excel 2016	QuickBooks 2017	macOS Sierra	LinkedIn	Windows 10
9781119311041	9781119255796	9781119293439	9781119281467	9781119280651	9781119251132	9781119310563
USA $24.99	USA $39.99	USA $26.99	USA $26.99	USA $29.99	USA $24.99	USA $34.00
CAN $29.99	CAN $47.99	CAN $31.99	CAN $31.99	CAN $35.99	CAN $29.99	CAN $41.99
UK £17.99	UK £27.99	UK £19.99	UK £19.99	UK £21.99	UK £17.99	UK £24.99

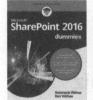 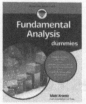 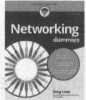 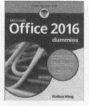   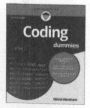

SharePoint 2016	Fundamental Analysis	Networking	Office 2016	Office 365	Salesforce.com	Coding
9781119181705	9781119263593	9781119257769	9781119293477	9781119265313	9781119239314	9781119293323
USA $29.99	USA $26.99	USA $29.99	USA $26.99	USA $24.99	USA $29.99	USA $29.99
CAN $35.99	CAN $31.99	CAN $35.99	CAN $31.99	CAN $29.99	CAN $35.99	CAN $35.99
UK £21.99	UK £19.99	UK £21.99	UK £19.99	UK £17.99	UK £21.99	UK £21.99

Learning Made Easy

ACADEMIC

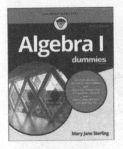

9781119293576
USA $19.99
CAN $23.99
UK £15.99

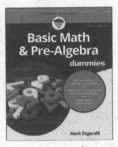

9781119293637
USA $19.99
CAN $23.99
UK £15.99

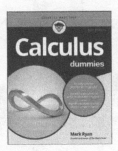

9781119293491
USA $19.99
CAN $23.99
UK £15.99

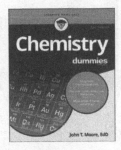

9781119293460
USA $19.99
CAN $23.99
UK £15.99

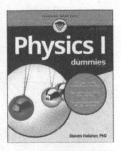

9781119293590
USA $19.99
CAN $23.99
UK £15.99

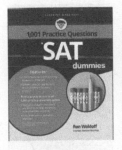

9781119215844
USA $26.99
CAN $31.99
UK £19.99

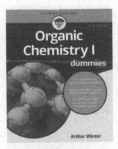

9781119293378
USA $22.99
CAN $27.99
UK £16.99

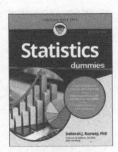

9781119293521
USA $19.99
CAN $23.99
UK £15.99

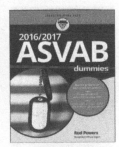

9781119239178
USA $18.99
CAN $22.99
UK £14.99

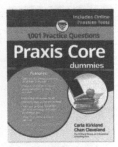

9781119263883
USA $26.99
CAN $31.99
UK £19.99

Available Everywhere Books Are Sold

dummies.com

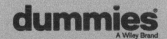

Small books for big imaginations

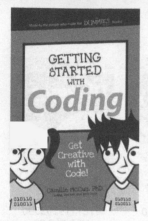
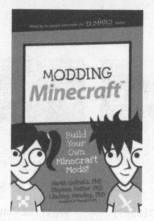
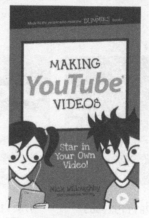
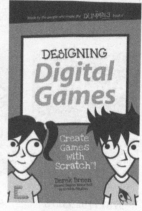
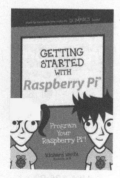
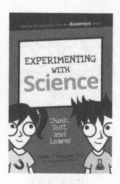
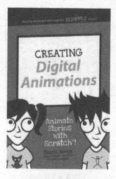
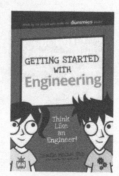
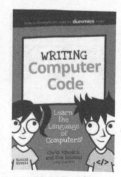